Ron

Thank you for your leadership in helping to eliminate the single greatest cause of premature death in our great nation.

Jonathan

■ Public Health Practice: What Works

Public Health Practice

What Works

EDITED BY

Jonathan E. Fielding, MD, MPH
Steven M. Teutsch, MD, MPH

MANAGING EDITOR

Stephanie N. Caldwell, MPH

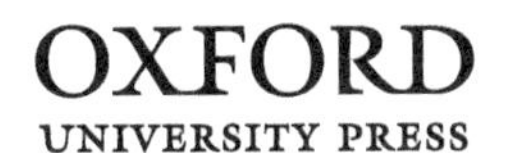

OXFORD
UNIVERSITY PRESS

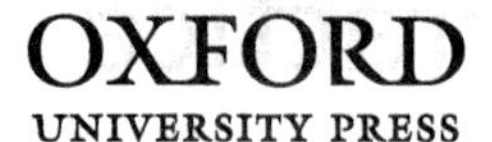

Oxford University Press is a department of the University of Oxford. It furthers the University's objective of excellence in research, scholarship, and education by publishing worldwide.

Oxford New York
Auckland Cape Town Dar es Salaam Hong Kong Karachi
Kuala Lumpur Madrid Melbourne Mexico City Nairobi
New Delhi Shanghai Taipei Toronto

With offices in
Argentina Austria Brazil Chile Czech Republic France Greece
Guatemala Hungary Italy Japan Poland Portugal Singapore
South Korea Switzerland Thailand Turkey Ukraine Vietnam

Published in the United States of America by
Oxford University Press
198 Madison Avenue, New York, NY 10016, United States of America
www.oup.com

Library of Congress Cataloging-in-Publication Data

Public health practice: what works / edited by Jonathan Fielding, Steven Teutsch;
managing editor, Stephanie Caldwell.
p.; cm.
Includes bibliographical references.
ISBN 978-0-19-989276-1 (hardcover: alk. paper)
I. Fielding, Jonathan E. II. Teutsch, Steven M. III. Caldwell, Stephanie N.
[DNLM: 1. Public Health Practice—Los Angeles. 2. Health Services—Los Angeles.
3. Local Government—Los Angeles. WA 100]
362.109794'94—dc23
2012019464

9 8 7 6 5 4 3 2 1
Printed in the United States of America
on acid-free paper

■ FOREWORD

GEORGES C. BENJAMIN, MD
Executive Director, American Public Health Association

If we want to look at how well we have done as a society to improve health, we can take heart from the unprecedented gains in the twentieth century. Life expectancy grew by 30 years, due in large measure to public health actions at the community level across the country. It didn't happen by accident, but was the result of concerted action by people who created a shared vision of what was possible and used an evidence-based approach to implement programs through strategic partnerships to translate that vision into reality.

While the principles and science of public health are well taught in schools of public health and presented in many excellent textbooks and journals, they do not fully convey the complexity and challenges of public health practice in states and local health departments. As a field, effective public health requires the practical application of a wide variety of skills from careful assessment, analysis, and reevaluation; to policy development, program planning, and implementation; to effective assurance strategies such as community organization and mobilization, risk communication, and quality improvement. Combining these skills together into effective public health action requires leadership, good management, scientific expertise, and political competency.

Until now, it has been difficult for students, academics, and policy makers to learn about on-the-ground public health practice without actually working extensively in a state or local public health department. This book fills that need. The case studies in *Public Health Practice: What Works* portray the richness of real-world public health practice and are filled with the array of health problems, resource constraints, partnerships, and solutions that can be brought to bear on many of the most serious health problems in the nation. From substance abuse to maternal and child health; from environmental health to the social determinants; and from control of infectious disease to responding to chronic conditions like the obesity epidemic, these case studies deliver insights from one of the country's most innovative public health departments.

While not an academic treatise, these case studies deliver insights into how to assess problems, plan and implement solutions, build partnerships, craft informational and policy infrastructure, and assess impacts. These real life examples are valuable insights to students, public health professionals, and policy makers.

In my career as the Health Commissioner for our nation's capital, as the Secretary of Health for the State of Maryland, and in my current role as Executive Director of the American Public Health Association, I have learned firsthand that the real work of improving the public's health occurs on the ground in our states and localities. Finding meaningful ways to share these experiences is an important effort that this text does very well. It is a valuable resource for all those who aspire to improve the public's health.

PREFACE

The health of the public is central to our well-being and prosperity as individuals, as communities, and as a nation. Our health is determined more by our social and physical environments, our communities and families, than by the health care system. Public health has the primary responsibility for assuring these conditions—the conditions that together keep people healthy. Despite the importance of the mission, the public and even many public health and public policy professionals who have never worked in a local or state public health jurisdiction may have little sense of what grass-roots public health entails. Hence this book.

Public health practitioners receive extensive training. Many have clinical training and even more have advanced degrees in public health. They have solid academic grounding in public health science, theory, and management. Yet missing from much of public health training is exposure to the day-to-day challenges of public health practice. This book seeks to fill that gap by providing real-world examples of public health challenges, the context in which those challenges occur and the results of each effort. These short stories of actual experiences are intended for practitioners, students, and others interested in understanding how to translate public health theory and experience into effective action at the local, regional, and state level. We see the book being used to inject reality for those without local public health experience and to provide examples that can help practitioners working on similar health problems. It should have similar value for public policy students and professionals.

Why case studies from Los Angeles County? Los Angeles is a microcosm of the diverse settings where public health is practiced in the United States. It has an urban core, yet large areas of the county are rural. The population is among the most diverse in the nation. In many ways, Los Angeles County—the most populous county in the country with its 88 cities—is as complex as a state. In sum, the public health issues found in almost any local, regional, or state jurisdiction can be found here.

The chapters in this volume illustrate innovative and conventional ways that we have addressed a wide range of population health problems facing local and state health departments. They have been selected to convey the scope of a local or state health department while providing practical lessons from real-world situations. The chapters that follow illustrate the core functions of public health and the essential public health services, including the value of planning, the necessity of careful program and policy development, the importance of evidence-based practice, and the need for effective partnerships to improve population health outcomes and reduce health disparities. The chapters also cover major common challenges, and why we are not always completely successful in meeting them.

Of necessity, case studies reflect past activities. Yet permeating the chapters is a vision for the future. The health equity and the social and physical environmental determinants are addressed in many chapters and are the focal point of several. In the current fiscal environment, resources are becoming scarcer while public health challenges are not. This demands greater attention to efficiency, organizational energy, policy, and innovation. Lessons from the case studies should be applicable to new challenges.

The book is organized into five main sections. The first provides historical context for the evolution of public health in Los Angeles as well as information about the public health department itself. It also covers many of the cross-cutting core capacities that every public health department needs. The second focuses on health promotion—how to affect the underlying determinants of health and the individual behaviors that largely determine our overall health and well-being. The third section is about health protection, the activities that reduce exposures to deleterious harms from infectious and toxic agents. The fourth section concerns emergency response, the capacity to address natural and other emergencies. The final section addresses the delivery of clinical and other services to prevent and control disease and injury over both the short term and over the entire life cycle. Since many case studies do not fall neatly into a single category, pertinent examples for a topic may be found in more than one section. Each case study begins with a description of the problem and the relevant contextual information, followed by the approach to the problem, how the solution was implemented, the qualitative or quantitative evaluation, and lessons learned.

This book would not have been possible without the help of many people. First and foremost, we must recognize the Los Angeles County Board of Supervisors (Michael D. Antonovich, Don Knabe, Gloria Molina, Mark Ridley-Thomas, and Zev Yaroslavsky) and their health deputies (Richard Espinosa, Phillip Chen, Elan Shultz, Yolanda Vera, and Amy Luftig Viste) for their commitment to the health of the people of Los Angeles County. We see that commitment every day in the strength of our Department and the Board's leadership. This book would not have been possible without their unwavering support for which we are most grateful. The County's Chief Executive Officer William Fujioka and Deputy Chief Executive Officer Sheila Shima have always encouraged departmental innovation and leadership. Robert Ragland, Principal Deputy County Counsel, provided wise guidance and reviewed content at every step of the process. The breadth and depth of this book are due to the diversity and skills of our colleagues in the Department. We express our appreciation to all the authors, and the staff who helped with manuscript preparation, graphics, and organization. Elizabeth Bancroft and Mark Malak made important contributions. Elishia Nelson, Filip Bartnik, Aisha Carter, Ligia Galvan, James Teng, Beverly Ware, Boyd Jackson, Summer Nagano, Maria Agosta, Patricia Gibson, Chris Foster, Carolyn Brown, Aura Wong, Wayne Sugita, Tim Duenas, Lana Skylar, Donna Sze, and Angelo Bellomo all played important supporting roles. Many other Los Angeles County departments and organizations contribute enormously to the work of the Department of Public Health and to this volume. We are grateful to them all. Financial support for initial editing of the book was provided by the Centers for Disease Control and Prevention (CDC) cooperative agreement number CD001274-02, though the contents are solely the responsibility of the authors and the Los Angeles County Department of Public Health and do not necessarily represent the official views of the CDC. Lastly, we want to thank the team of editors at Oxford for their encouragement and guidance.

S.M.T.
J.E.F.
Los Angeles, California
January 2012

CONTENTS

ACRONYMS

AA	1. African Americans, 2. Alcoholics Anonymous
AAEP	African American Engagement Project
AAR	After Action Report
ACDC	Communicable Disease Control Program
ACLAC	Asthma Coalition of Los Angeles County
ADA	American Diabetes Association
ADP	Alcohol and Drug Programs
ADPA	Alcohol and Drug Program Administration
AFI	Adult Film Industry
AHF	AIDS Healthcare Foundation
AHO	Area Health Office or Officer
AIM	Adult Industry Medical
ALbD	Active Living by Design
AMCHP	Association of Maternal and Child Health Professionals
AOC	Administrative Office of the Courts
APHSS	Adult Production Health and Safety Services
APIC	Association for Professionals in Infection Control
APNCUI	Adequacy of Prenatal Care Utilization Index
ART	Antiretroviral Therapy
AV	Antelope Valley
AVPH	Antelope Valley Partners in Health
BIH	Black Infant Health
BMI	Body Mass Index
BPTF	Border Puppy Task Force
BRFSS	Behavioral Risk Factor Surveillance System
BSO	Bureau of Special Operations
CAA	Certified Application Assistants
CADHS	California Department of Health Services
CAFA	Community Action to Fight Asthma
CAHAN	California Health Alert Network
Cal/OSHA	California Occupational Safety and Health Administration
Cal-EMA	California State Office of Emergency Services
CBO	Community-Based Organization
CBP	Customs and Border Protection
CCJCC	Countywide Criminal Justice Coordination Committee
CCR	California Code of Regulations
CCS	California Children's Services
CDC	Centers for Disease Control and Prevention
CDCI	Comprehensive Drug Court Implementation
CDCR	California Department of Corrections and Rehabilitation
CDPH	California Department of Public Health

CEO	1. Chief Executive Office, 2. Chief Executive Officer
CFH	Certified Food Handler
CFHC	California Family Health Council
CFM	Certified Farmers Market
CHDP	Child Health and Disability Prevention
CHOI	Children's Health Outreach Initiative
CHS	Community Health Services
CI	Confidence Interval
CIA	Central Intelligence Agency
CLPHN	Community-liaison Public Health Nurse
CMS	Centers for Medicaid and Medicare Services
COOP	Continuity of Operation Plans
COPM	Canadian Occupational Performance Measure
CPPW	Communities Putting Prevention to Work
CPSP	Comprehensive Perinatal Services Program
CRA	Countermeasures Response Administration
CRKP	Carbapenem-Resistant *Klebsiella Pneumoniae*
CTCP	California Tobacco Control Program
CTS	Consultation & Techinical Services
CVU	Credentialing Verification Unit
DCMIS	Drug Court Management Information System
DCP	Drug Court Program
DDT	Dichlorodiphenyltrichlorothane
DHS	Department of Health Services
DME	Durable Medical Equipment
DOC	Department Operations Center
DOPE	Drug Overdose Prevention Education
DPH	Department of Public Health
DPSS	Department of Public Social Services offices
DSE	Bureau of District Surveillance and Enforcement
DSW	Disaster Service Worker
ECC	Emergency Command Center
ED	Emergency Department
EH	Environmental Health
EHD	Environmental Health Division
EISO	Epidemic Intelligence Service Officer
EOC	Emergency Operations Center
EPA	Environmental Protection Agency
EPRP	Emergency Preparedness and Response Program
EPTEC	Emergency Preparedness Training and Exercise Committee
ExComm	External Relations and Communications
FBI	Federal Bureau of Investigation
FCEC	Fish Contamination Education Collaborative
FDA	Food and Drug Administration
FEMA	Federal Emergency Management Agency
FIMR	Fetal Infant Mortality Review
FISC	Functional Improvement Score
FM	Food and Milk Program

FPL	Federal Poverty Level
FRO	First Responding Officers
FWS	Fish and Wildlife Services
GAO	Government Accountability Office
HAU	Health Assessment Unit
HEA	Health Education Administration
HEPA	High-Efficiency Particulate Air
HIA	Health Impact Assessment
HIPAA	Health Insurance Portability and Accountability Act
HIV	Human Immunodeficiency Virus
HOU	Hospital Outreach Unit
HPV	Human Papillomavirus
IAP	Incident Action Plan
IC	Incident Command or Incident Commander
ICP	Infection Control Practitioner
ICS	Incident Command System
IDUs	Intravenous Drug Users
IEP	Individualized Education Planning
IIPP	Injury and Illness Prevention Program
IND	1. Improvised Nuclear Device, 2. Investigational New Drug
IRB	Institutional Review Board
IRT	Incident Response Team
ISD	Internal Services Department
JCAHO	Joint Commission on Accreditation of Healthcare Organizations
JITT	Just-in-Time Training
JRIC	Joint Regional Intelligence Center
LA HOPE	Los Angeles Health Overview of a Pregnancy Event
LAC	Los Angeles County
LACHS	Los Angeles County Health Survey
LAIV	Live-Attenuated Influenza Vaccine
LAMB	Los Angeles Mommy and Baby
LAUSD	Los Angeles Unified School District
LAX	Los Angeles International Airport
LBW	Low Birth Weight
LEA	Local Enforcement Agency
LHD	Local Health Department
LM	*Listeria monocytogenes*
LRN	Laboratory Response Network
MAA	Medi-Cal Administrative Activities
MARRP	Multi-Agency Radiation Response Plan
MCAH	Maternal, Child, and Adolescent Health
MCH	Maternal Child Health
MIHA	Maternal and Infant Health Assessment
MLC	Multi-State Learning Collaborative
MOU	Memorandum of Understanding
MPOC	Measure of Processes of Care
MRSA	Methicillin Resistant *Staphylococcus aureus*
MTC	Medical Therapy Conference

MTP	Medical Therapy Program
MTU	Medical Therapy Unit
MUH	Multi-Unit Housing
NAAT	Nucleic Acid Amplification Testing
NFP	Nurse Family Partnership
NHIS	National Health Interview Survey
NHSN	National Healthcare Safety Network
NIOSH	National Occupational Safety and Health Administration
nPEP	Non-occupational Post-Exposure Prophylaxis
NPHPSP	National Public Health Performance Standards Program
NPL	National Priority List
OAPP	Office of AIDS Programs and Policy
OCR	Optical Character Reader
ODT	Office of Organizational Development and Training
OEHHA	Office of Environmental Health Hazard Assessment
OII	Owner Initiated Inspection
OPIM	Other Potentially Infectious Materials
OR	Odds Ratio
OSHA	Occupational Safety and Health Administration
OSHSB	Occupational Safety and Health Standards Board
OT	Occupational Therapist
PAIM	Policy Adoption and Implementation Model
PAM	Policy Adoption Model
PASS	POD Assignment Staff System
PBAS	Performance-based Accountability Systems
PCBs	Polychlorinated biphenyls
PCR	Polymerase Chain Reaction
PDSA	Plan-Do-Study-Act
PEDIM	Partnership to Eliminate Disparities in Infant Mortality
PEP	Post-Exposure Prophylaxis
PHC	Preconception Health Collaborative
PHEERF	Public Health Employee Emergency Readiness Framework
PHEP	Public Health Emergency Preparedness
PHEPTC	Public Health Emergency Preparedness Training Collaborative
PHER	Public Health Emergency Response
PHN	Public Health Nurse
PI	Performance
PILC	Performance Improvement Learning Collaborative
PIO	Public Information Officer
PLACE	Policies for Livable Active Community Environments
PMHTF	Perinatal Mental Health Task Force
POD	Points of Dispensing
PPOR	Perinatal Periods of Risk
PR	Public Relations
PRAMS	Pregnancy Risk Assessment Monitoring System
PrEP	Pre-Exposure Prophylaxis
PREPARE	Promoting Emergency Preparedness and Readiness
PT	Preterm

PT	Physical Therapist
PV	Palos Verdes
QAC	Quality Assurance & Compliance
QT	Quarantine Station
RCI	Rapid-Cycle Improvement
RDD	Radiation Dispersal Device
RED	Radiological Exposure Device
RENEW	Renewing Environments for Nutrition, Exercise and Wellness
RFP	Request for Proposals
RM	Los Angeles County Radiation Management
RM	Radiation Management
RWJF	Robert Wood Johnson Foundation
RWQCB	Regional Water Quality Control Board
SAPC	Substance Abuse Prevention and Control
SARS	Severe Acute Respiratory Syndrome
SCHIP	Statewide Children's Health Insurance Program
SCoV	SARS coronavirus
SFDPH	San Francisco Department of Public Health
SHS	Secondhand Smoke
SIDS	Sudden Infant Death Syndrome
SKOOP	Skills and Knowledge on Opiate Overdose Prevention Project
SME	Subject Matter Expert
SNAP-ED	Supplemental Nutrition Assistance Program Education Program
SNS	Strategic National Stockpile
SPA	Service Planning Area
SRO	Single Room Occupancy
STD	Sexually Transmitted Diseases
SUD	Substance Use Disorders
TAG	Technical Advisory Group
TALC	Technical Assistance Legal Center
TCE	The California Endowment
TCPP	Tobacco Control & Prevention Program
TEW	Terrorism Early Warning Group
TIV	Trivalent Influenza Vaccine
TJC	The Joint Commission
UC	Unified Command
UCLA	University of California, Los Angeles
USDA	U.S. Department of Agriculture
USPSTF	U.S. Preventive Services Task Force
VAERS	Vaccine Adverse Events Reporting System
VPH-RCP	Veterinary Public Health & Rabies Control Program
WebCMR	Web-based Confidential Morbidity Report
WHO	World Health Organization
WIC	Women's, Infants and Children
WMDs	Weapons of Mass Destruction
WOW	WIC Offers Wellness

CONTRIBUTORS

Linda M. Aragon, MPH
Director, Tobacco Control and Prevention Program
Los Angeles County Department of Public Health

Jean Armbruster, MA
Director, PLACE Program
Los Angeles County Department of Public Health

Dee Ann Bagwell, MA, MPH
Director, Policy & Planning
Emergency Preparedness and Response Program
Los Angeles County Department of Public Health

Susie B. Baldwin, MD, MPH
Chief, Health Assessment Unit
Office of Health Assessment and Epidemiology

Noël Bazini-Barakat, RN, MSN, MPH
Director, Office of Organizational Development and Training and Acting Nursing Director
Los Angeles County Department of Public Health

Joshua M. Bobrowsky, JD, MPH
Policy and Planning Analyst
Los Angeles County Department of Public Health
Planning, Evaluation, and Development

Suzanne Bogert, MS, RD
Project Director, RENEW LA County
Los Angeles County Department of Public Health

Michelle Bosshard, MPH
Emergency Preparedness Training Coordinator
Office of Organizational Development and Training
Los Angeles County Department of Public Health

Suzanne Bostwick, BS
Director, Children's Health Outreach Initiatives
Maternal, Child and Adolescent Programs
Los Angeles County Department of Public Health

Benjamin Bristow, MD, MPH
Global Health Teaching Fellow
Mount Sinai School of Medicine
Formerly Preventive Medicine
Los Angeles County Department of Public Health

Rebecca Butler, AB
Public Health Fellow
STD Program
Los Angeles County Department of Public Health

Stephanie N. Caldwell, MPH
Special Assistant to the Director
Los Angeles County Department of Public Health

David Caley, RN, PHN, MPA
Community Health Consultant
Former Deputy Division Manager, Community Health Services
Los Angeles County Department of Public Health

Nancy Cappel, PT
Therapy Manager
Children's Medical Services
Los Angeles County Department of Public Health

Shin Margaret Chao, PhD, MPH
Chief, Research, Evaluation, and Planning Unit
Maternal, Child, and Adolescent Health Programs
Los Angeles County Department of Public Health

Michael Contreras, MA
Director, Emergency Operations Unit
Emergency Preparedness and Response Program
Los Angeles County Department of Public Health

Desiree Crevecoeur, PhD
Research Psychologist
UCLA Integrated Substance Abuse Programs

David E. Dassey, MD, MPH
Acute Communicable Disease Control
Los Angeles County Department of Public Health

Deborah Davenport, RN, PHN, MSPA
Director, Community Health Services
Los Angeles County Department of Public Health

Hector Dela Cruz, MS, REHS
Chief EHS
Bureau of Specialized Surveillance & Enforcement
Los Angeles County Environmental Health

Dickson Diamond, MD
Director, Threat Assessment Unit
Los Angeles County Department of Public Health

Giannina Donatoni PhD, MT (ASCP)
Staff Analyst
Maternal, Child, and Adolescent Health Programs
Los Angeles County Department of Public Health

Karen Ehnert, DVM, MPVM
Acting Director, Veterinary Public Health and Rabies Control
Los Angeles County Department of Public Health

Marian Eldahaby, BA
Research Analyst
Maternal, Child, and Adolescent Health Programs
Los Angeles County Department of Public Health

Jonathan E. Fielding, MD, MPH
Director and Health Officer
Los Angeles County Department of Public Health

Wesley L. Ford, MA, MPH
Director
Children's Medical Services
Los Angeles County Department of Public Health

Louisa Franco, MPH
Policy Analyst, PLACE Program
Los Angeles County Department of Public Health

Bernard Franklin, BS
Chief Environmental Health Specialist
Recreational Waters Program
Los Angeles County Environmental Health

Jonathan E. Freedman, MSPH
Chief Deputy Director
Los Angeles County Department of Public Health

Gary P. García, MPH
Research Analyst
Division of HIV and STD Programs
Los Angeles County Department of Public Health

Robert A. Gilchick, MD, MPH
Medical Director, Child and Adolescent Health Program and Policy
Los Angeles County Department of Public Health

Rachel Gonzales, PhD, MPH
Research Psychologist
UCLA Integrated Substance Abuse Programs

Jeffrey D. Gunzenhauser, MD, MPH
Medical Director
Los Angeles County Department of Public Health

Gayle Haberman, MPH
Policy Analyst, PLACE Program
Los Angeles County Department of Public Health

Cynthia A. Harding, MPH
Director
Maternal, Child, and Adolescent Health Programs
Los Angeles County Department of Public Health

Kim Harrison Eowan, MPH, CHES
Chief of Staff, Emergency Preparedness and Response
Los Angeles County Department of Public Health

Maxanne Hatch, MPA
Board Liaison
Los Angeles County Department of Public Health

Julia Heinzerling, MPH
Policy and Advocacy Specialist, Immunization Program
Los Angeles County Department of Public Health

Chandra Higgins, MPH
Epidemiologist
Maternal, Child, and Adolescent Health Programs
Los Angeles County Department of Public Health

Ernesto O. Hinojos, MPH
Emergency Preparedness Training Manager
Office of Organizational Development & Training
Los Angeles County Department of Public Health

Angel Hopson, RN, MSN, MPH
Program Specialist PHN
Maternal, Child, and Adolescent Health Programs
Los Angeles County Department of Public Health

Virginia Huang Richman, MPH, PhD
Chief of Policy, Analysis and Coordination
Planning, Evaluation, and Development
Los Angeles County Department of Public Health

Dawn Marie Jacobson, MD, MPH
Director Strategy and Development
Public Health Institute
Former Director, Performance Improvement
Los Angeles County Department of Public Health

Kathleen Kaufman
Director, Radiation Management (retired)
Los Angeles County Department of Public Health

Peter R. Kerndt, MD, MPH
Director, STD Program
Los Angeles County Department of Public Health

Sinan Khan, MPH, MA
Epidemiologist,
Emergency Preparedness and Response Program
Los Angeles County Department of Public Health

Moon Kim, MD, MPH
Medical Epidemiologist
Acute Communicable Disease Control Program
Los Angeles County Department of Public Health

Robert Kim-Farley, MD, MPH
Director, Communicable Disease Control and Prevention
Los Angeles County Department of Public Health

Sarah M. Kissell, MPA
Public Information Officer
Los Angeles County Department of Public Health

Catherine Knox, RN, MSN
Program Specialist, Community Health Services
Los Angeles County Department of Public Health

Raphael J. Landovitz, MD, MSc
Assistant Professor of Medicine
UCLA Center for Clinical AIDS Research & Education
David Geffen School of Medicine at UCLA

Janice Lewis, REHS
Chief Environmental Health Specialist
Los Angeles County Department of Public Health

Amy S. Lightstone, MPH, MA
Supervising Epidemiologist, Health Assessment Unit
Office of Health Assessment and Epidemiologist
Los Angeles County Department of Public Health

Anna Long, PhD, MPH
Chief of Staff
Los Angeles County Department of Public Health

Debra S. Lotstein, MD, MPH
Adjunct Health Services Researcher,
RAND Health
Santa Monica, CA
Associate Clinical Professor of Pediatrics
UCLA David Geffen School of Medicine
Los Angeles, CA

Laurene Mascola, MD, MPH
Chief, Acute Communicable Disease Control
Los Angeles County Department of Public Health

Mark Roy McGrath, MPH
Public Health Policy Consultant
AIDS Healthcare Foundation

Kenneth Murray, BA
Director, Environmental Protection Bureau
Los Angeles County Department of Public Health
Environmental Health Division

Tess Jens O'Hern, PT
Therapy Manager
Children's Medical Services
Los Angeles County Department of Public Health

Margot Ocanas, MBA, MIA
Policy Analyst, RENEW LA County
Los Angeles County Department of Public Health

Michelle T. Parra, PhD
Director, Immunization Program
Los Angeles County Department of Public Health

Mario J. Pérez, MPH
Director
Division of HIV and STD Programs
Los Angeles County Department of Public Health

Alonzo L. Plough, PhD, MPH
Director, Emergency Preparedness and Response Program
Los Angeles County Department of Public Health

Terrance Powell, BS, REHS
Director
Bureau of Specialized Surveillance & Enforcement
Los Angeles County Environmental Health

Diana Ramos, MD, MPH
Director, Reproductive Health Programs
Maternal, Child, and Adolescent Health Programs
Los Angeles County Department of Public Health

Richard A. Rawson, PhD
Associate Director
UCLA Integrated Substance Abuse Programs

Rose Anne Rodriguez, JD
Director, External Relations and Communications
Los Angeles County Department of Public Health

Sidney Roth, PhD
Research Analyst
Children's Medical Services
Los Angeles County Department of Public Health

Debra Ruge, PT
Director, Medical Therapy Program
Children's Medical Services
Los Angeles County Department of Public Health

Sharon Sakamoto, RN, MSN/MPH, CNS
Acute Communicable Disease Control Program
Los Angeles County Department of Public Health

Marita B. Santos, RN, MSN
Public Health Nurse
Los Angeles County Department of Public Health

Jennifer N. Sayles, MD, MPH
Medical Director, Quality Improvement & Health Assessment
L.A. Care Health Plan
Former Medical Director
Division of HIV and STD Programs
Los Angeles County Department of Public Health

Wendy K. Schiffer, MSPH
Director, Planning, Evaluation and Development
Los Angeles County Department of Public Health

Janet M. Scully, MPH
Staff Analyst, Maternal Child and Adolescent Health Programs
Los Angeles County Department of Public Health

Margaret Shih, MD, MPH
Chief, Office of Health Assessment and Epidemiology
Los Angeles County Department of Public Health

Elan Shultz, MPH
Health Deputy to Supervisor Zev Yaroslavsky
Los Angeles County, Third District

Paul Simon, MD, MPH
Director, Division of Chronic Disease and Injury Prevention
Los Angeles County Department of Public Health

Jeanne Smart, RN, MSN
Program Administrator, Nurse-Family Partnership
Maternal, Child and Adolescent Health Programs
Los Angeles County Department of Public Health

Kathleen Smith, RN, PHN, MSN, MPH
Assistant Nursing Director (retired)
Los Angeles County Department of Public Health

Jane Steinberg, PhD, MPH
Director, Programs and Policy
STD Program
Los Angeles County Department of Public Health

Dawn Terashita, MD, MPH
Acute Communicable Disease Control Program
Los Angeles County Department of Public Health

Steven M. Teutsch, MD, MPH
Chief Science Officer
Los Angeles County Department of Public Health

John Viernes, Jr., MA
Director
Substance Abuse Prevention and Control
Los Angeles County Department of Public Health

Mark D. Weber, PhD
Chief Epidemiologist, Tobacco Control and Prevention Program
Los Angeles County Department of Public Health

S. Benson Werner, MD, MPH
Chief, Disease Investigations Section
California Department of Health Services (retired)

1 Introduction and History of Public Health in Los Angeles County

JONATHAN E. FIELDING, JONATHAN FREEDMAN, AND STEPHANIE N. CALDWELL

Public health is what we, as a society, do collectively to assure the conditions for people to be healthy.

—*Institute of Medicine, 1988 (1)*

Public health has the broad responsibility to protect and promote health in all its dimensions. To fulfill this responsibility, a public health agency mission must be sufficiently broad to address the full range of factors that contribute to health and health disparities in various populations and their many subgroups. The public health agency must not only understand how to produce health and prevent disease and injury, but also capitalize on multiple targets of opportunity to advance health. It works to protect the entire population from health threats: communicable diseases, food-borne diseases, natural and man-made disasters, toxic exposures, and preventable illness and injury. On parallel tracks, its goals are to prevent both the occurrence and progression of chronic diseases such as heart disease, cancer, and diabetes, which collectively comprise over 75% of the burden of ill-health (2, 3). Minimizing chronic diseases requires intervention to reduce contributing risk factors and individual behaviors; these can include poor nutrition, inadequate physical activity, tobacco use, and the use and abuse of other legal and illegal drugs. However, to achieve significant improvements, the underlying determinants of our collective health burden must be addressed with equal vigor; these include the underlying physical, social, and economic environments.

Many objective and subjective judgments knit together the agenda for any state or local public health department. Given the panoply of potential opportunities for disease prevention and health protection and promotion, how should priorities be set? How should the mix of direct service programs, policy advocacy, health education and promotion, and community engagement be decided? The approach in Los Angeles County (LAC) is not unique. The department assesses and analyzes its populations, their health problems and prevention and mitigation opportunities; it determines where lies the greatest potential for impact, including analysis of gaps; it takes advantage of natural opportunities; and it continually monitors the performance of its activities. Underlying department planning is the assumption that there are always ways to become more efficient and effective. Staffs need to remain cognizant that they are public servants entrusted by taxpayers who deserve the best health returns on their investment of tax dollars. The planning process must factor in serious financial constraints, both limited resources and strictures on how money from various sources can be spent.

The chapters that follow illustrate innovative ways in which the department has addressed a range of local and state population health problems. This sampling of case studies conveys the scope of issues that a local health department can address, as well as providing practical lessons from real-world examples of challenges and opportunities. They illustrate the value of planning, the necessity of program and policy development, the importance of evidence-based practice, and the significant influence of effective partnerships for improving population health outcomes.

HISTORY OF PUBLIC HEALTH IN LOS ANGELES COUNTY

Like many states, California historically relied on localities to perform substantial public health functions. In fact, local involvement in public health in California predated the forming of the United States itself and also the formal establishment of public health departments as we know them today.

For more than 70 years under Spanish and Mexican colonial rule (1769 to 1847), municipal functions such as public safety were performed by a variety of local administrative entities. These included the system of religious missions throughout California, private land grant areas known as "ranchos," and formal government structures known as "pueblos" that held legal powers derived from Spain or Mexico.

This governmental history may appear irrelevant because today's American public health system first appeared in the late nineteenth century, and became fully developed in the early twentieth century. However, it is important to recognize that societal structures in California grappled with public health problems such as communicable disease, adequate food supplies, sanitation, and potable water long before formal public health agencies were formed. While the history of water supply in arid Southern California is well documented (4, 5), less well known is that the designated local "water master" or *zanjero*, charged to oversee the delivery of water, played a precursor role to what is known today as a public health officer (6). After colonial rule ended in California, the role of the *zanjero* endured; the *zanjero* was often among the highest paid municipal officials, with broad powers to control and regulate public and private water systems.

By 1850, following the end of the Mexican-American War, entry into the Union set the legal foundation for public health in California. As under Spanish and Mexican rule, the California Constitution assigned roles for local government to be carried out under state authority. Among such roles, the public health function was assigned to cities—and, where there were no cities, counties—to operate under the authority of the state public health apparatus. While this model is not unique in the United States, California's local public health agencies have a high degree of local control, with weak central state oversight, as under former Spanish and Mexican rule.

In 1857 the City of Los Angeles established its public health department and began to address issues of disease control in its growing populace. Due to slower population growth outside the City of Los Angeles, the Los Angeles County (LAC) public health department was established in 1903 primarily to focus on rural health issues.

From 1900 to 1920, public health in Los Angeles developed similarly to public health agencies in other major U.S. cities, namely by providing greater scientific and laboratory capability, increased regulatory authority, increased direct delivery of disease control and preventive services, and sometimes health care services. During this time, other cities within LAC began to develop public health departments or contract with the County to provide services. By the 1920s, local LAC policy makers began to understand the need for improved regional coordination for public health, as well as the challenge and cost of maintaining separate public health departments. In 1922 only nine cities had contracted with LAC, but by 1924 that number had increased to 19 and the populations served had grown from 107,000 to 325,000. From that time, as new cities were incorporated, contracting with the County for public health services became routine. In 1964 the City of Los Angeles public health department merged with that of LAC.

In the early 1970s, LAC consolidated four departments—public health, hospitals, mental health, and veterinary health—into a single department under the mantle of a comprehensive, "all in one" agency. Soon thereafter, mental health separated from the department as its professionals and constituencies contested that needed services were not receiving sufficient priority against other areas in the merged agency.

From the mid-1970s to 1984, the merged agency was divided into regional areas, which in effect created mini-agencies throughout the County. Tension became clear between two functions of public health: population health and health care provision to low-income populations. Paralleling the earlier contentions of the mental health constituency, public health professionals and advocates expressed concerns that public health needs were being subordinated to the demands of the public hospitals. To remedy this and related concerns, the regional system was dismantled to favor an organization with health care services in one division and public health in another. In effect, public health remained a department within a department until 2006, when the County Board of Supervisors created a separate department of public health.

The path of public health's development in Los Angeles cannot be separated from the overall context of governmental development. Throughout the mid- and late twentieth century, governmental organization in California became increasingly complex. More incorporated cities emerged, as did new school districts and many special and separate governmental entities, such as vector control districts, sewer and sanitation districts, regional air quality districts, and regional water quality districts. In addition, the role and reach of the federal government at the local level increased through entities such as the Food and Drug Administration, the Environmental Protection Agency, and the Department of Agriculture. This governmental complexity in Los Angeles heavily affects how public health functions are organized and accomplished, and more important, affects how new public health problems and challenges are framed and acted upon.

LOS ANGELES COUNTY TODAY

Today, California vests primary responsibility for public health in 58 counties and three cities; while in other parts of the country, city or city-state hybrid agencies have these responsibilities. LAC's governing body is a five-member elected Board of Supervisors who exercise both executive and legislative authority, and oversee all county government agencies and functions. Each supervisor serves a separate diverse constituency in urban, suburban, and rural areas.

As the nation's most populous county, LAC has more residents than does each of 42 respective states (7). Over 26% of Californians reside in LAC; over 9.8 million people live in LAC's approximately 4,000 square miles (8). The county encompasses 88 incorporated cities (9); 65% of the county's physical area is unincorporated, much of it rural, and the one million residents living in rural areas receive municipal services directly from the county government (10). To provide appropriate services and target initiatives to the specific health needs in different areas, for planning purposes the county is divided into eight geographic regions called Service Planning Areas (SPAs) (see Figure 1–1).

In addition to being large and populous, LAC is diverse in notable ways. Fifty-six percent of the population speak a language other than English at home (8), and as many as 224 languages are spoken by significant numbers of residents (11). Sixteen percent of the entire population and 23% of children live below the federal poverty level (8, 12).

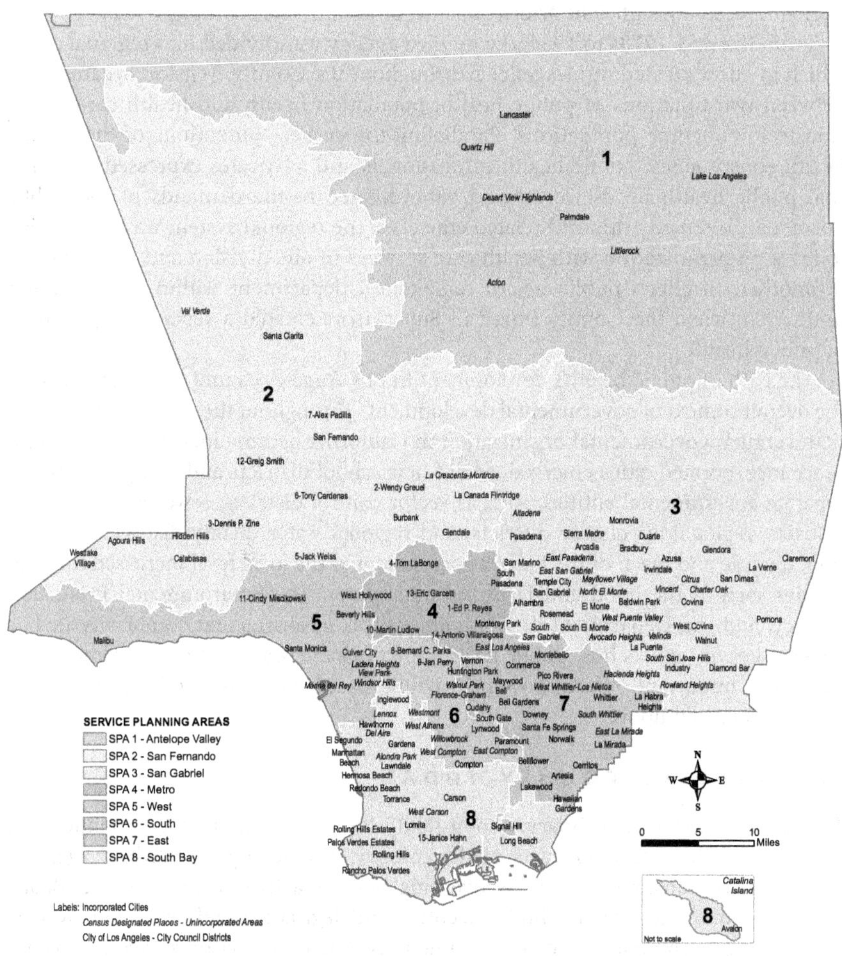

Figure 1–1 Cities and Communities of Los Angeles County, by Service Planning Area (SPA)

The county is also racially and ethnically diverse. In the 2010 census, 48% of the population reported being Hispanic or Latino, 28% White, 14% Asian/Pacific Islander, 9% Black, and 1% American Indian/Alaskan Native (8). Significantly, over 1,065,000 residents are aged 65 and over—nearly 11% of the population (8). Cultural values and social influences within subgroups defined by race, ethnicity, culture, education, and age contribute to disparate patterns of health and influence how the Department must work to improve health outcomes.

To address existing complexities and the range of community needs, LAC Department of Public Health's (DPH) 39 programs and 14 public health centers support its mission to protect health, prevent disease and promote the health and well-being of all county residents (see Figure 1–2). Chapter 3 details the elements of LAC DPH's strategic plan, including vision, mission, and priorities.

A crosscutting theme among programs, projects, and policies highlighted in this volume is the importance of their underlying scientific evidence (see Chapter 4). As responsible stewards of public funds, DPH consults the *Guide to Community Preventive Services*, *Guide to Clinical Preventive Services*, the Cochrane Collaboration, and other carefully performed systematic reviews. Where the evidence base for addressing a public health problem is insufficient but there is a need to act, DPH adds to that literature by carefully evaluating and publishing the results of its interventions.

Health Problems in Los Angeles County

Life expectancy has been slowly increasing in LAC and nationally. As of 2007, average life expectancy at birth was 80.7 years (13). But this longevity average hides persistent glaring differences among racial/ethnic groups. In 2007 Asian/Pacific Islanders lived an average of 84.9 years, while Blacks lived on average only 74.2 years (13). Disparities in life expectancy are largely due to differences in underlying social, environmental, and economic conditions in which people live. An inverse relationship exists between life expectancy and the level of economic hardship in LAC neighborhoods (see Figure 1–3).

As expected with an aging population, and similar to national trends, chronic diseases and related conditions constitute a majority of LAC's burden of ill-health. The leading cause of death and of premature death is coronary heart disease (see Figure 1–4) (14). Emphysema, pneumonia/influenza, and Alzheimer's disease are also among the top ten causes of death and disproportionately affect elderly populations (14). Mortality statistics only partially reveal the toll of chronic diseases. Their effect on quality of life, productivity, and functional capacity is even more widespread.

Yet chronic disease is just one element of the mortality puzzle. If we ask what cause of death is associated with the greatest foreshortening of life, homicide comes to the fore. Only the fourteenth leading cause of death, it ranks second among causes of premature death (14). An average of 44 years of life was lost for each homicide death, compared to four years for each coronary heart disease death (14). And, leading causes of death differ greatly by race/ethnicity (see Figure 1–5) (14).

Table 1–1 reflects some key health trends (15). Obesity, diabetes, and related conditions pose significant challenges for public health practitioners. Obesity among adults rose from 14.3% of the population in 1997 to 22.2% in 2007 (15), while those overweight increased from 34.4% to 35.9% (15). Largely due to these increases, the

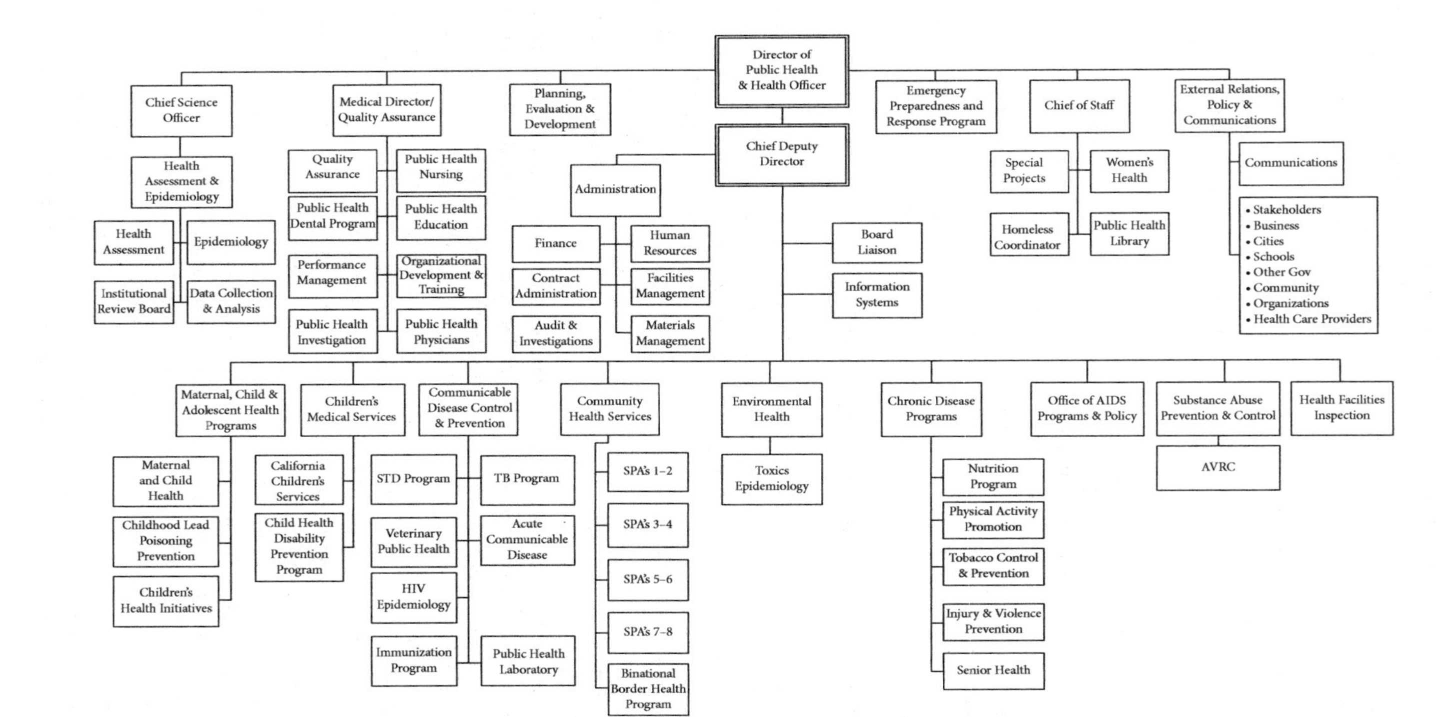

Figure 1–2 Los Angeles County—Department of Public Health

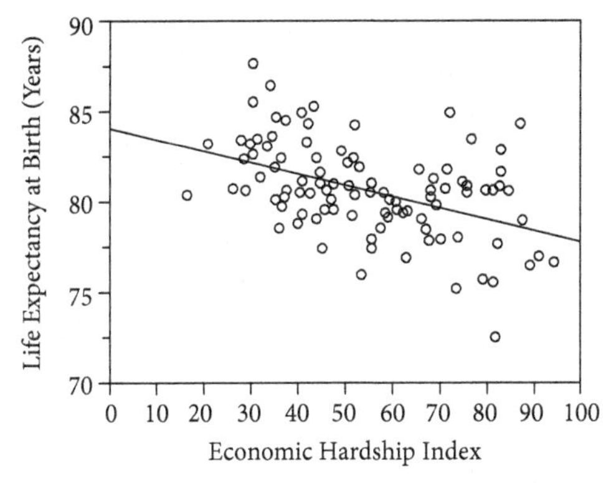

Figure 1–3 Association of Life Expectancy and Economic Hardship in Los Angeles County Cities and Communities, 2006 (13)

prevalence of adults diagnosed with hypertension, high cholesterol, and diabetes also rose over that time (15), with diabetes increasing from 6.6% to 9.1% (16).

Substance use and abuse in its multiple forms, including tobacco (see Chapter 13), illegal drug use, and misuse of prescription medications constitute the greatest preventable health burden. In LAC, drug overdose, including unintentional alcohol poisoning, is the sixth leading cause of premature death and the nineteenth leading cause of death (14). In 2009, drug offenses caused over 32,000 felony arrests (17). Sixteen percent of adults in LAC report binge drinking (5 or more drinks on one occasion for men, 4 or more drinks for women) in the last 30 days (18). In addition to driving under the influence offenses, alcohol is implicated in falls, suicide, poisoning, and occupational injuries (19).

Los Angeles County
58,043 total deaths and 461,838 years of life lost*

	Leading Causes of Death			Leading Causes of Premature** Death			
Rank	Cause of Death	No. of Deaths	Premature Death Rank	Rank	Cause of Death	Years of Life Lost	Death Rank
1.	Coronary heart disease	13,428	1.	1.	Coronary heart disease	59,821	1.
2.	Stroke	3,280	9.	2.	Homicide	37,087	14.
3.	Lung cancer	2,910	7.	3.	Motor vehicle crash	8,195	15.
4.	Emphysema/COPD	2,889	13.	4.	Suicide	22,177	16.
5.	Diabetes	2,190	8.	5.	Liver disease	19,749	9.
6.	Pneumonia/Influenza	2,171	22.	6.	Drug overdose	19,269	19.
7.	Alzheimer's disease	2,121	45.	7.	Lung cancer	16,862	3.
8.	Colorectal cancer	1,365	11.	8.	Diabetes	15,650	5.
9.	Liver disease	1,134	5.	9.	Stroke	15,197	2.
10.	Breast cancer	1,079	10.	10.	Breast cancer	12,346	10.

*Excludes infants less than 1 year of age and persons of unknown age.
**Death before age 75 years.

Figure 1–4 Ten Leading Causes of Death and Premature Death in Los Angeles County, 2008 (14)

Race/ethnicity Number of deaths Age-adjusted death rate	#1 cause Number of deaths Age-adjusted death rate	#2 cause Number of deaths Age-adjusted death rate	#3 cause Number of deaths Age-adjusted death rate	#4 cause Number of deaths Age-adjusted death rate	#5 cause Number of deaths Age-adjusted death rate
White 30,149 643 per 100,000	Coronary heart disease 7,596 154 per 100,000	Emphysema/COPD 1,955 41 per 100,000	Lung cancer 1,687 38 per 100,000	Stroke 1,552 31 per 100,000	Alzheimer's disease 1,487 27 per 100,000
Hispanic 13,591 500 per 100,000	Coronary heart disease 2,536 108 per 100,000	Diabetes 764 30 per 100,000	Stroke 749 31 per 100,000	Liver disease 594 18 per 100,000	Homicide 458 8 per 100,000
Black 7,697 879 per 100,000	Coronary heart disease 1,804 209 per 100,000	Stroke 469 55 per 100,000	Lung cancer 377 43 per 100,000	Diabetes 359 41 per 100,000	Emphysema/COPD 318 37 per 100,000
Asian/Pacific Islander 6,354 438 per 100,000	Coronary heart disease 1,437 99 per 100,000	Stroke 496 34 per 100,000	Lung cancer 406 28 per 100,000	Pneumonia/Influenza 297 21 per 100,000	Emphysema/COPD 258 18 per 100,000
Los Angeles County Total 58,043 601 per 100,000	Coronary heart disease 13,428 139 per 100,000	Stroke 3,280 34 per 100,000	Lung cancer 2,910 31 per 100,000	Emphysema/COPD 2,889 31 per 100,000	Diabetes 2,190 23 per 100,000

Figure 1–5 Comparison of the Leading Causes of Death, by Race/Ethnicity in Los Angeles County, 2008 (14)

Table 1–1 Los Angeles County Trend Data 1997–2007, percent and 95% CI (15)

LA COUNTY					
	1997	**1999**	**2002–03**	**2005**	**2007**
Percent of adults diagnosed with **hypertension**	15.8 (15.0–16.7)	19.1 (18.1–20.1)	20.1 (19.1–21.1)	23.4 (22.3–24.4)	24.7 (23.5–25.8)
Percent of adults diagnosed with high **cholesterol**	N/A	16.1 (15.2–17.0)	N/A	23.7 (22.7–24.8)	29.4 (27.8–30.3)
Percent of children in grades 5, 7, & 9 who are **obese**	N/A	18.9	21.9	23.3	22.9
Percent of adults who are **obese**	14.3 (13.5–15.1)	16.7 (15.8–17.7)	18.9 (17.9–19.9)	20.9 (19.8–22.0)	22.2 (20.9–23.5)
Percent of adults who are **overweight**	34.4 (33.3–35.6)	35.6 (34.3–36.8)	35.4 (34.2–36.6)	35.5 (34.2–36.8)	35.9 (34.4–37.4)
Percent of adults who **smoke** cigarettes	N/A	N/A	14.3 (13.5–15.2)	13.9 (12.9–14.8)	14.3 (13.2–15.4)
Percent of adults who obtain recommended amount of **exercise** each week	N/A	N/A	48.0 (46.8–49.2)	51.8 (50.6–53.1)	53.2 (51.7–54.6)
Percent of adults who are **minimally active or inactive**	N/A	N/A	41.8 (40.7–43.0)	37.5 (36.3–38.7)	36.2 (34.8–37.6)

(*continued*)

Table 1-1 (Continued)

LA COUNTY					
	1997	**1999**	**2002–03**	**2005**	**2007**
Percent of children ages 0–17 years with **current asthma**	N/A	N/A	8.1 (7.4–8.9)	8.8 (8.0–9.6)	7.9 (7.0–8.7)
Percent of adults ever diagnosed with **depression**	N/A	8.8 (8.1–9.5)	9.7 (9.0–10.4)	12.9 (12.0–13.8)	13.6 (12.5–14.6)
Percent of adults diagnosed with **diabetes**	5.7 (5.1–6.2)	6.7 (6.0–7.3)	7.0 (6.4–7.7)	8.1 (7.4–8.7)	8.7 (8.0–9.4)
Percent of adults who **binge drink**	N/A	15.7 (14.7–16.6)	17.0 (16.1–18.0)	17.3 (16.3–18.4)	16.2 (15.0–17.3)
Percent of adults who consume 5+ servings of **fruits/ vegetables** a day	N/A	11.6 (10.9–12.4)	12.3 (11.5–13.1)	14.6 (13.7–15.5)	15.1 (14.1–16.1)
Percent of women (40+ yrs) who had a **mammogram** within the past 2 yrs	70.6 (68.8–72.5)	73.7 (71.7–75.6)	73.5 (71.5–75.5)	70.6 (68.6–72.6)	73.7 (71.8–75.7)
Percent of adults (50+ yrs) vaccinated for **influenza** in the past year	N/A	N/A	N/A	40.7 (38.8–42.6)	51.9 (50.1–53.8)
Percent of adults (65+ yrs) ever vaccinated for **pneumonia**	N/A	54.9 (51.6–58.2)	55.7 (52.2–59.2)	57.7 (54.7–60.7)	60.5 (57.6–63.3)

ADDRESSING THE HEALTH PROBLEMS OF LOS ANGELES COUNTY

LAC DPH's strategic plan (see Chapter 3) addresses the preventable toll of illness and injury at multiple levels. In some instances, such as vaccine-preventable diseases, disease can be prevented from occurring. In others, it is necessary to ameliorate risk factors, such as tobacco use or poor nutrition, that in turn cause disease or injury. The newest and broadest objectives aim to modify underlying social and physical environmental determinants contributing to a range of health problems. To be effective across this broad spectrum of opportunities, DPH emphasizes proactive, policy-driven actions to modify social and physical environments. A common theme is to make healthy behavior the easy choice for all residents.

To accomplish health goals requires understanding the health problems, implementing evidence-based practices in collaboration with external partners, and using effective communication strategies. The case studies in the following chapters provide concrete examples of these principles in action. While LAC is unique in layered complexity, the lessons are applicable to local jurisdictions everywhere.

REFERENCES

1. Institute of Medicine. *The Future of Public Health*. Washington, DC: National Academy Press; 1988.
2. Bodenheimer T, Chen E, Bennett H. Confronting the growing burden of chronic disease: Can the U.S. health care workforce do the job? *Health Affairs*. 2009;28(1):64–74.
3. Lopez AD, Mathers CD, Ezzati M, Jamison DT, Murray CJL, editors. *Global Burden of Disease and Risk Factors*. New York: Oxford University Press; 2006. p. 89.
4. Hundley N. The *Great Thirst*. Berkeley: UC Press; 2001.
5. Gumprecht B. *The Los Angeles River*. Baltimore: Johns Hopkins Press; 1999.
6. Anton M. A way of life drying up. *Los Angeles Times*. Mar. 14, 2008.
7. Mackin P, Wilson S. *Population Distribution and Change: 2000 to 2010, 2010 Census Briefs*, issued March 2011 by U.S. Department of Commerce, Economics and Statistics Administration, U.S. Census Bureau.
8. U.S. Census Bureau. State and county quickfacts, Los Angeles County, California 2010. Available from: quickfacts.census.gov/qfd/states/06/06037.html (accessed Aug. 25, 2011).
9. Chief Executive Office, County of Los Angeles. Cities within the County of Los Angeles. 2010. Available from: http://ceo.lacounty.gov/forms/09–10%20Cities%20Alpha.pdf (accessed Aug. 25, 2011).
10. Unincorporated Areas, County of Los Angeles. Available from: http://lacounty.info/wps/portal/!ut/p/c5/04_SB8K8xLLM9MSSzPy8xBz9CP0os3gLAwgw8vcNNDMw8vHxcnUPMjcGigDlI5HkLUwC3YDyrhahnqbGRgaBZgR0h4Psw6PflIC8GUTeAAdwNMCv38xI388jPzdVvyA3wiDTU9cRAPAotzw!/dl3/d3/L2dJQSEvUUt3QS9ZQnZ3LzZfODAwMDAwMDAyT01RNjAyTExKRUdSNzMwSzA!/ (accessed Aug. 25, 2011).
11. Residents, County of Los Angeles. Available from: http://lacounty.info/wps/portal/lac/residents/ (accessed Aug. 25, 2011).
12. Annie E. Casey Foundation. *2011 KIDS COUNT Data Book*. Available from: http://datacenter.kidscount.org/data/bystate/Rankings.aspx?state=CA&ind=412 (accessed Aug. 25, 2011).
13. Los Angeles County Department of Public Health, Office of Health Assessment and Epidemiology. *Life Expectancy in Los Angeles County: How Long Do We Live and Why? A Cities and Communities Health Report*. July 2010.
14. Los Angeles County Department of Public Health. *Mortality in Los Angeles County 2008: Leading Causes of Death and Premature Death with Trends for 1999–2008*. December 2011. Available from: http://publichealth.lacounty.gov/dca/data/documents/2008%20Mortality%20Report%20web.pdf (accessed June 19, 2012).
15. Los Angeles County Department of Public Health. *Key Indicators of Health by Service Planning Area*. June 2009.
16. Los Angeles County Department of Public Health. *Trends in Diabetes: A Reversible Public Health Crisis*. November 2010.

17. California Department of Justice. *California Criminal Justice Profile 2009—Los Angeles County.* Available from: http://stats.doj.ca.gov/cjsc_stats/prof09/19/3A.htm (accessed Sept. 20, 2011).
18. Los Angeles County Health Survey, 2007. Available from: http://publichealth.lacounty.gov/ha/hasurveyintro.htm (accessed Aug. 10, 2012).
19. Los Angeles County Department of Public Health, Substance Abuse Prevention and Control. *Facts and Figures: Alcohol in Los Angeles County.* October 2010.

PART ONE
Core Capacities

2 Measuring Population Health

The Los Angeles County Health Survey

SUSIE B. BALDWIN AND AMY S. LIGHTSTONE

THE NATURE OF THE PROBLEM

Assessment is a core function of all public health agencies, as localities must be able to monitor population health status to identify and mitigate community problems. Assessment drives evidence-based public health practice by informing and supporting the other core public health functions, policy development and assurance (1). California state regulations require that "[t]he health department shall offer at least the following basic services to the health jurisdiction which it serves: (a) Collection, tabulation and analysis of all public health statistics, including population data, natality, mortality (1)." Fulfilling this obligation necessitates data collection.

In the twenty-first century, the need for population health data extends beyond traditional public health surveillance. Historically, infectious diseases posed the greatest threats, so most public health surveillance systems developed around communicable disease reporting. Now that chronic diseases and injuries represent the leading causes of morbidity and mortality, public health agencies require additional kinds of surveillance. Assessment of a population must capture the impact of these conditions by delineating their prevalence as well as the wide range of risk factors and protective factors that underlie or prevent them. Measurements of behaviors, access to care and preventive services and health-related quality of life have become essential indicators for public health. In addition, agencies must assess the social and environmental determinants of the health of their population (2–4).

Challenges arise in finding timely, population-based data to meet the assessment needs of a local public health department. Relevant information is most useful when it is available at the community level, but local health jurisdictions typically lack the resources to collect and analyze the broad range of data necessary for comprehensive assessment (5). National and state surveys, such as the National Health Interview Survey (NHIS) and the Behavioral Risk Factor Surveillance System (BRFSS), provide valuable data on health topics for large jurisdictions, but insufficient sample sizes prevent such surveys from thoroughly meeting the surveillance needs of local health jurisdictions (6). This is particularly true for a region as populous and diverse as Los Angeles County (LAC), in which the Department of Public Health (DPH) must maintain an understanding of the health status of numerous population subgroups.

CONTEXT

In 1997, the director of the LAC DPH (at that time part of the Department of Health Services) commissioned an independent review of the county's public health programs and services. This influential report concluded that there was no active assessment of the needs of the diverse LAC communities that could be used to define policies and goals, or to plan and execute programs to meet those goals (7). The report recommended creating a centralized assessment unit to monitor the health status of the entire LAC population, including chronic and communicable diseases, environmental health, and violence and injury prevention. Using information from these assessments, the DPH was to prioritize preventive actions; recommend integration of personal and clinical preventive services; identify areas for promotion and support of community-based preventive services; and propose allocation of County budget resources to achieve prevention priorities.

In response, the Los Angeles County Health Survey (LACHS) was inaugurated in 1997, and in 1998, the Office of Health Assessment and Epidemiology (OHAE) was created to house the Health Assessment Unit (HAU) that is responsible for all aspects of the survey. Since then, the LACHS has been performed every two to three years (see Figure 2–1).

APPROACH TO THE PROBLEM AND IMPLEMENTATION OF SOLUTIONS

In designing the LACHS, the DPH sought reliable population estimates for selected, key health indicators. The survey aimed to identify disparities across population subgroups, including subgroups based on gender, age, race/ethnicity, income, education, and geography; to track health trends over time; to compare the health of LAC residents with state and national data; and to benchmark them against national health objectives such as Healthy People. Over the years, the LACHS has become the foundation for evidence-based public health practice by DPH programs, generating needs assessment data to shape programs and policy, and allowing for the development of population health indicators that serve as performance measures.

In planning and designing the LACHS, epidemiologists and consultants emulated other established health surveys such as the NHIS and BRFSS. The questions from these national surveys have been validated for use in telephone surveys, so incorporating them allows LAC statistics to be easily compared with state and national data. For each survey iteration, HAU staff review questionnaires from the most recent

- Random digit-dial telephone survey
- Cell phone component
- Conducted every 2–3 years
- 6 Languages: English, Spanish, Mandarin, Cantonese, Vietnamese, Korean
- Weighted to reflect the non-institutionalized population
- Sample adequate to provide stable county and sub-county estimates
- Components
  - Adult: ~8,000; one adult randomly selected per household
  - Adult subsamples: mini-surveys administered to a subset of ~1,000 randomly selected adults from the main sample
  - Child: ~6,000 parents/guardians of children 0–17 years old
- Limitations
  - Self-reported data
  - Omits people without telephones and those living in group quarters, including college dormitories, nursing homes, jails
  - Declining response rates to telephone surveys nationwide
  - Increasingly expensive to reach the cell phone-only population

Figure 2–1 Characteristics of the LAC Health Survey

NHIS and BRFSS, along with other national, state, and local surveys on public health topics. This ensures that the LACHS approach remains current. LACHS questions on clinical care focus on the use of preventive services, are based on national guidelines such as the U.S. Preventive Services Task Force's Guide to Clinical Preventive Services (8), and are updated as recommendations change.

To be consistent with national statistics, such as those available from the Centers for Disease Control and Prevention (CDC), data collected through the LACHS use standard definitions. For example, some basic measures of public health, such as binge drinking, asthma, and cigarette smoking, have been refined, and guidelines have evolved for health-related activities such as Pap smear screening intervals. HAU staff monitor these changes to ensure that the survey questionnaires, as well as subsequent analyses and interpretation of the data, reflect up-to-date public health research and practice.

An advantage of designing and implementing a local health survey is that the DPH maintains flexibility to ensure that the survey meets the particular data needs of LAC. To this end, in designing the questionnaires, HAU staff meet with colleagues from many DPH programs, with key stakeholders in other county departments, and with partnering agencies. Generally, survey items must address a specific program goal, provide needed information for staff and constituents, or advance public health planning, evaluation, or policy. As the goals and priorities of the DPH shift over time, the LACHS also evolves; as many as half of the survey questions change from one survey to the next (see Figure 2–2).

The emergency preparedness questions provide a good example of shifting public health priorities and the LACHS's ability to capture them. Following the attacks on the World Trade Center of September 11, 2001, public health emergency preparedness efforts focused on bioterrorism, and survey questions in 2002 reflected this concern. However, because LAC is also vulnerable to a variety of natural disasters, including fires, floods, and earthquakes, the Emergency Preparedness and Response Program (EPRP) also needs data about residents' general level of preparedness. In some years, survey questions have focused on maintaining emergency home supplies (e.g., canned food, water, flashlights, and batteries) and whether families have a plan for contacting each other and meeting during or after an incident. After Hurricane Katrina, analyses focused on questions to quantify vulnerable populations and assess the public's level of trust in authorities. Later in the decade, as concerns about pandemic influenza increased, LACHS preparedness questions centered on flu preparedness and response and LAC residents' ability to "shelter in place." Today, as emergency preparedness efforts increasingly involve measuring and fostering community resilience, the LACHS is incorporating measures of neighborhood cohesion and interpersonal support.

ADMINISTRATION OF THE SURVEY

The DPH contracts with a survey research firm that performs sample design, administers hundreds of thousands of telephone calls, maximizes response rates, and delivers a weighted data set to the HAU. While staff salaries in the Health Assessment Unit derive from the county's general fund, the LACHS itself is not supported by any LAC monies. To pay the survey vendor, OHAE relies primarily on grant funds from programs and partners whose work requires high-quality population data collection. Over the years, key partners in funding the survey have included the DPH's Tobacco Control and Prevention Program, EPRP, and Substance

- Adults
  - Demographics and Social Factors
    - Gender
    - Age
    - Race/ethnicity
    - Income (% of Federal Poverty Level)
    - Educational attainment
    - Employment
    - Foreign-born vs. US-born
    - Language mostly spoken at home
    - Insurance Status
    - Disability status
    - Sexual orientation
    - Incarceration history
  - Chronic conditions
  - Health-related quality of life
  - Health behaviors
  - Health insurance & access to care
  - Preventive health services
  - Emergency preparedness
  - Caregiving
  - Environmental health
  - Neighborhood safety
  - Opinions on public health policy
- Children
  - Chronic conditions
  - Special health care needs
  - Health insurance & access to care
  - Biological mother's preconception knowledge
  - Breastfeeding
  - Child care
  - Parental routines
  - Nutrition
  - Physical activity
  - Screen time
  - Parental risk factors
  - Vaccination
  - Arts education

Figure 2–2 LAC Health Survey Topics

Abuse Prevention and Control. The Office of Aids Programs and Policy, Maternal Child Adolescent Health, and Environmental Health also have provided support. The LAC Department of Mental Health recently invested funds to collect more detailed data on mental health. Another major funding source is community partner First 5 LA, a child advocacy organization created by California voters that uses tobacco tax revenues to improve the lives of young children. First 5 LA generously supports the child portion of the LACHS to inform its work throughout LAC. In earlier years of the survey, funding also was provided by the California Department of Health Services, the Health Care Financing Administration (now the Center for Medicare and Medicaid Services), the LAC Medicaid Demonstration Project, and the LAC Department of Public Social Services.

CHALLENGES

The dependence on soft money to fund LACHS data collection presents significant challenges. Funders are not able to guarantee monies from one survey cycle to the next due to fluctuations in their own funding, competing needs, and the timing of their grant cycles. Beyond the need to raise money for the survey, the link between funding and questionnaire content impacts survey content. To receive enough money to conduct the survey, HAU must guarantee funders that the DPH will meet their data collection needs. However, the topics that funders favor must be balanced with other important health topics that lack well-funded constituencies, for example, the Immunization and Injury Prevention Programs. Because the entire survey lasts 25–30 minutes, important topics are almost always curtailed or omitted, and the process of striving for optimal content becomes pain staking.

The LACHS, like other telephone surveys, faces major challenges inherent to its design. Response rates to phone surveys are declining nationwide, and are lowest in urban areas like LAC. Rapid growth in the use of cellular phones, particularly growth of the population that depends exclusively on cell phones (known as "cell phone–only"), is forcing a change in the methodology of telephone surveys. When the LACHS began, in 1997, data collection via cell phones was not an issue. While a portion of the population was automatically excluded from the survey, such as the homeless and those too poor to afford telephone service, the survey could rely on landline contacts to reach a representative household sample. In 2002 an estimated 1.3% of Americans were classified as cell phone–only (9); by 2005 this number approached 10% (10). Recently published data from the National Health Interview Survey reveal that in the last half of 2010 three of every ten American homes (29.7%) had only wireless telephone service—an increase of 3.1 percentage points since the first half of 2010 (11). While exclusive cell phone use is increasing among Americans of all ages, rates of cell phone–only use are highest in families with children; in 2010, 31.8% of all U.S. children (more than 23 million children) lived in households with only wireless telephones. Data from a number of national studies reveal that people who rely on wireless phones differ from those who do not; they are more likely to be young adults, to live in or near poverty, to be Hispanic, and to rent rather than own their homes (10, 12, 13). Therefore, exclusion or limitation of the cell phone–only population biases telephone survey samples. The 2011 LACHS incorporates a cell phone component, which will improve the validity and generalizability of the resulting data, but which complicates survey administration and greatly increases its cost. As social media evolve, and younger generations increasingly use their phones as computers rather than as speaking devices, survey methodologies must adapt.

EVALUATION STRATEGY

The success of the LACHS is measured qualitatively, through the data's influence on program planning, evaluation, and policy making for the DPH and its government, community, and academic partners (see "Impact," below). LACHS data are widely shared through reports, community and conference presentations, peer-reviewed manuscripts, and through the DPH website, which houses dozens of standardized data tables and an interactive query system for the recent years of the LACHS (14). Quantitatively, the HAU receives five to eight customized data requests a month from stakeholders seeking data for use in grant applications, policy development, research, community outreach, and education.

In evaluating the representativeness of the LACHS, the DPH tracks survey response and cooperation rates. Response rates are defined as the number of completed survey interviews divided by the total number of phone numbers selected for the survey sample, including non-residential numbers, numbers where contact with a household member was never achieved, and numbers where the person who answered the phone did not wish to participate. The 2007 LACHS response rate was 18% for the Adult Survey and 15% for the Child Survey, including ineligible homes where no children lived. The 2007 LACHS response rates were lower than those achieved in earlier LACHS studies of 2005 (22.8% Adult, 26.0% Child) and 2002–2003 (31.1% Adult, 33.9% Child).

In 2007, the cooperation rates for the LACHS Adult and Child Survey both equaled 40%, meaning that 40% of the people who answered the phone and were determined to be eligible (because they lived in LAC and were 18 years of age or older) completed the health interview. Cooperation rates for the LACHS have declined from 49% for the adult portion of the survey in 2005 and 57% in 2002, and 78% for the Child Survey in both 2005 and 2002. (The steep drop in the cooperation rate for the Child Survey between 2005 and 2007 reflected a change in methodology for the calculation.)

The DPH also evaluates the LACHS by analyzing the quality of the sample. With lower-than-desired response rates becoming the norm for telephone surveys, HAU must ascertain if the sample of survey responders accurately represents the population from which they are drawn. Though the people who respond to a telephone survey may differ from those who do not, the LACHS sample closely reflects the non-institutionalized LAC population in terms of distribution of gender, age, income, race/ethnicity, language spoken at home, and percent foreign born, increasing confidence that data collected through the LACHS provide valid estimates of the health of the LAC population.

An informal measure of the survey's performance is its comparison with data collected by other validated LAC telephone surveys. Though the BRFSS collects a smaller sample, overall LAC estimates by the BRFSS and the LACHS generally align. Similarly, the California Health Interview Survey, the largest state-based survey in the United States, typically produces estimates similar to those of LACHS for variables that the surveys have in common.

IMPACT

Population-based data are essential to the core functions of public health. Such data are used in measuring a community's health (assessment); in establishing a community health improvement plan and related action steps via policies, programs, and guidelines (policy); and in evaluating the improvement plan and actions to provide feedback to the community (assurance) (15). LACHS data fulfill all of these functions for the DPH, providing a wealth of data at the county and sub-county level that are used for program planning and evaluation, policy development, workforce development, community assessment and outreach.

As an example, LACHS data have been used to identify areas of the county with the largest numbers of children who were eligible for public health insurance, but who were not enrolled. The Department of Health Services (DHS) used data from the LACHS to develop a needs-based formula to allocate funding for outreach and enrollment by Service Planning Area (SPA). The Children's Health Initiative, along with First 5 LA and other coalition partners, then worked to fund Healthy Kids, an expansion of California's Healthy Families (S-CHIP) program, to enroll and insure 65,000 children in the county. Figure 2–3 shows trends in children's health insurance coverage in LAC from 1997–2007 (see also Chapter 34).

LACHS findings showing higher rates of food insecurity among households with children led to policy recommendations and actions by the LA Collaborative for

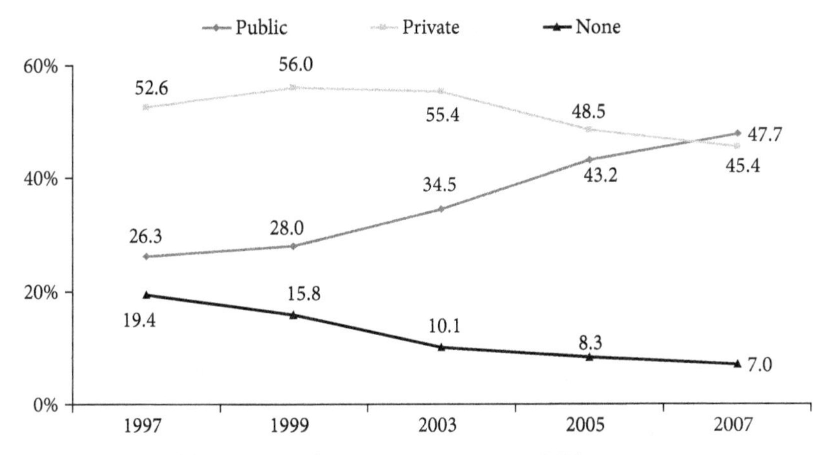

Figure 2-3 Child (0–17 years) Insurance Types, LACHS 1997–2007

Healthy Active Children, representing nearly 100 organizations. Because food insecurity impacted families with household incomes up to 300% of the federal poverty level, it was recommended that state and federal programs eliminate the "reduced-price" lunch category in favor of a free lunch program for all low-income students. The Collaborative launched the Healthy Breakfast Campaign, which included a media campaign to promote eating a healthy breakfast, the development of a teacher classroom tool kit about healthy breakfast, and assistance for school districts to reduce child hunger and improve nutrition within schools.

OHAE reports disseminate LACHS data to audiences within and outside LAC. Following each LACHS iteration, the DPH produces a Key Indicators of Health report, which presents data for the county's eight geographic SPAs and highlights health disparities and opportunities for improvement. Over 20,000 hard copies of these reports are distributed throughout LAC to people working on public health issues in local government, health care agencies, schools, academia, and community-based organizations. In cooperation with the LAC Office of Women's Health, HAU also creates a Women's Health Indicators report to highlight disparities among women by race/ethnicity, income, or insurance status.

"LA Health" briefs and Cities and Community reports also present LACHS data, providing local statistics regarding public health problems and recommendations for individual, community, and policy-level changes to address the issues (15). LA Health briefs identify disparities by age, gender, race/ethnicity, income, insurance status, and other underlying determinants of health, and typically involve collaboration across public health programs or with community partners. For example, in 2010 an LA Health brief on diabetes was produced in concert with the Division of Chronic Disease and Injury Prevention and with the local chapter of the American Diabetes Association (ADA). The report focused on the link between obesity and diabetes (see Figure 2-4 and Figure 2-5) and provided recommendations for confronting these related epidemics. The brief included one-page educational inserts in English and Spanish for the lay public, and the ADA used the materials extensively for outreach and education during National Diabetes Month and World Diabetes Day.

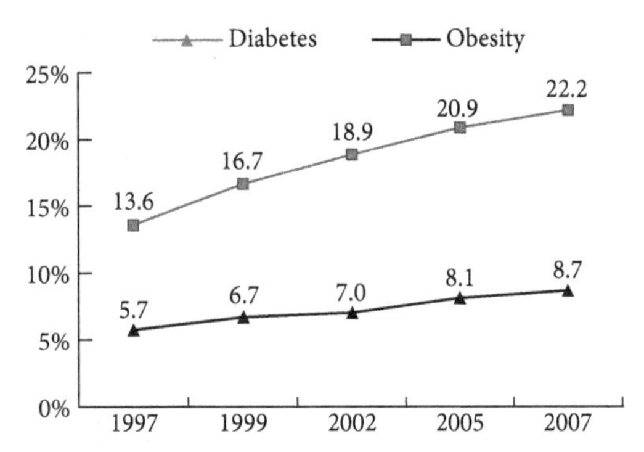

Figure 2–4 Adult Obesity and Diabetes Trends, 1997–2007 LACHS

Data from the LACHS have been used to model small area estimates for obesity and cigarette smoking. These estimates have been presented in OHAE's Cities and Communities reports as geographic indicators for the 88 incorporated cities and over 40 unincorporated communities that comprise LAC. Data from the Cities and Communities report on tobacco use have been cited by lawmakers to support tobacco control legislation in West Hollywood, Redondo Beach, and the City of Los Angeles. A DPH representative attending an LA City Council meeting in October 2010 reported that a "Councilman…held a copy of the cities tobacco prevalence report and frequently referred to it as he made the case for a citywide comprehensive smoke-free ordinance."

CONCLUSIONS AND KEY LESSONS

- Local health departments need data at the community level. Since 1997, the LACHS has provided key data for LAC.
- Well-designed population health surveys can identify disparities at the local level, including disparities by gender, age, race/ethnicity, income, education, nativity, languages spoken, and sub-county geography.
- The rapidly increasing prevalence of "cell phone–only" households and individuals necessitates a change from traditional landline-based sampling, but cell phone surveys are more difficult to administer and are much more expensive.
- Declining response rates to telephone surveys present a major challenge to telephone survey research. However, to date, the collection of a sample that closely reflects the LAC household population has enabled the LACHS to provide valid population estimates.
- As response rates for telephone health surveys decline, new methodologies will be required, possibly including web-based surveys, return to mail surveys, and mixed-methods surveys.
- As social e-media evolve, it will be necessary to adapt survey methodology to assure representative samples.
- Data from the LACHS improve community understanding of health issues and evidence-based public health policy.

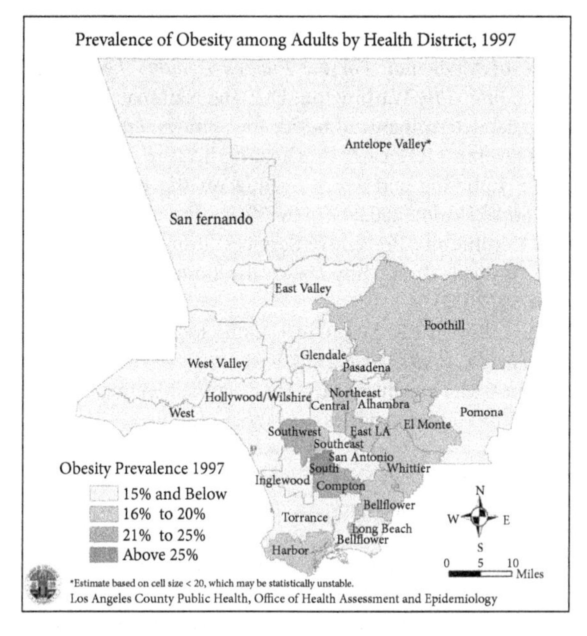

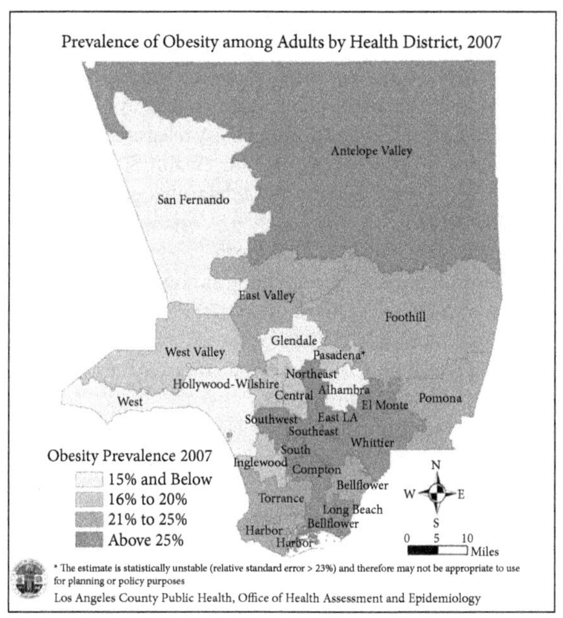

Figure 2–5 Prevalence of Obesity Among Adults in Los Angeles County, 1997 and 2007.

REFERENCES

1. IOM (Institute of Medicine). *For the Public's Health: The Role of Measurement in Action and Accountability*. Washington, DC: The National Academies Press; 2011.
2. Marmot M. Social determinants of health inequalities. *Lancet*. 2005;365:1099–104.
3. Srinivasan S, O'Fallon LR, Dearry A. Creating healthy communities, healthy homes, healthy people: Initiating a research agenda on the built environment and public health. *Am J Public Health*. 2003;93:1446–50.
4. The Guide to Community Preventive Services. Promoting health through the social environment. Available from: http://www.thecommunityguide.org/social/index.html (accessed June 19, 2012).
5. Luck J, Chang C, Brown ER, Lumpkin J. Using local health information to promote public health. *Health Affairs*. 2006;25:979–91.
6. Simon PA, Wold CM, Cousineau MR, Fielding JE. Meeting the data needs of a local health department: The Los Angeles County Health Survey. *Am J Public Health*. 2001; 91:1950–52.
7. UCLA School of Public Health Technical Assistance Group. *Report of Review of Public Health Programs and Services, Los Angeles County Department of Health Services*. July 1997.
8. U.S. Preventive Services Task Force. Available from: http://www.uspreventiveservices-taskforce.org/ (accessed June 19, 2012).
9. Piekarski L, Survey Sampling International. Cellular phones: Challenges and opportunities. *Survey Research Newsletter*, University of Illinois, Chicago, 2003;34.
10. Christian L, Keeter S, Purcell K, Smith A. Assessing the cell phone challenge, Pew Research Center. May 20, 2010. Available from: http://pewresearch.org/pubs/1601/assessing-cell-phone-challenge-in-public-opinion-surveys (accessed June 19, 2012).
11. Blumberg SJ, Luke JV. Wireless substitution: Early release of estimates from the National Health Interview Survey, National Center for Health Statistics. July-December 2010. Available from: http://www.cdc.gov/nchs/data/nhis/earlyrelease/wireless201106.pdf (accessed June 19, 2012).
12. Link MW, Battaglia MP, Frankel MR, Osborn L, Mokdad AH. Reaching the US cell phone generation: Comparison of cell phone survey results with an ongoing landline telephone survey. *Pub Opinion Quarterly*. 2007;71:814–39.
13. Currivan D, Roe D, Stockdale J. The impact of landline and cell phone usage patterns among young adults on RDD survey outcomes. American Association for Public Opinion Research Annual Meeting, 2008.
14. Los Angeles County Department of Public Health, Health Assessment Unit. Available from: http://publichealth.lacounty.gov/ha/ (accessed June 19, 2012).
15. Wisconsin Department of Health and Family Services, Division of Public Health. *Healthiest Wisconsin 2010: A Partnership Plan to Improve the Health of the Public* (PPH 0276). April 2002.

3 Strategic Planning

Visioning the New Public Health Agency

WENDY K. SCHIFFER,
VIRGINIA HUANG RICHMAN,
JOSHUA M. BOBROWSKY, AND
MAXANNE HATCH

NATURE OF THE PROBLEM

An understanding of the role of public health often eludes those not working in the field. The first thought associated with health is often medical care. From 1972 to 2006, public health in Los Angeles County (LAC) was a division of the Department of Health Services (DHS), which operated safety net hospitals and ambulatory care facilities in addition to its public health responsibilities. Patient care, with its immediate and urgent nature and chronic budget shortfalls, consumed most of the department's attention and financial resources. The mission and goals of public health were not widely articulated throughout the department, and often were eclipsed by higher visibility medical care issues.

Public health is complex. With work as diverse as laboratory sciences, environmental health inspections, infectious disease screening and treatment, health education, and policy analysis, as well as population-focused programs such as HIV prevention and children's health programs, public health staff and advocates often develop a narrow focus on a particular health issue or population. Categorical funding streams and statutory requirements reinforce this narrow approach.

Lack of a clear vision and a "silo" approach to health issues can lead to a weakly functioning public health department and a failure to capitalize on synergies that are less apparent to each subject area. A 1997 report on the state of public health in Los Angeles County, *Report of Review of Public Health Programs and Services, Los Angeles County Department of Health Services* (*Breslow Report*) (1), found that the DHS public health division was severely hampered in its ability to perform basic public health functions. The report cited deficiencies in staff morale, size and competency of the workforce, communication with communities, and long-term planning based on local needs. It also called for the appointment of a Health Officer with greater authority to lead population-level and preventive health activities, as required by California statute and county ordinance. At the time the report was written, the position within the DHS was only filled nominally. The *Breslow Report* provided the lever for major restructuring of the public health division and, years later, for creation of a separate Department of Public Health (DPH).

The restructuring created a need for strategic planning to set a direction and common vision for the department; a strategic plan for public health was completed in 2005. The DPH's establishment as a separate department in 2006 provided the impetus to create a new strategic plan, which built upon the 2005 plan. This plan, which covered the years 2008–2011, provided an excellent opportunity to increase awareness of the department, generate a shared identity among internal DPH divisions, and prioritize goals for the twenty-first-century public health department, including new initiatives to address the root causes of poor health.

CONTEXT

While prevention and control of infectious disease remain a major focus of public health, prevention of chronic disease merited greater attention if public health resources were to align with the greatest burden of disease. Chronic diseases, injuries, substance abuse, and mental health issues are the leading causes of mortality and premature death, as measured by years of potential life lost, and are largely preventable (2). Coronary heart disease, stroke, and lung cancer can be prevented to a significant degree through a healthy diet (see Chapter 11), exercise (see Chapter 12), and avoidance of tobacco (see Chapter 13); deaths from injuries due to homicide, suicide, motor vehicle crashes, and drug overdose can also be ameliorated. Obesity contributes to major causes of morbidity and mortality and requires public health action to address upstream determinants, such as creating environments that promote physical activity and affordable, accessible healthy food options.

In addition, emergency preparedness and response gained in importance after the events of September 11 and intentional anthrax attacks in 2001, Hurricane Katrina, and anticipated increases in natural disasters due to climate change. Public health staff have traditionally served as emergency responders; however, these highly visible events created a community and federal expectation that public health would play a greater response role. Public health departments needed to shift their organizational culture to inculcate all department employees with their responsibility in a public health emergency.

To address the public health threats and challenges of the twenty-first century, local health departments need to work with partners beyond the traditional health sector on issues such as land use, transportation, and environmental policies, as well as employment, education, and social cohesion (3). Attention to the physical and social environmental factors that affect health—making the easy choice the healthy choice—is redolent of the twentieth-century social progressive movement. Indeed, 25 of the 30-year gain in life expectancy during the twentieth century has been attributed to public health improvements such as sanitation and occupational and food safety (4).

Unfortunately, funding streams do not align well with the leading upstream determinants of morbidity and mortality. Three-quarters of the department's funding comes from categorical grants that focus on specific disease areas and have restrictive program requirements, restrictions that often increase as funding is reduced. Although the DPH has received tobacco control funding from the State of California since 1989, only with the recent creation of the 2010 Communities Putting Prevention to Work federal initiative has the DPH received significant funding to promote policies, systems, and environmental changes to address physical activity, nutrition, obesity, and tobacco use and exposure.

Factors other than funding affect DPH's priorities. Public health departments have statutory requirements, and the public and elected officials have expectations for what the DPH should address. DPH activities are also bounded by the capabilities of its staff. While the DPH has a highly capable staff, an insufficient number possess the skills to address underlying determinants, such as community engagement, policy analysis, and assessing preventable burden. The challenge was to develop a strategic plan that balanced a focus on determinants with the need to fulfill mandates and community expectations (e.g., increased attention to emergency preparedness), within the confines of categorical funding streams and staffing capabilities.

The DPH, as a public entity, has had to balance external stakeholder participation and transparency in the strategic planning process against the need to manage stakeholder expectations given the latitude a public entity has to transform within its jurisdiction, mandates, and resources. Stakeholder input for the 2005 plan was obtained via electronic surveys and key informant interviews conducted with public health staff and with external stakeholders, including elected officials, health care providers, community-based advocates, and federal and state representatives. Once the stakeholder data were analyzed, working groups developed elements of the plan, including the vision and mission, values, and organizational goals.

The 2005 plan focused on emerging issues such as obesity and emergency preparedness, and underlying determinants such as the physical and social environment. The plan also included goals to improve organizational effectiveness, workforce excellence, and fiscal accountability. Despite the plan's alignment with the pressing health needs affecting communities, it had difficulty gaining traction among DPH staff. There was not broad familiarity with the plan beyond the relatively small group of managers directly involved in its development, and consequently there was little buy-in. The plan focused on a few strategic areas rather than the full range of existing DPH activities, which resulted in some divisions feeling excluded. Infectious disease, for example, was excluded from the plan because it was not perceived to need a new strategic approach. The plan's focus on underlying determinants such as the physical and social environment also led to perceptions among some staff that the plan was irrelevant to their work. Most important, measurable goals and objectives were not developed for all priority areas, nor was lead responsibility assigned for many of the newest areas. Lessons learned from the 2005 plan informed the development of a strategic plan for the newly created DPH.

■ APPROACH TO THE PROBLEM AND IMPLEMENTATION OF SOLUTIONS

A Planning Division was created within the DPH, responsible for developing strategic plans, coordinating implementation, and monitoring progress. Planning staff worked with DPH leadership to create a plan that would clearly articulate DPH priorities and would be used to guide decision making. The new strategic plan, covering the years 2008–2011, built upon the foundation of the 2005 plan. However, the process was designed to avoid the implementation difficulties of the 2005 plan, specifically: 1) the plan was made more comprehensive to increase its applicability throughout the DPH; 2) goals and objectives were developed for all strategic priority areas; 3) readability was improved; and 4) planning staff actively taught the plan to all divisions within the DPH to increase familiarity and buy-in.

The DPH's plan, like most strategic plans, included vision and mission statements, values, and goals and objectives. The vision, mission, and values were kept brief and compelling so that they could be easily remembered, understood, and implemented. The DPH's vision, mission, and values are provided in Box 3–1.

The plan needed to balance a comprehensive approach, in which all or most of the department's programmatic areas are represented, with a more strategic approach,

BOX 3–1 ■ DPH Vision, Mission, and Values (2005 and 2008–2011 Plans)

Vision: Healthy people in healthy communities
Mission: To protect health, prevent disease, and promote health and well-being
Values:
Leadership
Customer Service
Quality
Collaboration
Accountability
Respect
Professionalism

in which goals and objectives primarily focus on the DPH's new or highest priority strategic initiatives. A comprehensive approach would increase buy-in because staff could see how the plan applied to their work. Since a strategic plan also serves as an education tool for the community, it should not exclude major programmatic areas. In response, the 2008–2011 plan included strategic priority areas (see Box 3–2) that spanned the DPH's broad range of responsibility. Priority areas encompassed programmatic as well as administrative areas. In this way, the DPH strategic plan aligned with LAC's strategic plan, placing the DPH's planning efforts within the context of its broader governmental structure. The LAC strategic plan, which was being updated in 2005 during the period that the DPH strategic plan was being developed, focused on priority areas that improved the county's internal capability to deliver services to the public. Priority areas included service excellence, organizational effectiveness, workforce excellence, and fiscal responsibility.

For each strategic priority area, goals and objectives were developed that were specific enough to be actionable, yet were still areas of strategic importance. For example, a health improvement priority area goal was to "address elements of the physical environment to improve population health and reduce disparities," and an objective under this goal was to "support cities in implementing land use, transportation, and organizational policies that protect and promote the health of residents and workers." Although this does not meet all the characteristics of a SMART objective (specific, measurable, achievable, realistic, and time-bound), it does specify a clear

BOX 3–2 ■ Strategic Priority Areas in the DPH Strategic Plan 2008–2011

1. Health Improvement
2. Health Protection
3. Preparedness
4. Organizational Effectiveness
5. Workforce Excellence
6. Fiscal Accountability

direction for the DPH. DPH planning staff worked with the responsible managers to ensure that the goals were a reach, yet achievable. As goals and objectives were being developed, planning staff regularly shared drafts with DPH leadership to ensure that the plan reflected DPH priorities. The process of DPH leadership working together to agree upon strategic priority areas and to develop specific goals and objectives created additional buy-in.

The strategic plan was designed to be easily used for internal planning. The text was reader friendly so that it would be accessible to staff at all levels in the organization. DPH communications staff designed the layout to make the plan attractive and easy to read; text was liberally interspersed with graphics and photos. Brief sections on LAC, demographics, health status, and descriptions of DPH programs were added. A feature entitled, "Today in the DPH..." highlighted activities that the DPH carries out every day. The layout and content served a secondary purpose—to educate external stakeholders about what the DPH does and its priorities for the future.

The plan was widely disseminated. A presentation tool kit included a one-page executive summary and an interactive slide presentation that served as a teaching module. The plan was sent electronically to all DPH employees, and presentations were made to every DPH division. The plan's content is included in training for all new employees and new supervisors. The plan was also sent to external stakeholders, including community advocates, elected officials, academics, and other county department heads, and is posted on the DPH website (5).

Strategic planning was not limited to the development of the DPH strategic plan. DPH planning staff assisted DPH divisions with their own strategic planning. A strategic planning tool kit was developed with materials and references, including a tip sheet on how to write a good strategic plan. Planning staff gave presentations, disseminated the tool kit, and provided reviews and comments on division-level strategic plans. Planning staff also facilitated the use of a prioritization tool for a division seeking to change focus, so that priorities would be informed by data and evidence-based practice.

■ EVALUATION STRATEGY

The 2008–2011 strategic plan was informed by evaluation findings from the 2005 plan. DPH planning staff obtained qualitative information on the 2005 plan through facilitated discussions with DPH managers and an electronic survey that evaluated their knowledge and use of the plan. The survey found that staff did not know where to find the strategic plan; did not know that a plan existed; saw the plan as having little relevance to their day-to-day work; and did not understand its purpose. These results influenced the development of the new plan.

Qualitative information was obtained to evaluate the 2008–2011 plan through facilitated discussions at several executive team meetings. More systematically, the plan's implementation was measured through departmental progress reporting. Sensitive to the reporting demands on DPH staff from funders, external agencies, and for other DPH initiatives, the Planning office opted not to create stand-alone, ongoing strategic plan progress reports. Rather, strategic plan progress reporting was integrated into the DPH performance improvement initiative (see Chapter 7). This approach established that implementation of the strategic plan and performance improvement should be integrated, and helped to assess how closely the work of the programs, as measured by their performance indicators, aligned with the strategic plan goals and objectives.

The strategic plan's goals and objectives were cross-walked to the division-level goals, performance measures, and population indicators to identify gaps. This revealed that some strategic plan objectives had no applicable performance measures. Most commonly this occurred for cross-cutting objectives that spanned multiple divisions. For example, the objectives associated with the goal "address elements of the social environment to improve population health and reduce disparities" had no performance measures. This goal area had no clear organizational home, and its implementation involved participation from the DPH director's office; Chronic Disease and Injury Prevention; Health Assessment and Epidemiology; Community Health Services; and other entities. The progress report led to recommendations around changes to divisions' measures, but more important, identified the need to develop crosscutting measures for objectives that applied to more than one division.

IMPACT

The strategic plan successfully articulated the department's strategic priorities for all employees and external stakeholders. The emphasis on the physical and social environment and obesity prevention provided the DPH with the impetus for addressing the underlying determinants of health, using tools such as community engagement and policy change. The department had been working on policy development around tobacco control for many years, and had recently established a program within the Chronic Disease division called PLACE (Policies for Livable Active Communities and Environments) that focused on using policy change to support the development of healthy, safe, and active communities (see Chapter 12). However, this strategy is not limited to the DPH's chronic disease division. The DPH's Community Health Services field staff are forging relationships with cities and advocacy groups to pursue policy change leading to healthier communities. When the federal Communities Putting Prevention to Work grants were released by the Centers for Disease Control and Prevention, the DPH was well positioned to implement grant activities focused on community determinants and policy development.

Numerous management practices have been aligned with the strategic plan priorities. High-level managers, including the department director, use the plan priorities to develop their annual management goals. The budget process considers strategic plan priorities in funding recommendations, as does the process for evaluating information technology projects.

The impact on staff is apparent. As planning staff continue to make presentations, employees now express familiarity with the plan and with the DPH's role in addressing underlying determinants of health. As the DPH embarks on creating a new strategic plan, planning staff will assess the existing plan, including repeating some of the questions from the earlier survey of staff knowledge and use of the plan.

A strategic plan, however, can only be as effective as the environment permits. Funding streams still largely dictate the DPH's activities. Ideally, health burden, preventability, and resource needs drive strategic actions. In reality, the department has limited discretionary funding, which frequently results in a mismatch between priority areas such as the physical and social environment and categorical funding streams that focus on particular diseases or risk factors. Fortunately, some new federal funding, such as the Communities Putting Prevention to Work grants and the Patient Protection and Affordable Care Act's Community Transformation Grants, support policy change for healthy communities that support important policy initiatives (see Chapters 12 and 13). Time will tell whether these become sustainable funding sources rather than time-limited pilot projects.

The department's organizational structure has also limited the plan's impact. For example, there is no obvious division to take responsibility for work around the social environment, and the DPH's niche remains to be more clearly defined, since primary responsibility for factors such as education and income lies in other organizations. This ambiguity has made progress difficult to measure and to achieve. The "silo factor" widely discussed in public health has also hindered progress. Divisions have few fungible resources and a full complement of existing activities, in some cases mandated by funders, which limits their ability to incorporate new activities to support strategic plan goals. Where strategic plan goals and objectives were cross-cutting, the diffusion of responsibility rather than the assignment of a single lead manager hindered progress.

The process of strategic planning has been almost as important as the product itself. A periodic process for strategic planning provides time for introspection and analysis of data and evidence-based practice, and establishes a learning organization. The process gauged organizational strengths and weaknesses, political and social environmental changes, and allowed leadership to identify the need for organizational transformations and the pace at which they should occur. Strategic plan goals and objectives provided a road map for program priorities and, therefore, day-to-day work and continuous quality improvement efforts; indeed, a strategic plan is a prerequisite for public health accreditation (6).

■ CONCLUSIONS

The strategic planning process provided a number of important lessons, including:

- A strategic plan must balance comprehensiveness and strategic vision in order to garner staff buy-in and applicability to all departmental divisions. The department's core functions or major lines of work should not be excluded; however, the plan's goals and objectives must be elevated above daily functions.
- Undergoing the process of introspection with staff, management, and community members is valuable. The visioning and prioritization processes create shared goals and a commitment to the road map for achieving the strategic plan's vision.
- Stakeholder input is essential to ensure that the plan reflects organizational and community needs; yet expectations must be managed throughout the planning process. Unrealistic expectations may arise when participants do not share a common set of guiding principles or a basic understanding of the department's mandated and categorically funded functions.
- Goals and objectives must be measurable to monitor progress over time, and performance measures should be developed for all strategic plan goals and objectives.
- The plan should be attractive and reader-friendly, to pique the interest of internal and external stakeholders.

- The plan should be presented to employees in an engaging, interactive manner, to generate understanding and buy-in among those who will be working on implementation of the plan's objectives.
- An implementation plan should be developed with specific strategies, responsible managers, and time frames to ensure accountability and to track progress.

■ REFERENCES

1. Breslow L, Luck J, et al., *Report of Review of Public Health Programs and Services, Los Angeles County Department of Health Services*. Los Angeles: UCLA School of Public Health Technical Assistance Group; 1997.
2. Los Angeles County Department of Public Health, Office of Health Assessment and Epidemiology. *Mortality in Los Angeles County 2007: Leading Causes of Death and Premature Death with Trends for 1998–2007*. 2010. Available from: http://www.publichealth.lacounty.gov/dca/data/documents/2007MortalityReport.pdf (accessed Aug. 22, 2011).
3. National Prevention Council. *National Prevention Strategy*. Washington, DC: U.S. Department of Health and Human Services, Office of the Surgeon General; 2011; p. 14–7. Available from: http://www.healthcare.gov/center/councils/nphpphc/strategy/report.pdf.
4. CDC. Ten great public health achievements: United States 1900–1999. *MMWR Weekly* 1999;48(12):241–3.
5. Los Angeles County Department of Public Health, Office of Planning, Evaluation, and Development. *Department of Public Health Strategic Plan 2008–2011*. 2008. Available from: http://www.publichealth.lacounty.gov/docs/StrategicPlan.pdf (accessed Aug. 22, 2011).
6. Public Health Accreditation Board. *Standards and Measures v. 1.0*. 2011. Available from: http://dl.dropbox.com/u/12758866/PHAB%20Standards%20and%20Measures%20Version%201.0.pdf (accessed Aug. 22, 2011).

4 Programs and Policies That Work

How Evidence Can Drive Action

STEVEN M. TEUTSCH

THE NATURE OF THE PROBLEM: THE MISSING EVIDENCE

Many of the largest and oldest parts of the Los Angeles County (LAC) Department of Public Health (DPH) are categorically funded programs, such as those addressing sexually transmitted diseases, substance and alcohol abuse, and tobacco control. Each evolved as the changing nature of disease and funding sources required. Their intervention strategies reflected the state of the public health sector based on accumulated experience, expert opinion, and best practices. Some had been critically evaluated but many were based instead on traditional public health models lacking validation. Many were forms of health education and individually oriented case findings or clinical care. Public health was called upon to address a burgeoning set of issues with chronically scarce resources as the need increased to assure resource allocation to interventions shown to be effective.

This reassessment of programmatic resources revealed that many well-entrenched clinical interventions were of little value or were downright harmful. The era of expert opinion, patient demand, and pathophysiologic reasoning slowly gave way to a demand for proof that interventions worked. Although belatedly, public health leaders realized that they had to follow the new path.

This realization coincided with the need to increase prevention and control of intentional and unintentional injuries, chronic diseases, and environmental harms. Decisions about which interventions to implement to reduce these problems required a stronger, scientific foundation. For example, was driver education sufficient to prevent automobile crashes due to distracted driving? If so, what solutions would be most effective: through schools, small or large media, or driver education courses and printed materials? How effective were laws outlawing the use of mobile telephones while driving? How necessary was stronger enforcement of those laws? If a combination of strategies was necessary, what combination? Given finite resources, what should a public health department do?

When confronting newly recognized problems, there is the opportunity to assess the literature to ground program and policy initiatives in state-of-the-art science. For existing programs, the challenge is greater. Whole infrastructures had been built around specific interventions, such as sex education or drug education in schools or partner tracing and notification for patients with sexually transmitted diseases. In many ways, changing existing patterns is even more daunting than starting anew.

CONTEXT

The blossoming of basic and clinical sciences in the twentieth century brought an explosion of new technologies. The professorial model of handing down the wisdom and experience of one generation of clinicians to the next was challenged by discoveries of wide variations in clinical practice across the country (1), yet limited understanding of the consequences. There was overuse in some areas and underuse in others. Literature reviews, the scientific standard of the day, were found to be subjective, prone to bias, and inefficient, leading to suboptimal recommendations. In the mid-1980s the U.S. Preventive Services Task Force (USPSTF) (2) began applying the principles of clinical epidemiology to assess the efficacy of clinical preventive services. By using a clear hierarchy of evidence, the USPSTF rated clinical preventive services on their level of methodologic rigor and effectiveness. One member of that task force was Jonathan Fielding, who subsequently became LAC DPH's Director and Health Officer. The wisdom of using evidence-based methods to assess the effectiveness of clinical services gradually made its way into mainstream practice, supplanting expert-opinion–based methods and non-systematic literature reviews. With this emerging paradigm, the need to apply similar evidentiary rigor to population-based interventions became clearer. As a field that prides itself on the use of science, public health needed to step to the plate. The Community Preventive Services Task Force, the population-based counterpart to the USPSTF, began in 1996, led by Fielding and myself. It adapted methods used for the development of clinical recommendations to population-based recommendations and then applied them to key areas of public health (3).

Although public health leaders were committed to adopt a more evidence-based approach, these concepts were often unappreciated by many public health workers, political leaders, the public, and other stakeholders. Thus the mandate for implementing evidence-based programs began with a narrow base of support.

■ APPROACH TO THE PROBLEM

Evidence-based strategies must be built on good information about burden of disease and relevant determinants of health in the population of interest. Such populations can be a geographic area; a community; an ethnic, social, or faith-based group; an income or education-attainment group; or based on sexual orientation. DPH programs conduct their own surveillance activities, many quite detailed. More generally, the DPH conducts the LAC Health Survey (see Chapter 2), which provides much of county's health relevant data and is supplemented by information from the California Health Interview Survey, vital records, and other sources (see Chapter 10 on social determinants). The DPH also produces a "Key Indicators" report with extensive comparative data across the county's eight Service Planning Areas and compares that data with other benchmarks such as Healthy People objectives (4). These data, along with causes of death and other information, are used to set priorities for attention that have led to the creation of units responsible for chronic disease and injuries, for example.

Programmatic accountability for investing resources in those strategies and tactics with good evidence that they improve the public's health and reduce health disparities is operationalized through the DPH's performance improvement plan (see Chapter 7). That plan establishes metrics to monitor progress toward goals and objectives. Intrinsic to being able to achieve those objectives is a logic model that describes how resources are allocated to specific processes and how those processes link to intermediate and health outcomes.

Drawing on evidence-based recommendations and reviews such as the Guide to Community Preventive Services and the Cochrane Collaboration (5), each program is asked to select interventions that have documented effectiveness (see Table 4–1). The menu of evidence-based guidelines for each program, however, varies substantially in completeness and quality. For some areas, such as immunizations, the menu is long and robust. Not only do highly effective intervention strategies address demand (such

TABLE 4–1 *Examples of Interventions Recommended by the Community Guide (CG) and How They Are Implemented in LAC*

CG Topic Area	CG Recommendation(s)	Implemented by
Alcohol Consumption	Regulation of alcohol density locations	Implemented by local cities, Alcohol and Beverage Control, and a few SAPC* contracted programs in selected communities
Asthma Control	Home-based multi-trigger, multicomponent interventions for children and adolescents	Asthma Coalition of Los Angeles County
Oral Health	Community water fluoridation	Oral Health Program with community partners
Vaccination to Prevent Disease: Universally Recommended Vaccines—and Targeted Vaccines	Provider and client reminder/recall systems Multi-component interventions include education, home visiting interventions, and assessment and feedback for vaccination providers.	CA Immunization Registry (CAIR), African American Immunization Collaborative Project, LAC IP* (Nursing Unit, Field Staff and AFIX* Implementation Team)
HIV/AIDS, STIs, and Pregnancy	Group-based comprehensive risk reduction interventions for adolescents	STD* Program: Don't Think, Know campaign and Health Awareness Project OAPP*: Contracts with external agencies provide group level interventions targeted at youth
	Partner notification by provider referral to identify HIV-positive people	OAPP and STD work collaboratively to ensure that PCRS* through provider referral is: (1) offered to every individual diagnosed with HIV and (2) completed quickly/efficiently
	Community-, group-, and individual-level behavioral interventions for MSM*	OAPP: Contracts with external agencies to provide the three levels of interventions targeted at MSM*
Cancer Prevention and Control: Breast and Cervical Cancer (Client-Oriented)	Client reminders	OWH*: print and telephone
	One-on-one education	OWH: health fair brochures, newsletters and quarterly e-mail
	Small media	OWH: telephone with risk assessment

* SAPC = Substance Abuse Prevention and Control; IP = Immunization Program; AFIX = Assessment, Feedback, Incentives, and eXchange; OAPP = Office of Aids Programs and Policy; PCRS = Partner Counseling and Referral Services; STD = Sexually Transmitted Disease; MSM = Men Who Have Sex with Men; OWH = Office of Women's Health

as school laws requiring vaccination), incentives (such as no or low co-pays), access (such as in WIC centers, walk-in clinics open after hours), and provider and patient education (e.g., reminders), but we also know that multiple interventions that address each of these areas are more effective than single interventions or interventions that address one issue in multiple ways (6, 7).

For other areas, the menu is sparse. Notably, strongly evidence-based interventions to staunch the obesity epidemic have only slowly emerged (8), so interventions showing less robust evidence have necessarily been selected. The Secretary's Advisory Committee on Health Promotion and Disease Prevention developed a framework for deciding when action is needed in the face of suboptimal evidence and how to select among interventions when that is the case (9). We know that social determinants, including education, income, and social cohesion, are among the most important contributors to health, but there is less clarity about which specific interventions can effectively change them or the role of public health in those areas (10). Indeed, most interventions lie outside traditional public health domains. Thus high school graduation rates are under the purview of educators, and the availability of healthy food depends on agricultural and food-processing practices as well as on food vendors and consumer demand. Both are complex social phenomena in which public health can play important, but often secondary roles. When programs select interventions where the evidence is weak, it is incumbent on them to provide a strong evidence-based rationale as well as a plan for a well-conducted evaluation.

Developing the evidence of effectiveness can sometimes be relatively straight forward. One can show that reminders for mammography increase the number of women screened. It is much more difficult and time-consuming to show that interventions to change diets, such as 5 a Day, actually alter rates of breast cancer (11). Thus we often are faced with the unfortunate anomaly that we have greater evidence for short-term, individually directed interventions, such as for mammography screening, than for interventions targeting the clinical care system or more fundamental population-health problems with the potential for greater impact affecting more people and a broader range of health outcomes.

Since it is unrealistic to wait decades for the results of careful studies of interventions to improve the underlying determinants of health (e.g., income and education), by which time the specific interventions undoubtedly would be less relevant, alternative methods are needed to prospectively assess impacts. To address this problem, the DPH uses other tools to identify the effectiveness of interventions. Among those are health impact assessments and modeling. Health impact assessment is a process for organizing and systematically examining the evidence of the health impact associated with policies, programs, or projects usually outside the health field, for example, a living wage law, a transportation project, or the Farm Bill (12). A health impact assessment of menu-labeling, for example, contributed directly to passage of a county ordinance, which was soon preempted by a state ordinance, which in turn was preempted by the Affordable Care Act (ACA; see Chapter 11) (13). These tools can provide important insight by synthesizing available information to provide estimates of the potential impact of interventions. The use of well-crafted sensitivity analyses can determine the upper and lower bounds of beneficial effects and harms. These assessments need to be followed by careful evaluations of the interventions implemented to assure that the findings of studies materialize in practice, as well as to learn the strengths and weaknesses of the models themselves.

Unlike many clinical services that use specific technologies, population-based interventions are commonly adapted to local circumstances. Thus tobacco taxes or clean air acts intended to reduce exposure to tobacco smoke may differ from one county jurisdiction to another. Programs always face the dual challenge of needing high fidelity with proven interventions, combined with the flexibility to adapt them to local circumstances.

■ CHALLENGES

Funding streams often require specific services to be rendered. These resources often have strong constituencies with little desire for change. A typical example is substance abuse rehabilitation that uses behavioral rehabilitation strategies. Only recently have some of those resources been designated within the LAC DPH for prevention rather than control. Similarly, on behalf of the state, the DPH operates what are essentially insurance plans for special needs children (see Chapter 34). The specifications of those programs' funding may provide some flexibility, such as in selection of specific therapies, but limited room for flexibility in others, such as the ability to use the resources to prevent the conditions in the first place. Thus program requirements may not be constructed based on evidence of the relative effectiveness of alternative ways to improve the health of their target audiences. Alternatively, some funding streams, typified by the Centers for Disease Control and Prevention's tobacco control or Community Transformation Grants, now provide clear guidance that proposed interventions need to be evidence based. Indeed, many funding announcements now include specific reference to evidence-based interventions and the Community Guide.

Although the Community Guide has published recommendations in journals and on the internet for over a decade, many LAC DPH staff had limited familiarity with evidence-based methods in general and Community Guide recommendations in particular. While they do not need to be expert in evidence-based methods, staff do need to be good consumers of evidence-based resources so that they can incorporate evidence-based interventions into their programs, as well as implementing them with fidelity. To bridge this gap, professional meetings such as the annual DPH Science Summit and regular staff meetings have been used to inform staff about evidence-based public health, so most staff now recognize the key resources for designing evidence-based programs. Nonetheless, change does not come easily. As noted above, the performance improvement process used throughout the DPH requires that programs incorporate evidence-based practices and metrics, an important lever for translating the principles of evidence-based public health into departmental practice (see Chapter 7).

The virtue of a stable, skilled workforce has its counterpart in reluctance to forgo familiar, traditional ways of doing things, particularly delivering the individual-level services that often provide the greatest personal satisfaction. Helping staff to understand which programs and policies have the greatest preventable burden has increased the acceptance of new directions captured in the strategic plan (see Chapter 3).

Policy change is among the most powerful interventions. Tobacco use in LAC is among the lowest in the nation (14.3%) (4), largely as a result of changes in social norms through policy change. Clean air laws have banished tobacco from public buildings, restaurants, and worksites. Restrictions on sales to minors and enforcement tied to vending licenses have been central to making tobacco use no longer acceptable. These changes, however, have not come easily. With 88 cities and 42 school districts, policy change is incremental. Chapter 13 shows how evidence-based policies are translated into practice through solid science and close collaboration with community partners.

CAPITALIZING ON OPPORTUNITY

At times of great change come new opportunities. Health reform will have a major impact on programs such as HIV, where the Ryan White Act provides funding to pay for HIV/AIDS services. As patient care becomes mainstreamed under the Affordable Care Act, there will likely be large changes in the HIV program. This provides unique opportunities to review current activities and evidence-based HIV prevention and control strategies to re-assess the portfolio of interventions. A process is underway to do just that. The program is building a logic model that examines upstream determinants, sexual behaviors, as well as clinical interventions including testing, counseling, and treatment. Understanding the effectiveness of strategies as different as stigma reduction and job programs to increasing adherence to highly active anti-retroviral therapy, as well as the magnitude of effect of each in isolation and combination, is expected to provide important insights into program priorities and resource allocation.

IMPACT

The use of evidence-based interventions has become an important underpinning of the department's basic work. It has become a demonstrable part of the department's planning and performance improvement processes. This planning builds on health assessments that identify the county's greatest health needs. Programs responsible for ameliorating those needs must then identify the appropriate mix of evidence-based interventions, capitalizing on core resources and available funding streams to develop the capacity for delivery.

Staff now understand the importance of doing "what works" rather than "what we have always done." We often say that the one unacceptable reason for continuing a particular intervention is because we have always used it. Nonetheless, most resources are earmarked for categorical programs and activities, so change is less speedy than perhaps desired. New funding provides ways to reshape programs and build requisite skills. For example, it can be challenging to transform a program whose job has been to implement and monitor health care contracts. New responsibility for innovative and effective prevention programs are slowly being implemented, and the ACA is providing the opportunity to shift resources from direct services to more effective population-based initiatives.

Community stakeholders also have begun to see the value of evidence-based practice to help move their agendas forward and to note the difference that these interventions can make in their communities, including changes in the food environment, walk-ability and bike-ability, tobacco use, and infant health (see Chapters 11, 12, 13, 32 and 33).

CONCLUSIONS

The department has undergone a significant transition from traditional public health programs built around epidemiologic investigation, health education, and direct services, to a more population-oriented approach focused on community action and policy change that harken back to the sanitation movement of the late nineteenth and early twentieth centuries. This requires firm grounding in evidence-based practice. Continued professional education, greater investment in evidence-based policy development, and better tools for public health practitioners are needed.

Important lessons learned:

- Staff need a common understanding of what constitutes evidence-based interventions—not simply what someone says works for them, or a single study, but the result of a systematic review of high-quality studies.
- Evidence-based practice requires data and information. It is built on sound surveillance, with descriptive and authoritative information about "what works."
- The Community Guide and Cochrane Collaboration are examples of scientifically based reviews and recommendations that can inform programmatic choices.
- A well-crafted performance system assures proper identification of problems, solutions, and metrics to monitor progress.
- It is feasible to build evidence-based public health principles into local public health action.
- Adherence to evidence-based practice often leads to more effective and sustainable policy-oriented initiatives.
- Integration of evidence-based individual and population-based interventions is required to maximally improve health outcomes.

■ REFERENCES

1. Wennberg J, Gittelsohn A. Small area variations in health care delivery. *Science.* 1973;182(117):1102–8
2. U.S. Preventive Services Task Force. Available from: http://www.uspreventiveservicestaskforce.org/index.html (accessed Aug. 4, 2011)
3. Task Force on Community Preventive Services. Available from: http://thecommunityguide.org/index.html (accessed Aug. 4, 2011).
4. Los Angeles County Department of Public Health, Office of Health Assessment and Epidemiology. *Key Indicators of Health by Service Planning Area.* June 2009. Available from: http://www.publichealth.lacounty.gov/docs/keyindicators.pdf (accessed Aug. 4, 2011).
5. The Cochrane Collaboration. Available from: http://www.cochrane.org/ (accessed Aug. 4, 2011).
6. Task Force on Community Preventive Services. *Vaccinations to Prevent Diseases.* Available from: http://www.thecommunityguide.org/vaccines/index.html.
7. Ndaiye SM, Hopkins DP, Shefer AM, et al. Interventions to improve influenza, pneumococcal polysaccharide, and hepatitis B vaccination coverage among high-risk adults: A systematic review. *Am J Prev Med.* 2005;28(5S):248–79.
8. IOM (Institute of Medicine). *Bridging the Evidence Gap in Obesity Prevention: A Framework to Inform Decision Making.* Washington, DC: The National Academies Press; 2010.
9. Secretary's Advisory Committee on National Health Promotion and Disease Prevention. *Evidence-based Clinical and Public Health: Generating and Applying the Evidence.* Available from: http://www.healthypeople.gov/2010/hp2020/advisory/EvidenceBasedClinicalPH2010.htm (accessed Aug. 16, 2011).

10. Commission to Build a Healthier America. *Beyond Health Care: New Directions to a Healthier America*. Princeton): Robert Wood Johnson Foundation; 2009.
11. Key TJ. Fruit and vegetables and cancer risk. *Br J Cancer*. 2011;104(1):6–11.
12. Cole BL, Fielding JE. Health impact assessment: a tool to help policy makers understand health beyond health care. *Annu Rev Public Health*. 2007;28:393–412.
13. Simon P, Jarosz CJ, Kuo T, Fielding JE. *Menu Labeling as a Potential Strategy for Combating the Obesity Epidemic: A Health Impact Assessment*. Los Angeles County Department of Public Health, 2008. Available from: http://publichealth.lacounty.gov/docs/Menu_Labeling_Report_2008.pdf (accessed Aug. 4, 2011).

5

From Direct Service to Community Orientation

Transformation of Nursing Practice

DAVID CALEY AND DEBORAH DAVENPORT

THE PROBLEM

Over the past century, the toll of chronic diseases has grown to account for 80% of all mortality in Los Angeles County (LAC), while the overall burden of communicable diseases has steadily decreased. These changes were not reflected in the role of LAC's district public health nurses (PHNs), who until recently mainly conducted communicable disease investigations and follow-up.

The impetus for change began in the 1990s when PHNs were assigned to neighborhoods or identifiable communities. Their focus was still on communicable disease control, but PHNs became very knowledgeable about local health issues by listening to community members discuss their concerns at community meetings. However, PHNs lacked the resources to intervene.

At this same time, the county was divided into eight Service Planning Areas (SPAs) to assure that all LAC family-related services departments applied the same geographic boundaries. The point was to foster interdepartmental cooperation and to reduce the number of "doors" required to access services. In 1999, the Health Officer created the SPA Area Health Offices reporting to the director of Community Health Services (CHS). Each Area Health Office employed an Area Health Officer (AHO), business administrator, medical director, nursing director, and field staff including district PHNs. The AHOs quickly realized that to address the large and growing chronic disease burden they needed to reach into respective communities. Thus began the concept of designated community "liaison" PHNs in LAC's urban core; these worked in partnership with a health advocacy group in the San Gabriel Valley region that developed women's health and nutrition projects. As these PHNs effectively increased the AHOs' "reach" into the community, other AHOs recognized the value and began identifying similar positions within their health offices. Initially, little coordination existed among them. For example, the AHO responsible for the high desert region of LAC engaged community partners to address a staggering infant mortality rate (see Chapter 33). The AHO used district PHNs to work with community support programs that could effectively identify and manage high-risk/at-risk pregnant women. "Community liaison PHNs" began to educate communities about their health status through existing city and community service organization networks or to help build new ones where there were none.

In 2008, the Health Officer directed CHS to systematize the community liaison role and to train a cadre of public health nurses and health educators to increase engagement with their local communities. They would do this by identifying and implementing evidence-based interventions, assuring that essential stakeholders participated in planning and implementation activities, fostering social cohesion, and expanding community resources.

■ CONTEXT

A 2007 assessment of the Area Health Offices recognized that the shift in burden from communicable diseases to chronic health conditions required a new approach. This report examined how services were delivered and distributed in relation to various community health needs. It showed that as communicable disease reporting decreased, so too did PHNs' workloads, creating windows of opportunity to identify PHNs able—or at least willing—to learn to work on community engagement and collaboration to improve the community's health overall. Thus the AHOs expanded the PHNs' "community liaison" role without jeopardizing communicable disease control. A smaller workforce could meet the immediate disease control need, while other staff could be devoted to community-level health improvement. Regardless of role, however, all staff still needed full training so that they could be mobilized rapidly for any public health emergency.

This new role was both intriguing and daunting for many district PHNs and the Area Health Offices. Many nurses who gravitate to public health work effectively in a social environment that includes the individual, family, workplace, and community. However, before the creation of a formal community liaison role, PHNs were uncertain how to add more population-based initiatives to their established day-to-day duties consisting mainly of communicable disease investigation, case management of children with elevated lead levels, and follow-up to sudden infant death syndrome cases, where they dealt primarily with individuals and families. Previously, with few exceptions, "helping out the community" had meant providing information on immunizations and communicable disease control at health fairs or community group meetings. The new role required the ability to address such diverse issues as school nutrition and walk-to-school programs, breastfeeding programs in hospitals, and preparing communities to respond to emergencies. These required a new set of competencies, such as the ability to analyze community health data to identify needs, to develop health improvement plans, to provide leadership, and to implement and evaluate programs. Many nurses had been with the public health department for years, some having received MPH or MSN degrees; but many others had attended nursing school decades ago, when population health was taught less rigorously than today, so the latter were not fully prepared to undertake community-level health improvement. Gebbe and Hwang outlined this issue and the skill areas required to carry out population-based work by PHNs (1).

In addition, some district PHNs did not feel comfortable making what salespeople refer to as "cold calls." In the PHNs' traditional role, nurses have defined reasons for a visit, such as a child with a high lead burden or a communicable disease report, and such visits are essentially scripted through the use of forms, procedures, and referral processes. In their new role, they needed to rely more on experience—their training and practice—to proactively address multiple disease prevention and control challenges that affect the community as a whole, not just individuals.

■ APPROACH TO THE PROBLEM

CHS chose PHNs as community liaisons (CLPHNs) to work closely with the AHO, who could build a community stakeholder network to address chronic disease.

Training and practice assured long-term program success and enhanced relevant skills of the CLPHNs.

Training

To build the necessary competencies, CHS held regular monthly training sessions to teach CLPHNs specific skills. The sessions also included a work documentation process to capture their knowledge of communities and stakeholders and to demonstrate how those relationships can be leveraged to address long-term health outcomes. Community advocates, local government officials, and academicians teach best practice and evidence-based approaches to community interventions. Desktop exercises require CLPHNs to apply their skills to address practical problems in their own communities, for example lack of places for physical activity, safe routes for children to walk to school, or access to affordable fresh fruits and vegetables. Each session includes "peer review" where staff present projects and updates collegially to garner new ideas.

Training sessions cover local government organization; data analysis and reporting; community engagement and resilience; change processes; developing messages and effective communication; project management; determinants of health; place-based interventions; community development and planning; as well as targeted health issues such as infant mortality. All PHNs continue to be trained in areas such as outbreak management, STD treatment and follow-up protocols, and disaster response, to assure that they are prepared for their communicable disease control and disaster response roles when needed.

Practice

Successful community practice starts with a firm grounding in the theoretical bases for nursing and public health practice. CLPHN activities are framed using a familiar nursing model, the LAC DPH PHN Practice Model (see Figure 5–1) (2), which integrates the Minnesota Association of PHNs and the Minnesota DPH PHN

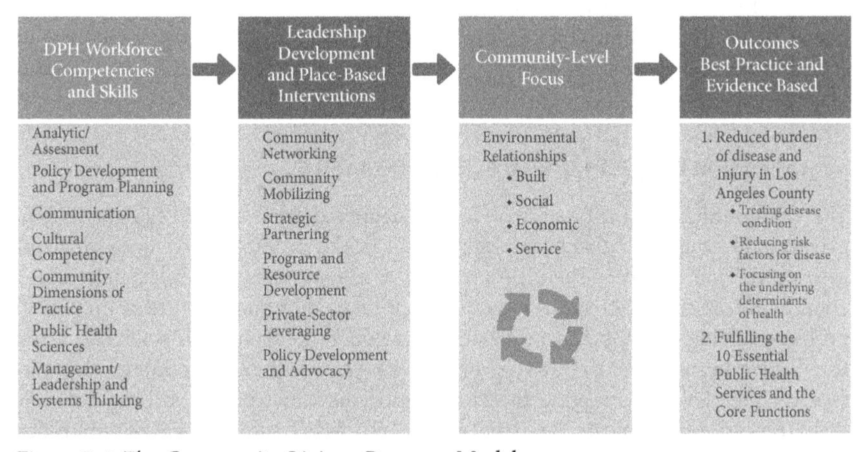

Figure 5–1 The Community Liaison Program Model.

framework Intervention Wheel (3) with other nationally recognized frameworks of PHN practice. Other plans include the Scope and Standards of PHN Practice (4), Essential Public Health Services, and Healthy People's leading health indicators (5). These link competencies with the leadership skills needed to implement place-based interventions and strong community focus. They use evidence-based programs to achieve better health outcomes.

The Council on Linkages between Academia and Public Health Practice (6) identified core competencies needed by public health professionals to protect and promote community health. The competencies build skills in several areas: analysis and assessment; policy development and program planning; communication; cultural competency; community dimensions of practice; public health sciences; financial management; and leadership and systems thinking. Training in each competency has been developed for three levels of instruction: entry level staff, supervisors, and senior staff and managers.

To track and analyze community interventions, the CLPHNs use the Community Engagement Project Tool (CEPT). Using the CEPT establishes a standardized approach to projects across LAC, building on the competencies already learned. It structures CLPHNs' work by requiring them to:

- State the purpose of the project;
- Assess the current political will in the community to take on the issue;
- Provide data to document or frame the community health issue;
- Document community concerns, both real and assumed;
- Document evidenced-based strategies that can be employed to achieve positive outcomes;
- Identify potential barriers to planned interventions;
- Determine the measurable and realistically achievable outcomes;
- Document available community and intradepartmental resources and assess their sufficiency to achieve the identified outcomes;
- Define short, intermediate, and long-term objectives;
- Define the evaluation process to determine success, lessons learned, and actual outcomes.

The CEPT format is also a project-tracking tool and a vehicle for management to assure that CLPHNs are targeting priority community health issues. An electronic reporting format under development will facilitate tracking and assist in evaluating liaison PHN's work.

IMPLEMENTATION OF SOLUTIONS

The Community Liaison Program (CLP) increases awareness and generates public, private, and nonprofit organization support of health promotion, wellness, and disease prevention services. The CLP leverages a group's strengths by capitalizing on community assets. A strength-based strategy takes advantage of the community's problem-solving capacity and motivates its members to apply their skills and assets to effective initiatives (7). This type of strategy helped to decrease infant mortality (see Chapter 33). By engaging the community, the effort produced programs and volunteers to communicate the issue to the faith-based and business communities. These efforts produced a broad regional network to support pregnant women at risk and to promote inter-conceptional health of women at risk.

Using competencies learned in their monthly trainings and working with supervisors and senior staff, CLPHNs engage communities to creatively address the complex built, social, and economic health determinants that they confront. CLPHNs provide data to help communities understand their health status and underlying problems. This information can be used for setting priorities, planning, taking action, and advocacy. CLPHNs are routinely challenged to find solutions to distinct yet interrelated problems. For example, by using the core competencies, CHS staff collaborated more effectively with the Chronic Disease Prevention Division and the Policies for Livable, Active Communities and Environments program. Together, these comprehensive community-level interventions addressed obesity issues through the natural and built environments. One SPA in LAC's urban core established projects that included highlighting healthy menu choices in local independent restaurants, conducting walking clubs in local parks, and developing health components for city General Plans.

■ EVALUATION STRATEGY

The CEPT is the primary tool for evaluating the CLP. It documents any given project's entire work continuum, often over many months or years, for example, a city's General Plan update. The CEPT has been used to assess a project's progress, how it was planned and implemented, whether time lines were achieved, as well as whether the intended intermediate and health outcomes were achieved. Participant questionnaires and key informant interviews in two SPAs demonstrated that the CLPHNs established valued relationships at once sensitive to time commitments and that celebrate reaching milestones and, ultimately, project completion.

■ IMPACT

The CLP provides the DPH with a direct conduit to key community stakeholders. Successful relationships with stakeholders and partners have been leveraged long after earlier projects were completed. For example, for the five years preceding the H1N1 pandemic, the DPH implemented point of dispensing (POD) events during the influenza vaccination season. When the pandemic occurred, the CLPHNs leveraged those relationships and cities' local staffing resources and multi-jurisdictional/city collaboratives, thus enabling many cities to independently implement their own PODs (see Chapter 27).

Of course, not every project goes as planned. Community priorities change, resources get diverted, elections replace key players who bring different agendas, staff turnover changes levels of commitment to projects, and funding may be exhausted. But awareness of these issues and their ramifications guides the day-to-day management of projects, as well as informing strategic planning for future projects.

It is frequently necessary to scale down initial projects to achieve more modest and achievable community goals. Then, once a proven track record is established, larger more sustained projects can be built on the successful working relationships of the initial projects. In many approaches to our communities, the initial focus was community access to primary care. The AHOs provided data to shift community focus from "personal care," that is, the number of available hospital beds or local community clinics, to looking at community-level data such as smoking, its impact on chronic disease, and the lack of available tobacco cessation programs. Communities successfully added such programs and moved on to further advocacy for non-smoking ordinances in several LAC cities.

The CLP also helped break down programmatic silos within the DPH by leveraging and integrating subject matter expertise of different DPH programs, addressing common concerns, and providing consistent messages with a single "face" to the community. In doing so, the CLP has achieved greater credibility with the community. This saves precious time when working with groups where relationship development can be lengthy yet critical to forming solid working partnerships.

Among the successful outcomes of the Community Liaison Program are:

- Specific health relevant objectives incorporated into General Plan updates and Master Plans—such as for parks or seeing to the needs of senior residents;
- Availability of improved and timely comprehensive prenatal care, reduced low birth weight and other poor birth outcomes that contribute to elevated rates of infant mortality in the African American community in northern rural LAC;
- Facilitated breastfeeding consortiums and Baby-Friendly Hospital designation in LAC hospitals;
- Collaboration with community stakeholders petitioning for joint use policies that allow community members to use school facilities for physical activity when otherwise unused;
- Multidisciplinary collaborations with school districts improving nutritional food content on campus (eliminating sugar-laden drinks, changing vending machine food content for increased nutritional value, improving cafeteria nutritional offerings); coordinated training for physical education instructors; assured minimum standards of physical activities; elimination of fund-raisers through sales of food with poor nutritional content;
- Policy adoption restricting use of tobacco;
- Collaboration on Safe-Routes-to-Schools programs;
- Targeted high-risk minority populations to influence and help groups with significant risk of diabetes, cardiovascular heart disease, hypertension, stroke and obesity through local community prevention initiatives;
- Improved community resilience in emergency preparedness planning by conducting readiness training and ICS for local cities;
- Collaboration between local school districts and faith-based organizations in a remote LAC area to increase education and awareness about high STD rates in their local high schools.

CONCLUSIONS

Acting as extensions of the AHO, and ultimately the Health Officer, CLPHNs build relationships with community stakeholders in more systematic and comprehensive ways by providing information and data to help residents create opportunities for civic engagement. This helps to prioritize potential and sustainable solutions through leveraging of local assets and resources and is in keeping with the IOM's 2010 report on the Future of Nursing (8). Garnering community engagement in identifying local health issues is critical for execution and sustainability, as are prioritizing strategies to address them, and leveraging their resources/assets when implementing community action plans. Thus:

- Routine competency-based training within the CLP expanded the capacity of staff. Initiatives now are more sophisticated in scope, more effectively use available resources and time, and achieve clearer outcomes.

- Message development and other aspects of communication strategies are essential components of community projects. The best-planned initiatives can be dismantled if sectors of a community perceive exclusion or alienation. Staff doing CLP work must understand and carefully use message development and the various levels of presenting appropriate information, including mass media and targeted communication, and how they can engage community members around issues. Communication must include community stakeholders who are engaged in projects as true partners and who play active roles essential to a project's success.
- Future strategic expansion of the CLP to increase DPH capacity to leverage relationships, resources, and assets with local community stakeholders helps to achieve mutually designed strategic goals addressing the Social Determinants of Health. These include:
    1. Developing a system for engaging and managing ongoing relationships with key stakeholders in cities and unincorporated areas;
    2. Enhancing staff skills and resources to promote effective engagement;
    3. Improving internal communication related to external engagement;
    4. Evaluating the effectiveness of engagement with cities and unincorporated areas.

■ REFERENCES

1. Gebbie KM, Hwang I. Preparing currently employed public health nurses for changes in the health system. *Am J Public Health*.2002;90(5):716–21.
2. Smith K,Bazini-Barakat N. A public health nursing practice model: Melding public health principles with the nursing process. *Public Health Nursing*. 2003;20:42–8.
3. Minnesota Department of Health. *Public Health Nursing Section: Public Health Interventions–Applications for Public Health Nursing Practice*. St. Paul: Minnesota Department of Health; 2001.
4. American Nurses Association. *Public Health Nursing: Scope and Standards of Practice*. Silver Spring, MD: American Nurses Association; 2007.
5. U.S. Department of Health and Human Services. *Healthy People 2020*. Available from: http://healthypeople.gov/2020/default.aspx (accessed June 14, 2012).
6. Council on Linkages Between Academia and Public Health Practice. *Core Competencies for Public Health Professionals*. Public Health Foundation. Available from: http://www.phf.org/resourcestools/pages/core_public_health_competencies.aspx (accessed Apr. 24, 2011).
7. Kretzmann JP, McKnight JL. *Building Communities from the Inside Out: A Path Toward Finding and Mobilizing a Community's Assets*. Evanston, IL: Institute for Policy Research; 1993.
8. Committee on the Robert Wood Johnson Foundation Initiative on the Future of Nursing, Institute of Medicine. *The Future of Nursing: Leading Change, Advancing Health*. Washington, DC: National Academies Press; 2011.

6 Assuring Competence

Credentialing and Privileging of Public Health Physicians

JEFFREY D. GUNZENHAUSER AND KATHLEEN N. SMITH

THE PROBLEM

The credentialing and privileging of physicians have long been familiar activities in hospital settings. This practice spread to outpatient settings in 1991 when the Joint Commission developed accreditation standards for ambulatory care (1, 2). In California, Title 22 of the Code of Regulations requires that every medical clinic use a system for credentials review, delineation of clinical privileges, and a peer review process (3). For the public health community, the Public Health Accreditation Board's proposed standards for local health departments includes verification and documentation that staff meet the qualifications for their positions (4).

Within local health departments, some physicians do not regularly see patients, but rather provide consultation, technical assistance, and "population medicine" services to specific communities. Even so, under special circumstances (e.g., in response to large-scale outbreaks or public health emergencies), all physicians may be called upon to provide hands-on, clinical care services. While these requirements and circumstances imply the need for a systematic approach to review credentials and grant privileges for all physicians in public health departments, no national public health organization has done so.

As with other local public health organizations, the Department of Public Health (DPH) in Los Angeles County (LAC) had not established a formal organization-wide credentialing and privileging system. The H1N1 influenza pandemic, in which all physicians were called to provide clinical services, prompted urgency to implement a system to review and authorize medical staff credentials and privileges.

CONTEXT

Physicians are key elements of the public health workforce but public health departments lack self-regulating structures akin to professional staff structures extant in traditional health care organizations. While personnel departments confirm state licensure and specialty certification for pay purposes, they seldom verify an individual physician's competence, scope of training, or prior work performance, and public health departments lack formal processes to do so. In other clinical organizations, processes to grant privileges based on thorough credential and performance reviews assure both baseline and ongoing levels of competence and accountability. Although credentialing takes time and expense, the investment can prevent adverse events and subsequent liability exposure (1, 2, 5, 6). Credentialing and privileging help to build a higher quality medical staff, not only by adhering to statutory requirements, but also by protecting the public interest (7, 8). These processes should not be considered perfunctory. They are a critical form of oversight requiring active department leader involvement and a commitment to quality improvement (9).

The terms *credentialing* and *privileging* are not widely understood within public health organizations. The LAC DPH uses standard definitions to differentiate the two terms. *Credentialing* assesses and confirms the qualifications of a health care practitioner. *Privileging* authorizes practitioners to provide specific services to patients (10). To our knowledge, no state or local health department "privileges" its public health physicians who provide population medicine services (11).

Within a public health organization, the medical services of physicians vary widely. Within the LAC DPH, only a minority provide direct, hands-on clinical care services for sexually transmitted diseases, tuberculosis and communicable diseases, or immunization. Others, such as the physicians in the California Children's Services program, review medical charts to determine eligibility for benefits and provide technical assistance to other clinical personnel. Still others, such as the Medical Director of the Immunization Program and the Director of Maternal Health, provide technical assistance and consultation to community providers. Numerous physicians oversee outbreak investigations, while many provide "population medicine" assessments of the health of various communities or supply medical input to the development, delivery, or evaluation of evidence-based essential public health services. This tremendous variation in the location and nature of medical services challenges any organization to "privilege" its physician workforce.

■ APPROACH TO THE PROBLEM: DEVELOPING THE SYSTEM

A team of physicians and nurses began by researching the organization and processes of credentialing and privileging LAC hospital medical staff. The team determined that a single "model" hospital in the LAC Department of Health Services was adaptable to public health settings. A site visit was conducted with the credentials staff at that hospital to learn more about its approach. Documents were obtained related to credentialing and privileging, including bylaws of the physician staff organization, application packets for newly hired physicians, re-application packets for current physicians, and checklists for procedures to manage the process. These materials required substantial revision to be adapted to a public health practice setting that included both individual patient care and population-level physician practice. The area of physician privileging was especially thorny. It was challenging to identify the privileges that all physicians needed, with subsets particular to those in patient care and those in population-based medicine. The team also conducted a literature review and produced a brief that was shared throughout the department and on the internet. This brief and subsequent discussion introduced the topic to the physicians and began their preparation for accepting and engaging in the process.

Resources did not exist at first for assessing the quality of physician workforce medical services and setting performance standards. While a "Physician Administration" unit appeared on DPH's organizational chart when it was begun in 2006, it had not been staffed. Under leadership of the Medical Director, a Medical Executive Committee was formed, including representatives of senior physicians from DPH divisions, and newly established subcommittees for continuing medical education, credentials, and interdisciplinary practice. A "Credentialing Policy" holdover from the time when the

DPH separated from the Department of Health Services was revised and adapted to public health practice. Bylaws from the model hospital were simplified and integrated into existing DPH personnel management processes. For newly hired physicians, new processes were established to expand the review of credentials to require letters of recommendation from medical peers with whom physicians previously worked, to authorize the release of information related to their medical performance from the organizations for which they previously worked, and to assure a query of the National Practitioner Data Bank. A new process also was established to administratively assign "proxy" physician supervisors (for medical practice) for physicians whose supervisor was a non-physician. This allows non-physician supervisors to independently review the adequacy of medical services and contribute to annual performance evaluations of physicians whom they supervise.

A core implementation team consisted of the Medical Director, the senior physician in the division providing clinical services (Community Health Services), an assistant nursing director from within the Office of the Medical Director, and a senior nurse from within the Communicable Disease Control and Prevention Division. A key new element was a process for physicians to request privileges. Previously it had been assumed that physicians were qualified to perform specific medical tasks, based on routine personnel hiring processes. The new process required physicians to request specific medical privileges and to simultaneously provide information on their training, background, and work experience to substantiate their competence. The core team adapted forms used in the hospital setting to develop new documents for physicians to request privileges relevant to public health practice. To gain organizational buy-in and ownership, the documents were widely shared. The new approach was discussed with the Department Director, the Chief Deputy Director, the Director of Human Resources, and all senior physicians through the Medical Executive Committee. The process and key issues also were discussed in an all-physician meeting. And the approach received legal review and was coordinated with the DPH physicians' union. Table 6–1 highlights the key steps in establishing the program.

■ IMPLEMENTATION

Implementation has at least three phases: preparation, accommodation of the existing workforce, and procedures to bring new physicians on staff while also periodically reappointing members of the current medical staff. A review of the credentialing and privileging process also must be included in new employee orientation (12, 13).

TABLE 6–1 *Key Steps in Establishing a System to Credential and Privilege Physicians*

1. Physician executive sponsor agrees to lead the process.
2. Establishment of core team to develop a policy, a procedure, application documents, and an implementation plan, to include accommodation of the existing physician workforce and procedures to rapidly on-board new appointments to the medical staff.
3. Identify resources to support the credentialing and privileging process.
4. Involve physician and other group leaders to assure organizational ownership and buy-in.
5. Coordinate implementation with Personnel Division, Legal Counsel, and Organized Labor.
6. Provide information to the physician workforce.

A credentialing verification unit (CVU) manages the actual process for individual physicians. The practitioner completes an application, for which verification is sought using primary source data. Then the CVU reviews the information and determines whether to authorize the requested privileges. If accepted, the CVU sends a letter to that effect. The privileges are usually approved for two years.

Establishing a credentialing and privileging system requires several key decisions. First is whether the system will reside within a medical staff committee structure or will include members of other disciplines in a professional staff organization structure with bylaws, policies, rules, and regulations. The DPH decided on a medical staff committee structure using policies and procedures rather than formal bylaws. Second is to define the minimum set of privileges, if any, for which each physician must apply. In the LAC DPH, all physicians in the workforce must maintain minimal, essential skills in clinical medicine, such as the ability to perform a history and physical examination, to provide consultation to other clinical providers, to be able to interpret the results of medical tests, and to be able to prescribe or administer certain medications. In addition to the essential skills in clinical medicine, physicians also must request additional privileges in either clinical medicine or in population medicine. Including population medicine privileges in the framework (i.e., those recognized by the American Board of Preventive Medicine) establishes the legitimate role of population medicine as medical practice. Third is to determine the means by which a physician will maintain competence (skills and knowledge) and the mechanism to monitor each physician's proficiency through a system of testing, such as a skills-lab approach or required demonstration. For physicians providing population-based medical services, this requires standards of practice to evaluate and assure the quality of services, such as conducting outbreak investigations, evaluating the adequacy of population health assessments, and designing systems to link individuals with needed clinical services. Since the Medical Director occupies the top position in a hierarchical organizational structure, a special process is needed to review his or her credentials and request for privileges. And, the relationship of the processes to assess performance (including peer review and evaluations of substandard performance) with the organization's overall performance evaluation and disciplinary processes must be defined. Within the LAC DPH, when issues of physician performance are identified that may rise to a level requiring disciplinary action, an ad hoc peer review team of physicians is established to formally review facts related to medical practice and to recommend to the physician's supervisor whether disciplinary action should be taken. The DPH process also includes:

- Peer review (especially for units with only one physician);
- Provision for modification, limitation, suspension, and revocation of privileges;
- Requirement for proof of participation in continuing medical education;
- Protection of confidentiality of credentialing decisions under peer review;
- Ensuring adherence to due process when making decisions related to privileges.

■ EVALUATION STRATEGY

What value does establishing a "credentialing and privileging process" provide to a local health department? First, it promotes professionalism within the medical workforce. Evaluating a physician's practice should validate the importance of work that is medical in content and enhances overall perception of the value of professional work. In the absence of such a process, physicians may feel isolated and disconnected from the profession for which they have trained. Physicians state that the new opportunities to connect DPH physicians in self-evaluation processes, to share results of scientific studies, and to discuss ways to improve medical practice foster learning from others about best practices. Second, the approach addresses potential risk management and liability issues by establishing procedures to assure that medical practitioners are evaluated in ways that are considered "standard practice" in clinical organizations. Third, the process should assure that physicians in the workforce perform services that are medical in nature.

By recognizing and formalizing privileges for population medicine as well as clinical medicine, the approach provides equal emphasis on each. Since the roles of the professional staff within a public health agency (e.g., physicians, nurses, and epidemiologists) may overlap, privileging delineates specific medical functions that distinguish physician services from those of other professional staff.

■ EVALUATION

The evaluation strategy being developed will include numerous domains. First, department executives and senior leaders will be queried periodically to assess their views of physician performance within their workforce, including the extent to which physicians provide services that are mainly medical (including both population and clinical services), as well as the overall quality of those services. Second, the evaluation will include an assessment of the competence of individual physicians through self-assessment, peer review, and observed testing. Competence assessment also is expected to formalize and establish clear performance criteria and standards of practice for medical privileges related to population medicine. Third, the evaluation will include assessment of the overall job satisfaction of physicians within the workforce. We anticipate that improvements in physician performance, development of a more socially integrated medical workforce, and increased awareness of the importance of medical professionalism will favorably impact the physicians' work environments and will also improve the quality of their services. Finally, the value of this approach will be assessed when the LAC DPH seeks accreditation by the Public Health Accreditation Board. Hopefully, the department's new approach will be recognized as a best practice by the Board.

■ IMPACT

Implementing a process to privilege the DPH physician workforce has yielded favorable impacts. Numerous physicians acknowledge that the process substantially increased their connection with other DPH physicians and that these connections are of practical day-to-day value (14). While quantitative data are not yet available to assess such assertions, confidential evaluations of department-wide physician meetings about medical practice reveal many anecdotal comments that such processes are valued for improving their performance. Simultaneous efforts to organize and improve the performance of other members of the professional DPH staff (nurses, health educators, public health investigators, and dentists) have increased awareness of the unique contributions of each professional discipline. Several programs recognize that employees with very different professional backgrounds (e.g., physicians, nurses, epidemiologists) are performing very similar work with no obvious variation in the quality of work performed. This has led administrators to question the relative value that each profession contributes and to consider more cost-effective ways to use or reorganize the existing workforce. As the evaluation is completed, it will allow greater organizational understanding of the effectiveness, quality, and value of the most costly element of the public health workforce. Organizational benefits will include better decision making about when to use unique services that only physicians can provide; the assurance that those services meet acceptable standards of practice; and the ability to choose less costly approaches supporting equal or greater impact.

CONCLUSIONS

Among the important lessons learned:

- "Credentialing and privileging of physicians" is a well-established best practice in clinical organizations and should be standard practice within public health departments.
- Medical skills of public health physicians who provide population medicine services for communities as defined by the American Board of Preventive Medicine should be accommodated by recognizing these as "privileges" requested by and approved for practicing public health physicians.
- Processes used in clinical organizations to assess physician competence and performance can be adapted to the environment of a local or state health department.
- The focus of the Public Health Accreditation Board on the competence of the public health workforce will likely encourage state and local health departments to develop or adopt best practices to assure competencies of public health physicians.
- The experience in the LAC DPH can serve as a model for other health departments.
- A deliberate, well-planned approach to review credentials and grant privileges to public health physicians can promote awareness that the medical services of population medicine physicians are an established form of medical practice and are amenable to evaluation for adherence to practice standards.
- Systems to assure public health physicians' competence can potentially increase public accountability and minimize organizational risk management liabilities.
- Efforts to organize and oversee medical practice in public health departments is likely to enhance a sense of professionalism, the quality of professional practice, the accountability of high-salaried workers, and an awareness of the unique and interlocking skill sets of the various professional workforces.

REFERENCES

1. Brott LB. Credentialing and its importance: Part one of two. *Community Health Forum*, 2001 Jul/Aug.
2. Brott LB. Credentialing and its importance: Part two of two. *Community Health Forum*, 2001 Sept/Oct.

3. State of California. California Code of Regulations, Title 22. Sacramento, CA. 1990.
4. Public Health Accreditation Board. *Proposed Local Standards and Measures for Public Health Accreditation Board.* 2009. Available from: http://www.phaboard.org/accreditation-process/public-health-department-standards-and-measures/ (accessed June 14, 2012).
5. Cassel CK, Holmboe ES. Credentialing and public accountability. *JAMA*. 2006;295:939–40.
6. Payne DE. Credentialing and privileging ensure skilled care. *Nurs Man.* 1999;30(8):8.
7. Hernandez AM. Trends in health care practitioner credentialing. *J Health Care Fin.* 1998;24(3):66–70.
8. Lumb EW, Oskvig RM. Multidisciplinary credentialing and privileging: A unified approach. *J Nurs Care Qual.* 1998;12(4):36–43.
9. LaValley D, editor. Credentialing, privileging, and patient safety. *Forum.* 2006;24(3):1–21.
10. U.S. Department of Health and Human Services, Health Resources and Services Administration, Bureau of Primary Health Care. *Policy Information Notice 2001–2016 and 2002–2022: Credentialing and Privileging of Health Center Practitioners.* 2002. Available from: http://bphc.hrsa.gov/policiesregulations/policies/pin200116.html and http://bphc.hrsa.gov/policiesregulations/policies/pin200222.html (accessed June 19, 2012).
11. Institute of Medicine. *Training Physicians for Public Health Careers.* Washington, DC: The National Academies Press; 2007.
12. Green J. It's a privilege: the board's role in physician credentialing and privileging. *Trustee.* 2008;4(3):8–11.
13. Wilson CN, Iacovella A. Physician credentialing. *Hosp Topics.* 2000;78(4):15–9.
14. Tilson HE, Gebbie KM. Public health physicians—an endangered species. *Am J Prev Med.* 2001;21:233–40.

7 Performance Improvement

Using Rapid-Cycle Improvement Techniques to Improve Public Health Services

DAWN MARIE JACOBSON AND DEBRA LOTSTEIN

THE NATURE OF THE PROBLEM

Over the past decade, public health leaders have experienced increased expectations for accountability and transparency from political leaders, external funding organizations, and the general public. This was due to calls for improved tracking and reporting of monies spent by government agencies, as well as requests by political leaders for documentation of return on investment for funded programs. In response, public health practitioners and their academic partners began exploring new performance measurement and improvement approaches applicable to local and state health departments (1, 2). This led to objectives of characterizing a common set of services that all local health departments should provide to their communities and identifying "high-performing" local health departments (LHDs) to serve as models that others could emulate.

Early efforts led to the National Public Health Performance Standards Program (NPHPSP) of the Centers for Disease Control and Prevention (CDC) (3) and a handful of state-led accreditation programs. These programs offered the opportunity for LHDs to complete an organizational self-assessment (4–6) and better understand how they organize and deliver essential public health services. To support these efforts, the Robert Wood Johnson Foundation (RWJF) funded and supported three learning collaboratives, called the Multi-State Learning Collaborative (MLC), which assessed the feasibility of accreditation and developed an initial set of "best practices" for using performance improvement tools, such as the Plan-Do-Study-Act cycle, within local and state health departments (7). At the same time, several city and county officials implemented programs for measuring, tracking, and reviewing performance data via reporting systems such as CitiStats (8, 9), and the Los Angeles County (LAC) Performance Counts! initiative that links performance metrics to the county budget (10).

Currently, three performance improvement (PI) initiatives[1] are available to LHDs: 1) voluntary accreditation; 2) development of performance-based accountability systems (PBAS) (11); and 3) adoption of performance improvement (PI) methods and tools for designing public health PI projects.

The first option focuses on performing an overall organizational assessment of core services with an emphasis on high-level infrastructure development (e.g., the presence of disease surveillance systems, emergency response capabilities, and a department strategic plan). The second focuses on the selection of priority process and output measures that are linked to population-level health outcomes.

Data for these measures are routinely collected, analyzed, and reviewed by executives. The third option focuses on selecting data-driven priority improvement projects. Such projects may address issues common to the overall organization (e.g., efficient processing of contracts and grants, maximizing collection of revenue), or a specific public health program (e.g., timeliness in completing outbreak investigations, increases in the number of city ordinances that promote tobacco-free and healthy food environments, and improvements in referrals of low-income persons to primary and specialty health care services).

These initiatives are not mutually exclusive. Indeed, several LHDs have simultaneously pursued a combination of these PI activities. However, each initiative requires the commitment of a large amount of staff time and resources, and the decision of LHDs to participate in any of them is highly dependent on local/regional leadership. No approach has clearly established itself as the primary means to assess services delivered by LHDs or to define "high-performing" LHDs.

■ CONTEXT

The LAC Department of Public Health (DPH) is pursuing all three PI initiatives. Primary emphasis has been directed toward developing a robust PBAS and implementing rapid-cycle improvement projects across the department. The department is taking steps to prepare for voluntrary accreditation, which launched nationwide in 2011 (13).

Performance-Based Accountability System

In the early 2000s, the LAC Chief Executive Office implemented a county-wide performance measurement initiative called "Performance Counts!" using the results-based accountability (RBA) approach (14). This approach is designed for use by any public agency, not just LHDs. It links program-level processes (e.g., percent of people reached through a public program) with jurisdiction-wide outcomes (e.g., percent of county residents who achieve a particular outcome related to education, health, transportation, or child protective services).

The LAC DPH modified the RBA approach to create a conceptual framework that distinguishes population-level health from program-specific performance. To emphasize this distinction and avoid confusion, the term *population indicator* is used to describe measures of population health, whereas the term *performance measure* is used to describe measures of program performance (e.g., processes and outputs). Details on the framework and features of the DPH PBAS have been described elsewhere (12).

The DPH also developed an agency-wide approach to efficiently collect, analyze, and share performance data. Implementation of an online data entry and reporting system with real-time dashboard capability is proceeding as time, funding, staffing, and political momentum allow.

Rapid-Cycle Performance Improvement Projects

After establishing a robust PBAS, the DPH began exploring the best application of PI tools and methods. Of central importance was the selection of a formal

PI method that is both readily understood by all levels of DPH staff and easily integrated into the existing PBAS.

The LAC DPH reviewed various PI methods used by the MLC, the National Association of County and City Health Officials (NACCHO), and the RAND Corporation "Promoting Emergency Preparedness and Readiness (PREPARE)" project, which was based on the method used in the Institute for Healthcare Improvement's Breakthrough Series Learning Collaborative (15–16). Ultimately, the simple application and clear steps of the PREPARE approach made it seem best-suited for the LAC DPH to integrate with its PBAS.

■ APPROACH TO THE PROBLEM

The DPH prioritized organization structural changes and team-based approaches to enable transformation to a PI culture where opportunities to improve business practices are seen as a part of everyone's job.

Operations and Implementation Time Line

A Division of Quality Improvement was established to oversee agency-wide PI activites (see note 1). A Director of Performance Improvement was hired and an interdisciplinary Performance Improvement Team (PI Team) was created to guide the development of PI activities. This team includes representatives from each of the DPH divisions that are required to participate in PI efforts.

Key activities and their periodicity based on staff time and availability include: 1) collecting performance data biannually; 2) requesting updates to the core set of performance measures (e.g., add, modify, or drop) annually; 3) writing and reviewing performance reports annually with additional brief reports as needed; 4) providing training as needs are identified; and 5) implementing rapid-cycle improvement projects based on performance data trends and department priorities.

Measuring Performance

The LAC DPH identified approximately 74 population indicators and 227 performance measures. To allow for benchmarking, efficiency of data collection, and timely reporting of results to parties at all levels of government, the LAC DPH integrated tracking and reporting of performance with existing frameworks. Population indicators are aligned with the health outcomes found in Healthy People (17) where applicable. Performance measures are a mix of structure, process, and output measures and are organized under the PHAB accreditation domains (18). They are also aligned with federal, state, and local grant monitoring and evaluation requirements, when feasible.

Rapid-Cycle Improvement Projects: A Learning Collaborative Approach

Given the large size and organizational complexity of the LAC DPH, programmatic units tend to function independently in the absence of structure and incentives to collaborate. To address this challenge, a Performance Improvement Learning

Collaborative (PILC) was established to: 1) allow staff to identify common processes with the greatest potential for influencing performance improvement; 2) empower staff members through peer-level discussions on "what works"; and 3) generate enthusiasm and support for PI leaders throughout the department.

The PILC format brings teams of public health practitioners together to learn PI methods and share their experiences while working on an improvement project of importance to their specific program. The PILC teams were taught a four-step improvement model: 1) identify an aim for improvement; 2) map the process to be improved; 3) identify and collect data for performance measurement; and 4) make changes for improvement. This last step involves adapting promising ideas for change to the local environment using small-scale, rapid-cycle tests of change and PDSA cycles. The four-step model was integrated into the existing DPH PBAS to allow continuity of instruction and implementation of projects into priority program activities.

■ IMPLEMENTATION OF SOLUTIONS

Eight units, broadly representative of LAC DPH services, participated in the PILC. A mix of managers, senior staff, and administrators was encouraged to work together to create the most effective teams and to increase the chance for successful implementation of their rapid-cycle improvement project. Each PILC team leader was required to be an active member of the PI Team.

The PILC team projects covered a wide range of public health services. These included performance-based contracting, improving access to prevention and treatment services, and targeting educational outreach for maximum reach and effect (see Table 7–1). Specific aims for improvement centered on programmatic processes prioritized by senior management, with an emphasis on areas with ongoing data collection

TABLE 7–1 *Targeted Areas for Improvement, Los Angeles County*

Division or Unit	Target Area (Population Impact)[a]	Process Improvements (Program Impact)[b]
Children's Medical Services	Increase access to specialty medical care for children with special health care needs	Improve timeliness and completeness of referral paperwork processes by contracted providers
Office of Senior Health	Decrease the prevalence of chronic disease in persons age 65 years and older	Improve online dissemination of health alert messages and health promotion materials by community organizations
Office of Women's Health	Decrease the prevalence of heart disease in women ages 40–65	Improve completion rates of a Heart Health assessment tool via a health information hotline
Tobacco Control and Prevention Program	Decrease prevalence of tobacco use for adolescents and adults	Increase successful policy campaigns and passage of anti-tobacco city ordinances through improving technical assistance to contracted providers

a. *Population impact* refers to the countywide health outcomes targeted by each project.
b. *Program impact* refers to structural, process, or output objectives targeted by each project that are *linked* to the project's countywide health outcomes. Linkages are determined by review of current best evidence and accepted public health principles.

efforts. When existing data was less robust or not reflective of a priority process step, project teams developed new metrics and designed new data collection methods or instruments. Teams were encouraged to develop promising practices for improvement based on evidence, such as the systematic reviews from the Community Guide to Preventive Services (19).

Over a 12-month time frame, the PILC participants attended three in-person learning sessions led by the DPH PI Director and an outside consultant from RAND corporation. In an environment of collegiality, the teams worked together to learn the four-step model, develop skills to apply PI tools to their rapid-cycle improvement projects, and share lessons learned. The sessions included didactic education, small group discussion, and direct application of the technique. Four PI tools received particular emphasis for use: brainstorming, process maps, run charts, and Pareto charts (20).

Teams submitted monthly progress reports and were provided technical assistance between the in-person sessions. Required monthly PILC team reports ensured that the teams stayed engaged over the course of the one-year project. The reports also provided a window of opportunity to catch gaps in team member knowledge and to make mid-course corrections, if needed. Individual team coaching sessions provided opportunities for just-in-time tailored training unique to each project and for troubleshooting project issues related to PDSA design, implementation, and interpretation. Each team had roughly four individual coaching sessions.

At the end of the 12-month collaborative period, the PILC teams provided an overview of their projects at a final sharing session. Each PILC team presented its project in a storyboard, and presentations focused on overall lessons learned from the experience. A number of interactive activities during the three-hour session were designed to encourage the senior managers in attendance to begin planning new PI projects.

■ EVALUATION STRATEGY

The goal of the PILC was to develop an effective model in which multiple ongoing PI projects could be implemented across the department. Evaluation methods included a pre-test and post-test survey of PILC participants, a baseline senior manager survey (n = 81), and semi-structured interviews with selected executives (n = 10). The evaluation questions were:

1. How do knowledge, attitudes, and use of PI methods by DPH staff change as a result of PILC participation?
2. What is the impact of PILC participation on selected DPH performance measures and associated health outcomes?
3. What are the key facilitators and challenges to the introduction and application of a structured PI process within the DPH?

■ IMPACT

Change in PILC Participants' PI Knowledge, Attitudes, and Practices

Changes in PI knowledge, attitudes, and practices were collected using a validated survey that was distributed to all participants at the beginning of the PILC and at the end of the working period one year later.

Knowledge of PI methods increased significantly among PILC participants. Statistically significant improvements were seen using a PI knowledge scale, in which respondents rated their knowledge of 14 different PI methods using a three-point Likert scale (0 = no knowledge, 1 = some knowledge, 3 = proficient). Overall, respondents increased their knowledge from a baseline average of 9/14 items to an average of 13/14 items ($p<0.0008$). There were no improvements in the ratings of PI-supportive organizational culture (21), organizational change readiness (22), or department-wide PI practices.

PILC participants were asked to rate their experience with the PILC and their likelihood to use PI methods in the future. The majority of participants felt that they had received the right amount of training and coaching in PI methods. The PILC participants reported that an experiential, "hands-on learning" approach was helpful.

Participants reported that using the four-step model helped to engage their whole team and other division members. In particular, they felt that using process maps and PDSA cycles was especially helpful in focusing group efforts. Notably, 79% of respondents felt that their team was successful or very successful in reaching their project goals, and 84% said they were likely to use the methods they learned in their future work.

Impact of PILC Participation on the Teams' Performance Measures and Health Outcomes

The results of each PILC teams' self-reported performance measures showed one team with breakthrough improvement (see Box 7–1), four teams with incremental improvement, and three teams with no change in performance.

BOX 7–1 ■ Strategies to Improve Performance of a Heart Disease Risk Factor Assessment Tool Using a Multilingual Telephone Hotline

Situation

Heart disease is the leading cause of death for women. The DPH Office of Women's Health (OWH) developed a Heart Healthy Risk Assessment tool to help educate women on how to decrease their risk factors for heart disease. The OWH integrated use of the tool into their exisiting multilingual hotline call system. Monitoring is ongoing, and a database to track the number of hotline calls and client activities is the foundation for evaluation.

Step 1. Identify the Aim (Aim Statement)

By June 30, 2010, increase awareness of cardiovascular disease and its risk factors in low-income women of color in LAC and ultimately decrease the prevalence of heart disease by:

- Exploring effective methodologies that result in increased utilization of the multilingual hotline and increased client completion of the Heart Healthy Risk Assessment

(*continued*)

BOX 7–1 (*Continued*)

Step 2. Map the Process

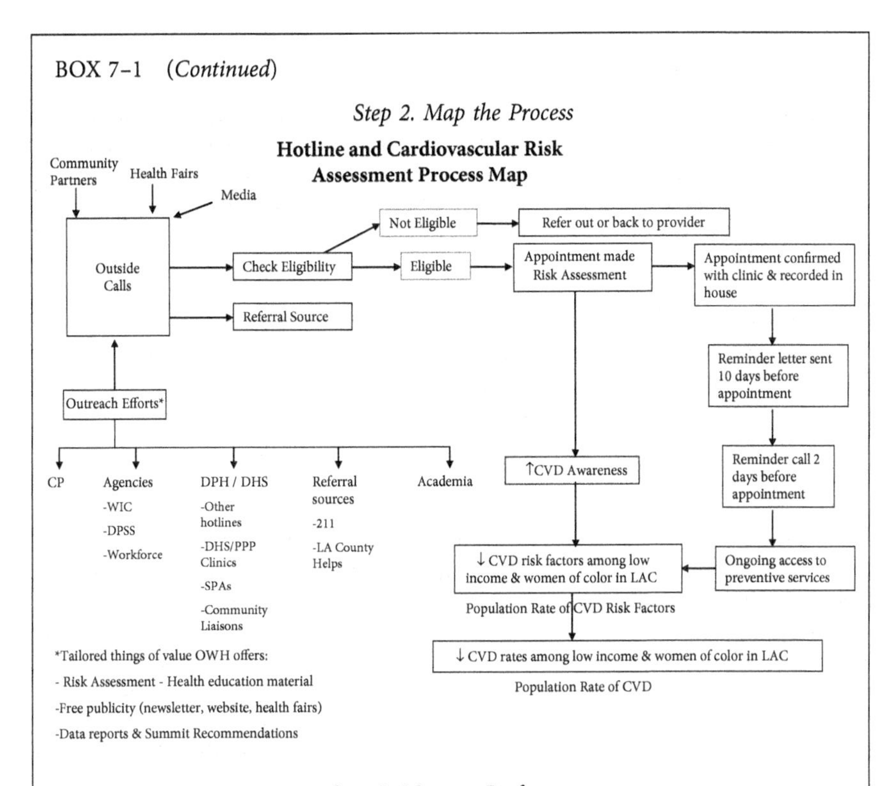

Step 3. Measure Performance

A. Population Indicator
   Percent of women below 200% federal poverty level, age 40–64 years, diagnosed with heart disease in LAC
   Baseline: 6.7% Target: 6.5%
B. Performance Measure
   Percent of hotline callers who completed the Heart Healthy Risk Assessment
   Baseline: 29% Target: 50%
C. PI Team Project Measures
   Percent of completed Heart Healthy Risk Assessment questionnaires mailed to low-income women
   Baseline: 71% Target: 100%

Step 4. Make Changes for Improvement (Plan-Do-Study-Act Cycles)

Recruitment of Participants at a Foreign Consulate (February 2010)
Selected one foreign consulate for in-person outreach to increase awareness of OWH hotline services and recruit participants for the Heart Healthy Risk Assessment. Clearance by the department communication office was required and took longer than expected. Daily visits to the consulate for one week resulted in no hotline calls.

Recruitment of Participants at Community-Based Organizations (4 cycles; March and April 2010)

(*continued*)

BOX 7–1 (*Continued*)

Using the results of a literature review, OWH staff used a variety of recruitment strategies tailored to Korean communities, an African American clinic, a community library of Chinese women, health fairs for Chinese and Mexican communities, and a free medical clinic that serves all ethnicities. Recruitment was considered adequate and several subsequent hotline calls were completed.

Overall Results

Over the PILC one-year period, the number of hotline callers increased (data not shown), the percent of women completing the Heart Healthy Risk assessment increased from 29% to 39% and women receiving their results by mail increased from 71% to 88%. This is considered breakthrough improvement by the PILC leaders.

Unsurprisingly, changes in health outcomes were not seen over the one-year period of the PILC. Despite the lag time in attempting to associate process level improvements with improved community health outcomes, the PILC leaders concluded that the linkages between the two levels of performance were extremely important. This is because public health practitioners who lead PI projects often make one of two major errors: 1) set their aim too "high" and including only a population-level health outcome as the sole emphasis for short-term improvement (for example, to improve the prevalence of physical activity in the community); or 2) setting their aim too "low" and focusing exclusively on a small internal process improvement step without clearly understanding the larger context in which improvements in population-level health are linked to their project. Including both population indicators and performance measures throughout the PI project reminds the project participants that both are needed to improve overall performance.

Key Facilitators and Challenges to the Introduction of a Structured PI Process

Facilitators

The PILC four-step model was readily understood and absorbed by the PILC project teams. This allowed team members to view rapid-cycle PDSA activities as "doable" and as a positive set of skills and knowledge that they could feasibly use in their daily work. In general, teams that made the most progress implemented higher priority projects, had managers as team members, identified feasible performance measures early in the project period, and used measures with frequent data collection.

Senior managers supported and provided time for teams to meet and work on projects, prepare for coaching sessions, and attend the in-person learning sessions. All interviewed DPH executives supported substantially increasing the use of PI methods in the department. The majority felt that PI activities should become a routine part of staff's jobs, and not as an "extra" special project. The majority of senior managers reported knowledge and use of PI methods; however, fewer reported knowledge or use of specific methods used in the PILC (e.g., PDSA cycles and other aspects of the four-step model).

PILC participants rated individual team coaching as very helpful. Planning for more of this resource-intensive type of coaching means possibly limiting the number of projects the PI Director can oversee with current staffing levels.

Challenges

Standard, "off the shelf" metrics were not available for the majority of PILC projects. This delayed the selection of performance measures and the assessment of baseline data until mid-project for several project teams.

Project leaders and team members are much more familiar with the principles and steps of *program evaluation* and were not as adept at implementing small-scale steps for change in a rapid-cycle improvement process.

The PILC participants identified an inadequate understanding of PI methods by senior leaders and frontline staff as a major barrier to planning and completing PI projects. Participants noted that due to the lack of common understanding, extra time was needed to explain their projects to other division members. In some cases they were not able to get the full buy-in needed to test and make changes.

A particular challenge in LAC is that there are 88 cities, each with its own, largely autonomous, health policy and decision-making structure. This makes county-wide interventions coordinated by the DPH and its partners challenging to implement and the effects on county-level health outcomes harder to influence. Thus, success is at times defined by sub-county analysis showing health improvement for a particular region or city within the county (depending on data availability and validity).

■ CONCLUSIONS AND LESSONS LEARNED

A dedicated PI initiative has proven valuable to the DPH. It encourages accountability through the identification of priority departmental activities linked to population-level health outcomes; the creation of a data measurement system that allows routine data collection for a subset of prioritized services; and the use of evidence to select the most effective intervention strategies. These activities are important due to the call for increased efficiency in government agencies and the emergence of large public health threats (e.g., pandemic influenza, the obesity epidemic, a built and social environment that incentivizes less healthy behavior choices) during a time of shrinking budgets.

The DPH PILC experience demonstrates that PI methods and tools taught through a multidisciplinary collaborative approach can be successfully applied in a local public health department. A recurrent theme was the need to integrate PI activities more closely with the department's strategic plan, and to select priority rapid-cycle improvement projects using measures taken from the DPH PBAS. Executives also emphasized actively publicizing and disseminating the results of rapid-cycle improvement projects throughout the department.

Using population health indicators (e.g., prevalence of tobacco use, up-to-date childhood immunization rates) as the only measures of success for a PI project is not recommended. This is because data may not be available at a similar sub-county level. For example, a PI project that aims to improve use of a tobacco quit line might focus its outreach efforts and measure its impact in several small neighborhoods within a county, whereas data on the prevalence of tobacco use might only be available at the county level. In addition, the time to see changes in population health outcomes as a result of an intervention may be many years. One way to address this challenge is through the use of process maps that identify measurable steps along the way to health impact.

This initiative also encourages public health entrepreneurship (23) by executives, senior managers, and frontline staff who strive to be innovative leaders within their spheres of influence. To fully capture cost-saving and revenue-generating opportunities, a clear understanding of the key steps of service delivery (e.g., process mapping) and how they can be *measured over time* is required for data-driven management decisions and implementation of change concepts for streamlining operations and improving overall delivery of services. We have found that this is best achieved through a collaborative, team-based approach in which all levels of staff participate in the identification of processes, metrics, and change concepts and are allowed opportunities for the implementation of rapid-cycle improvement projects without fear of blame or failure.

■ NOTES

1. As per Gunzenhauser et al. (12), the term *quality improvement* is considered a broad effort that includes three key areas: 1) development of professional standards and competencies; 2) identification and implementation of evidence-based practices; and 3) design and management of performance improvement systems. The term *performance improvement* encompasses the selection of measures of performance, the routine collection and analysis of performance data, and the use of Plan-Do-Study-Act cycles to improve performance in priority areas.

■ REFERENCES

1. Final recommendations for a voluntary national accreditation program for state and local public health departments. Summary Document, September 12, 2006. Available from: http://www.phaboard.org/wp-content/uploads/ExploringAccreditationFullReport.pdf (accessed June 14, 2012 4).
2. IOM (Institute of Medicine). *For the Public's Health: The Role of Measurement in Action and Accountability*. Washington, DC: National Academies Press; 2011. Available from: http://www.iom.edu/Reports/2010/For-the-Publics-Health-The-Role-of-Measurement-in-Action-and-Accountability.aspx (accessed July 20, 2011).
3. National Public Health Performance Standards Program. *State and Local Public Health System Performance Assessment Instruments* (Version 2). Available from: http://www.cdc.gov/nphpsp/TheInstruments.html (accessed July 20, 2011).
4. State of Missouri Voluntary Public Health Agency Accreditation Program. Available from: http://www.michweb.org/accred.htm (accessed July 20, 2011).
5. North Carolina Local Health Department Accreditation. Available from: http://nciph.sph.unc.edu/accred/ (accessed July 20, 2011).
6. The Michigan Local Public Health Accreditation Program. Available from: http://accreditation.localhealth.net/index.htm (accessed July 20, 2011).
7. The Multi-State Learning Collaborative: Leading States in Public Health Quality Improvement. Available from: http://www.nnphi.org/programs/mlc (accessed July 20, 2011).

8. Baltimore Citistats. Available from: http://www.baltimorecity.gov/Government/AgenciesDepartments/CitiStat.aspx (accessed July 20, 2011).
9. Perez T, Rushing R. *The Citistats Model: How Data Driven Government Can Increase Efficiency and Effectiveness*. Washington, DC: Center for American Progress; April 2007. Available from: http://www.americanprogress.org/issues/2007/04/pdf/citistat_report.pdf (accessed June 14, 2012).
10. Los Angeles County Performance Counts! Available from: http://performancecounts.lacounty.gov/ (accessed July 20, 2011).
11. RAND Corporation. *Toward a Culture of Consequences: Performance Based Accountability Systems for Public Services*. Santa Monica, CA, Arlington, VA, and Pittsburgh, PA; 2010. Available from: http://www.rand.org/pubs/monographs/MG1019.html (accessed July 22, 2011).
12. Gunzenhauser J. et al. The quality improvement experience in a high-performing local health department: Los Angeles County. *J Public Health Man*. 2010;16(1):39–48.
13. Accreditation: Why It Is Important Now. Available from: http://www.phaboard.org/ (accessed July 21, 2011).
14. Friedman M. *Trying Hard Is Not Good Enough: how to Produce Measurable Improvements for Customers and Communities*. Victoria, BC: Trafford Publishing; 2005.
15. Lotstein D, Seid M, Ricci K, Leuschner K, Margolis P, Lurie N. Using quality improvement methods to improve public health emergency preparedness: PREPARE for pandemic influenza. *Health Affairs*. 2008;27(5):w328–39. Available from: http://content.healthaffairs.org/cgi/reprint/27/5/w328 (accessed July 22, 2011).
16. The Breakthrough Series: IHI's Collaborative Model for Achieving Breakthrough Improvement. IHI Innovation Series white paper. Boston: Institute for Healthcare Improvement; 2003. Available from: www.IHI.org.
17. *Healthy People 2020: Topics and Objectives*. Available from; http://www.healthypeople.gov/2020/topicsobjectives2020/default.aspx (accessed July 22, 2011).
18. Public Health Accreditation Board (PHAB). *Standards and Measures: Version 1.0* (May 2011). Washington, DC. Available from: http://www.phaboard.org/index.php/accreditation/standards/ (accessed July 22, 2011).
19. The Guide to Community Preventive Services. Available from: http://www.thecommunityguide.org/index.html (accessed July 22, 2011).
20. Memory Jogger 2: Tools for Continuous Improvement and Effective Planning. 2nd edition. 2010. GOAL/QPC, p. 53, 122, 182. Available from: www.goalqpc.com.
21. The Baldrige Assessment and Criteria. Available from: http://www.baldrige.com/baldrige/baldrige_process/baldrige-faqs-the-baldrige-assessment/ (accessed July 22, 2011).
22. Caldwell D, et al. Implementing strategic changes in a health care system: The importance of leadership and change readiness. *Health Care Manage R*. 2008;33(2):124–33.
23. Jacobson P, personal communication. Public health entrepreneurship. 2011.

8 The Medium and the Message

Strategies for Effective Communication

ROSE ANNE RODRIGUEZ AND
SARAH M. KISSELL

THE PROBLEM

In today's world, few escape bombardment from a variety of daily, even hourly, messages from multiple sources, representing a range of intentions. Information and misinformation are readily available on nearly every subject through the internet at the touch of a button. Advertising and marketing continue to evolve, surrounding the public with both subtle and obvious messages. Twenty-four-hour news cycles present the latest information at a rapid rate. So when the Los Angeles County (LAC) Department of Public Health (DPH) creates and disseminates health-related messages, multiple factors determine how those messages can best penetrate the media clutter to reach, be meaningful to, and be retained by the intended audience.

In addition to concerns over competition for the public's attention, the LAC DPH is aware of the perception that many associate a department of public health with an organization that primarily provides health care services to those without health insurance and the indigent. This perception limits the effectiveness of the department's population-wide initiatives to improve and protect the public's health. This erroneous perception also can affect funding allocations and can undervalue the critical role of the LAC DPH in a disaster or emergency.

CONTEXT

Communicating with the public is essential to the LAC DPH's mission "to protect health, prevent disease, and promote health and well-being." Health messaging plays a vital role in improving population health outcomes, whether through health promotion messages, such as calls to action for a hand-washing campaign, or a sexually transmitted disease prevention campaign, or health protection messages such as food product recall information, guidance on vaccination, or a "boil water" order following a natural disaster that risks contamination of the water supply. One of the challenges for the LAC DPH has been to unite in the public's mind the work of the department's 39 unique and diverse programs as all emanating from a single trusted authority.

Some residents experience public health through community or clinic outreach. Programs like Acute Communicable Disease Control, Community Health Services (which oversees the LAC DPH's 14 health centers), Office of Women's Health, and Chronic Disease and Injury Prevention, among others, have a strong presence in many LAC communities. Other programs provide key data and analysis or serve primarily administrative functions having lower visibility. Public messages from these different types of programs generally were developed by subject matter experts with deep knowledge and experience, but less familiarity with providing information in plain language and through optimal channels to reach target populations. Audiences could be very narrow (e.g., those that ate recently at a particular restaurant associated with a food-borne outbreak) or very broad (e.g., the importance of routine hand washing) (1). Until recently, there was limited planning about priorities for public messaging and no systematic review process to assure accurate, understandable, and timely messaging.

After the LAC DPH became a separate department in 2006 (see Chapter 1), it focused more resources on establishing itself as both a trusted source of information for the public, and as an advocate for consumer health and well-being. To present a clear identity, all communications from the LAC DPH needed a consistent look, feel, and quality—a "brand," if you will—to meet the public expectation of authoritative, accurate, and clear messaging.

■ APPROACH TO THE PROBLEM

Branding is the visual representation of the DPH's personality and presence in the community; it conveys a level of trust in the unique roles, core responsibilities, and authorities of our local public health department (2). Through proactive communication and outreach, the LAC DPH has defined its brand to solidify its image as a consumer-oriented department relevant to all residents, every day. Its appeal is designed to address a range of situations—from restaurant and beach water inspections and tuberculosis control practices to food-borne illness investigations and mass vaccination during a public health emergency. In many situations, the DPH magnifies the effect of its communications by teaming with partner agencies and stakeholder groups. Within the LAC DPH, media engagement and management is centrally coordinated. Its many audiences include elected officials and their field offices, public- and private-sector stakeholders, cities and other local public health departments, health care providers, those with particular health problems or health risks, news media, and the general public (1). Each audience has unique needs and requires functional relationships with the department for its official communications to be maximized for reach and authority.

The public face of the LAC DPH is its Health Officer. The Health Officer's role carries legal responsibilities in health protection, such as the authority to close a school following an illness outbreak or to inspect all restaurants for conformance with the health code. The broader roles of the Health Officer are (a) to promote the health and well-being of all residents, such as providing advice on healthful nutrition or avoidance of recalled foods; and (b) to deliver actionable guidance in times of crisis. While the LAC DPH is fortunate to have a large number of excellent program directors, medical, nursing, epidemiologic, and laboratory professionals, field staff, and other administrators, having a consistent authority figure and spokesperson helps to establish the department's presence as a professional, people-oriented organization with a clear and consistent mission.

Some public health efforts elicit more media coverage than others. In general, what is "new" trumps ongoing problems. For example, media are more likely to broadcast details of a sudden food-borne illness at a popular restaurant and are less likely to cover a news report tracking continuing high levels of obesity. "Selling" non-breaking news stories requires the LAC DPH to be aggressive in pushing stories that otherwise might not get sufficient media attention. Doing this involves knowing the particular interests and priorities of different media channels and reporters (3). Responding quickly to media inquiries is also critical, calling for 24/7 availability of media-savvy personnel.

On major health issues, the DPH regularly connects with other local public health providers to build a coherent message with optimized reach and intensity. It also works collaboratively with the LAC Board of Supervisors, other LAC departments, city leaders, and health officials at the state and federal levels to build support for many initiatives, such as controlling tobacco use, reducing childhood obesity, and reducing drug-related harms.

An established brand, a trusted voice, and a face of authority are essential for effective risk communications (4). Particularly during health emergencies, people expect public health organizations to provide credible and accurate information (5). Each new emergency may evoke an air of familiarity—either in training scenarios or to past events—but each is unique in populations affected, stakeholders involved, and time frames in which events unfold. The objectives in each situation are to (a) reassure the public that a threat is recognized and that appropriate timely actions to minimize it are authorized and underway; (b) provide almost continuous availability for media to report on developments and thus establish the DPH as a reliable, timely source of information; and (c) rapidly respond to any misinformation that may be spread via mass or social media.

Important in maintaining credibility in crises is a willingness to answer, "We don't know at this time" to insistent questions, regardless of the gravity of a situation (6). In these situations, demonstrating a calm demeanor helps stanch the overreaction which almost invariably accompanies public health crises.

To better serve media, the DPH builds trusting relationships by understanding and responding to their needs. The DPH provides opportunities to satisfy reporters working on specific stories as conveniently as possible. For example, when coordinating a press conference on a new recommendations for Tdap (tetanus, diphtheria, pertussis) vaccine for minors, attending media received images of immunizations from a clinic, interviews with doctors from a major private health care provider, and the opportunity to capture a testimonial from a parent whose unvaccinated child had pertussis. Media events are supplemented with handouts featuring key messages, local data, and information about the importance of media coverage of the topic. By consistently providing high-quality information from relevant spokespeople, the LAC DPH endeavors to respond to reporters' needs and has cultivated valuable relationships that help to ensure that public health messages are shared accurately, understandably, and broadly (6).

For communication partnerships to be effective, partners need to appreciate the department's roles and responsibilities. Public health investigations are usually mysteries with unclear end dates and shaded, emerging clues; they are not clear-cut puzzles with defined pieces that neatly fit together. Illness investigations can take months and may yield only unclear diagnoses. Cause and effect are often indefinable at the onset of an outbreak investigation. Initial reports of symptoms may point to several plausible illnesses, but final diagnoses sometimes differ from original suspicions. Understanding that investigations take time and often involve multiple agencies, and that it is often inappropriate to speculate on alternate possibilities, can support more collaborative relationships with media. In addition to media partners, elected officials and others who might be asked about an investigation need to understand these issues and not prematurely opine on causes or consequences.

IMPLEMENTATION

The LAC DPH Office of External Relations and Communications (ExComm) oversees three core functions: public information, multimedia services, and legislative affairs (see Box 8–1 for staff responsibilities).

BOX 8–1 ■ ExComm Responsibilities

- Public Information and Community Outreach:
  The Public Information Officer (PIO) coordinates education and risk communication messaging, media interviews, press outreach and translation services, and maintains the department's social media pages. The PIO works with other agencies, such as other local health departments, fire and law enforcement, and hospital partners, to ensure that accurate and non-conflicting public health information is distributed.

  Community outreach liaisons analyze and provide technical expertise and analysis to the department on communicating effectively to ethnic and multi-language communities. They oversee projects to improve health outcomes and emergency readiness in special populations, including the disabled, seniors, businesses, schools, and other special populations.
- Communications: Publications, Design, and Multimedia Services
  Staff handle a variety of functions related to maintaining the LAC DPH's brand throughout all internal and external print and electronic communications. This includes publications, such as the annual report, newsletters, fact sheets, program reports, and briefs; slideshow presentations and poster presentations; and the LAC DPH website. Brand uniformity is achieved through several methods: the creation and dissemination of brand guidelines, which are posted on LAC DPH's intranet and, therefore, are accessible by all staff; the development of pre-branded templates, which may be used by all programs; and the use of project consultations, ideally before design and layout commence.

  Writing, editing, design, photography, and videography are the key skills offered by the communications staff. In addition to producing the monthly internal employee newsletter for nearly 4,000 staff, communications staff project-manage and edit an external clinical newsletter for 10,000 physicians. The unit provides audiovisual support for press outreach, social media videos, and event coverage. Further, staff assist the LAC DPH's 39 programs with their writing, editing, and photography needs.
- Legislative Affairs:
  The Legislative Branch of ExComm is responsible for communicating directly with community, city, county, state, and federal partners. It does this through meetings and workshops and whenever there is need to analyze legislation that will have an impact on the public's health. It also maintains strong relationships with nine of the county's Latin American consulates, including those for Mexico, El Salvador, Columbia, Costa Rica, Ecuador, Guatemala, Honduras, Nicaragua, and Peru.

ExComm established a consistent look for all materials produced by LAC DPH programs, from clinic handouts and press releases to web design and PowerPoint presentations. ExComm ensures clear, appropriate language for each audience. Plain language efforts entail writing of press releases, web posts, fact sheets, and other documents at a fourth-grade reading level. This ensures basic accessibility and facilitates translation into multiple languages.

The department's communication response during the 2009 H1N1 pandemic (H1N1) exemplifies the use of the LAC DPH's emerging brand to clarify local guidance. When the pandemic started, information, recommendations, and instructions poured from all levels of government. The guidance documents mixed information for the general public and for health care providers, sometimes in the same document. The complexity and incompletely defined nature of H1N1 caused responding agencies to disagree, which became apparent as conflicting guidance documents reached the media, stakeholders, and the public. Through it all, the LAC DPH consistently assured stakeholders that the local health officer is vested with authority to parse dissonant guidance, to assess what is in LAC's best interest, and to determine next steps such as whether to declare a local health emergency or to close schools (see Box 8–2).

While pandemic influenza preparedness exercises hinted at a voracious media appetite for news, at the start of H1N1 a virtual onslaught of inquiries came from reporters internationally, from the general public, health care providers, hospitals, other local public health departments, and elected officials. For weeks, the department's media phone line received hundreds of calls daily. Notwithstanding the amount of guidance, the number of press conferences, and the provision of alternate hotline phone numbers, residents wanted more continuous and more personal attention from the DPH to calm their fears.

BOX 8–2 ■ Managing Media Needs during Pandemic H1N1 2009

During the H1N1 response, the Health Officer had to balance responding to significant media demand with departmental response to the pandemic. One-on-one requests for interviews stopped almost immediately once it became apparent that H1N1 was no ordinary flu strain. The LAC DPH switched to a press conference format, holding at least one press conference daily for almost two weeks. An LAC DPH Spanish-language spokesperson was made available for nearly all press conferences. One notable press conference, led by the LAC DPH, combined representatives from the LAC Emergency Medical Services division, Los Angeles World Airports, the Los Angeles Unified School District, the LAC Office of Education, and the LAC Department of Health Services. This one-stop-shopping approach for the media was immediately effective in calming fears about airline and seaport travel, the status of school closures, guidance for the medical community, the status of emergency rooms, and general guidance for the public. In addition to the press conferences, simultaneous press call-ins were held where members of the media, staff from political offices, first responders, other departments and agencies, health care providers, and other stakeholders could make contact to hear the same, unedited guidance. These call-ins were then made available via phone replay.

The LAC DPH seeks to assure that each stakeholder group receives appropriate local messages, from the Health Officer and from state and federal documents. Tailored messages went to schools, colleges and universities, first responders, faith-based and community-based organizations, hospitals, physicians, long term care facilities, and the general public. Each required nuanced language shaped to its needs, but the general design and the guidance itself remained consistent and recognizable as emanating from and approved by the LAC DPH. Tailored messages gave partners and residents confidence that the LAC DPH and the Health Officer could respond to their unique needs, providing timely, vetted information. If the LAC DPH had not already established its brand of trusted leadership prior to H1N1, effective communications with unique stakeholders could have been insurmountable.

The LAC DPH's leadership and communications capacity was further tested by its response to the nuclear crisis following the March 2011 tsunami and earthquake that struck near Sendai, Japan. The DPH and several other agencies monitored LAC air quality amid concerns over airborne radioactive material, quickly providing assurances that Los Angeles was unlikely to experience an increase in radioactive exposure, and also advising the public against taking potassium iodide. Initially, this guidance was met with skepticism because it denied residents actionable options to protect themselves. The Health Officer reinforced overall reassuring messages in interviews and press conferences with local elected leaders and first responders. Daily updates that the Japanese radiation would not affect exposure in LAC helped to calm fears. Quickly aligning the message with elected leaders and health care professionals was possible in part because trusting relationships had already been built with these stakeholders.

ExComm has developed relationships with all active LAC media. This includes roundtable discussions with mainstream print journalists and broadcasters, ethnic media outlets, and editors or owners of blogs. In 2011 at least 110 print newspapers served ethnic groups or geographically defined communities, and at least 10 television stations broadcast in languages other than English. An early ExComm priority was reaching out to ethnic media, and during the pandemic H1N1 response the LAC DPH furthered its reputation as a viable resource among these communities.

The LAC DPH is also active on social media as one of the first public health departments to establish a Facebook page in Spanish in addition to English, and to issue bilingual messages on Twitter. Its YouTube channel features videos in English, Spanish, and other languages such as Mandarin Chinese. The internet's capacity to reach broad segments of the population expands message delivery options and permits video messaging to better reach low literacy audiences (7).

Aside from standardizing material and presentation formats and creating protocols for use of the logos and graphics, ExComm prompts LAC DPH leaders to review educational materials, public reports, and campaign literature. This high-level review aims to assure quality and consistent branding. Additionally, all media inquiries are routed to the Public Information Officer for vetting, approval, and assignment to the Health Officer or a designated spokesperson.

These efforts come with challenges. One is program staff management of inquiries from the public. Typically, mainstream reporters connect to the department through its established media phone line. Yet bloggers may call a program office and ask questions about initiatives, campaigns, or other resources without identifying themselves as media. Employees may respond informally, not realizing that their comments may be reproduced online and picked up by still other media. One role of ExComm is to heighten program staff awareness, advising them about proper questions for screening callers and how to refer possible media callers, like bloggers, to the media line.

Another example stems from the H1N1 response. LAC DPH conducted mass vaccination clinics (see Chapter 27) when the vaccine first became available, though supplies were limited. Public expectations of the populations that the LAC DPH could serve during the initial period of constrained supply had to be managed, given that most of the vaccine was allocated to private providers and community clinics for their regular patients. Media expectations of unfettered access to DPH vaccination dispensing sites (PODs) had to be managed, as their interests collided with federal requirement to observe Health Insurance Portability and Accountability Act (HIPAA) privacy guidelines. It was decided to restrict media access at the PODs to intake and provision-of-care areas. Prominently posted signs prohibited videography, photography, or documentation of POD-related activity. Discussions with station managers and editors reiterated the restrictions and, more important, why restrictions were needed.

To maintain good media and public relationships and to provide transparency to the mass vaccination process, alternate media opportunities for access included walk-throughs of clinics with reporters and cameras before operating hours, and photo and interview opportunities with pre-selected patients who represented the demographics of a media outlet's audience and/or a vaccine priority group who agreed to be interviewed or photographed. Transparency, consistency, planning, and appropriate exercise of authority again were critical to manage public and media expectations.

Technology expands media landscapes. Any reporter or private citizen can post a video clip, send a Tweet, or maintain a blog. As proactive public health communicators, the LAC DPH considers daily the benefits and drawbacks to such broad access. Messages increasingly have to be more strategic, clear, and plain in language to accommodate the various methods by which that message is disseminated.

Public health communication needs to provide context and perspective. Public health scientists and epidemiologists handle complex and sensitive information routinely and can become desensitized to how it is perceived by lay people. For example, epidemiologists started seeing cases of a pathogen known as carbapenem-resistant *Klebsiella Pneumoniae* (CRKP) in a small sample of patients from several hospitals. CRKP was newly seen here, but had been identified elsewhere in the country. The epidemiologists intended to present their limited findings as an observational study at a professional conference at Atlanta's Centers for Disease Control and Prevention (CDC). An embargoed abstract went to select media representatives across the nation. They immediately noted the CRKP presentation, raising increasingly alarmist questions. CRKP was dubbed "the new superbug" by some who speculated that it could be a killer-pathogen lurking in nursing homes.

Challenges arose quickly. Local health care providers heard reports of this "new superbug" and claimed that the LAC DPH failed to keep them informed. The LAC DPH determined that the best response was education through matter-of-fact explanation of the minimal data available. Controlled access to LAC DPH personnel also was quickly implemented.

A press conference call, with no camera access, featured the Health Officer, the lead epidemiologist, the department's Spanish-language spokesperson, and the Public

Information Officer. A separate conference call engaged local hospitals, health care agencies, and hospital associations to offer the same reassurance. Concise answers were factual, offering lots of perspective. And the LAC DPH website featured a statement by the Health Officer (see Box 8–3, which repeats the statement's main elements). Addressing the facts and context directly helped to prevent widespread panic and unnecessary public avoidance of necessary health care services and facilities.

The LAC DPH continues to expand its messaging to solidify its reputation as a trusted source of timely, accurate communications. Moving forward, ExComm plans to strengthen its relationship with media through roundtables, forums, and educational discussions that highlight important public health issues. ExComm also created an online portal for local city and community leaders to share vital information,

BOX 8–3 ■ Communication Statement Elements: Carbapenem-Resistant *Klebsiella pneumoniae*

- What is the issue and when did LAC DPH find out about it?
  Recent news reports have covered a data analysis by the LAC DPH of a health-care-associated, multiple-drug resistant pathogen called carbapenem-resistant *Klebsiella pneumoniae* (CRKP). Following reports of cases of CRKP at local hospitals in spring 2010, Public Health required for the first time that all laboratories for health care facilities report cases of this disease. Between June and December 2010, laboratories countywide reported a total of 356 cases.
- How did this come to light?
  A summary of DPH's first analysis of data was developed for presentation at a national epidemiology conference on April 4, 2011. As part of the promotion for the conference, the conference organizers released this data to the media on March 23, 2011.
- What does this mean for the residents of Los Angeles County?
  This survey is intended to establish a baseline for the overall frequency of CRKP infections in LA County. It is important to note that 356 cases represent a very low percentage of health care–associated infections and CRKP is only one of a growing number of multiple-drug resistant organisms.
- What is LAC DPH doing about this issue?
  All multiple-drug resistant organisms are a concern to Public Health. We will continue surveillance to assess trends in the number of cases of CRKP in Los Angeles County. The department is notifying physicians about the study findings regarding this organism and providing continuing education about the problem of multiple-drug resistant bacteria as well as the role of appropriate antibiotic use in combating the continuing problem of resistance development.
- What can the public do about this issue?
  Patients can help prevent the spread of antibiotic resistant bacteria by fully completing the course of treatment for any prescribed antibiotics and not insisting on antibiotic therapy for a health problem unless recommended by their physician. Finally, both health care staff and patients can reduce the spread of CRKP and other pathogens through frequent hand washing or use of a waterless alcohol-based hand rub.

create a venue for dialogue between cities and the department, and provide resources that agencies can pass on to their constituents. These strategies are designed to engage partners in the department's broad spectrum of activities while increasing messaging efficiency to key stakeholders when the next public health crisis occurs.

EVALUATION AND IMPACT

Assessing the impact of these communications initiatives has been primarily qualitative. The frequency of requests for information and coverage of press conferences, health alerts, and other activities to protect and promote public health confirms the LAC DPH as a regular, authoritative source of health information for the media. Often, especially during emergencies such as the Japan nuclear crisis response and the pandemic H1N1 response, other public health departments adapt LAC DPH materials for their own outreach, either through co-branding or with (and even without) permission to reissue. Social media postings often are reissued by stakeholders with reference to the LAC DPH. The frequency and nature of requests help the department to gauge how its materials are received, used and understood by various audiences (such as the general public) and organizations (such as the state health department). Fulfilling these requests also helps ExComm expand the department's reach and presence to other jurisdictions.

CONCLUSION

The scope of LAC DPH responsibilities and authority, coupled with rapid change in communication distribution channels, requires a constant and varied flow of information from the department to all stakeholders. The objective is to gain and maintain public trust in the DPH's ability to respond to crises by providing useful information safeguarding the public's health. Communicating with the public is a multifaceted task requiring both consistency and innovation to meet expectations.

Some key lessons learned show that it is important to:

- Centrally coordinate disparate message delivery and standardized formats to promote the collective work of a broad professional staff, while simultaneously establishing a recognizable department "brand."
- Take time to create a recognizable and respected brand—a constantly evolving process. Branding efforts need the support of relationship building with community partners and media, and staff buy-in as well.
- Partner with all stakeholders, including the media—vital in large and diverse jurisdictions such as LAC. Though time-consuming and sometimes frustrating, the benefits far outweigh any drawbacks. Partnerships also enhance credibility and provide support, particularly in emergency incidents.
- Do advance planning for crisis communication, but remain flexible, as is essential to communicating effectively during an emergency.
- It is sometimes more effective to think outside the press box: substitute a press call-in or alternate means of communicating with media for a press conference when images may distract from the technical importance of a message.
- Monitor blogs, Twitter feeds, consumer forums, and other online media and respond to them as to traditional media. Monitoring online sources also can indicate how publics perceive health-related information.

- Regard bloggers as reporters and give them the same consideration as any other journalists, with the same access and/or restrictions.
- Maintain credibility and authority by giving attention to managing expectations of all partners, stakeholders, media, and publics.
- Establish a brand, a trusted voice, and a face of authority for the local public health department—all critical in any risk communication scenario.

■ REFERENCES

1. Nelson DE, Brownson RC, Remington PL, Parvanta C, editors. *Communicating Public Health Information Effectively: A Guide for Practitioners*. Washington, DC: American Public Health Association; 2002.
2. Evans WD, Blitstein J, Hersey JC, Renaud J, Yaroch AL. Systematic review of public health branding. *J Health Commun*. 2008;13(8):721–41.
3. Park H, Reber B. Using public relations to promote health: A framing analysis of public relations strategies among health associations. *J Health Commun*. 2010;15(1):39–54.
4. Shore DA. Communicating in times of uncertainty: The need for trust. *J Health Commun*. 2003;8:S1,13–4.
5. Avery EJ, Kim S. Preparing for pandemic flu while managing uncertainty: An analysis of the construction of fear and uncertainty in press releases of major health agencies. *J Health & Mass Commun*. 2010;1(3/4):177–93.
6. Brunner W, Fowlie K, Freestone J. Using media to advance public health agendas. Contra Costa Health Services, Public Health Division Brief, March 2011. Available from: http://www.cdph.ca.gov/programs/cclho/Documents/UsingMediaToAdvancePHAgendas.pdf (accessed Sept. 26, 2011).
7. Cassell MM, Jackson C, Cheuvront B. Health communication on the internet: an effective channel for health behavior change?, *J Health Commun*. 1998;3:1,71–9.

9

Understanding Birth Outcomes and Adverse Birth Events

LAMB and LA HOPE

SHIN MARGARET CHAO, GIANNINA DONATONI, CHANDRA HIGGINS, MARIAN ELDAHABY, AND CYNTHIA A. HARDING

THE NATURE OF THE PROBLEM

Infant mortality is an indicator of community health (1). The infant mortality rate in Los Angeles County (LAC) has declined from 8.0 deaths per 1,000 live births in 1990 to 4.9 deaths per 1,000 live births in 2000. There was no decline, however, between 2000 and 2005, and the rate increased slightly in 2002 (2).

Between 2000 and 2007 some 150,000 births and 1,500 fetal and infant deaths occur in LAC annually. The county faces racial/ethnic and geographic disparities in maternal and infant morbidity, mortality, and birth outcomes. These arise from causes ranging from differential access to health care and health behaviors, to psychosocial factors, nutritional status, environmental exposures, poverty, and racism (3).

Historically, the LAC Department of Public Health (DPH) Maternal, Child, and Adolescent Health (MCAH) Programs lacked basic surveillance data on the maternal population. MCAH used vital records data to monitor infant mortality rates, implement programs, and plan services. These data, however, did not identify the multifaceted reasons for differences across groups or county regions. The California Department of Public Health (CDPH) requires MCAH Programs to review fetal and infant deaths annually. This review is conducted using the Fetal Infant Mortality Review (FIMR) approach, which is designed to determine why the deaths occurred and to recommend means for preventing future deaths. The MCAH FIMR program provided data on the medical and social circumstances of each death, but the results did not aid population surveillance or planning. The materials reviewed—autopsies, medical charts, and maternal interviews—varied in quality, completeness, and availability. Reviews usually indicated the same material medical conditions as the causes of death. Only 45 cases were reviewed each year, and by year-end there was no time left for recommendations. New tools were needed to understand and monitor the causes of infant mortality and to engage community stakeholders in finding solutions to lower the risks. An increase in infant mortality in one LAC region gave MCAH the opportunity to use the new tools (see Chapter 33).

CONTEXT

MCAH evaluated the feasibility of developing more comprehensive and systematic perinatal surveillance data for the county. At first, staff considered two established surveys that addressed some limitations of vital records and FIMR data. California's Maternal and Infant Health Assessment (MIHA) and the Centers for Disease Control and Prevention's Pregnancy Risk Assessment Monitoring System (PRAMS) surveyed (in English and Spanish) women who recently gave birth on their experiences before, during, and soon after their most recent pregnancy (4, 5). MCAH reviewed the surveys and protocols and decided that MIHA and PRAMS data were useful for tracking progress toward state and national objectives, but that greater flexibility was needed to assess the complex causes of infant mortality in LAC, the most populous and diverse county in the country (6, 7). Public and community stakeholders gave input on questions. MCAH developed the Los Angeles Mommy and Baby (LAMB) project for LAC residents who had recently delivered live infants. A complementary survey, the Los Angeles Health Overview of a Pregnancy Event (LA HOPE) was framed for women who had recently lost a fetus or infant. LA HOPE was meant to replace the traditional data collection process for the state-mandated FIMR program. LA HOPE did not increase costs because existing MCAH staff conducted the survey.

■ APPROACH TO THE PROBLEM

The LAMB and LA HOPE projects provide comprehensive information on preconception health, prenatal care, medical conditions during pregnancy, psychosocial factors, risk factors, postpartum health, and infant care for women, data not readily available elsewhere.

Instrument Development

Developing the survey instrument involved reviewing the literature on birth outcomes and infant mortality, identifying available data and what was still needed to meet the requirements of all interested stakeholders, conducting focus group meetings, and piloting the survey. The final instrument contained over 80 mostly pre-validated questions. In-depth literature reviews and PRAMS and MIHA questionnaires identified the primary areas addressed for LAMB: preconception health, prenatal care, medical conditions during pregnancy, psychosocial factors, risk behaviors, postpartum health, and infant care. MCAH staff met with DPH and community stakeholders to ensure that the information collected would be useful. Where appropriate, questions were added to meet their specific needs. A pilot instrument was tested in LAC's Antelope Valley (AV) region during an infant mortality investigation there (see Chapter 33). Staff held focus groups with African American, Hispanic, and white mothers to confirm the survey instrument's cultural and linguistic appropriateness. Questions were added to address transportation barriers to prenatal care, discrimination, and neighborhood conditions to assist community partners in developing solutions to improve birth outcomes.

The revised survey was translated into Spanish and Chinese, and a telephone translation service provided access in 88 languages. The survey was approved by the DPH Institutional Review Board.

LA HOPE, a companion survey to LAMB, was developed to monitor the health of women who have suffered an infant or fetal death. We believe that it is unique. Mothers are sampled from fetal and infant death certificates. Death certificate information is linked to birth certificate information and then linked to survey responses. The linkage provides a robust picture of events. The major content areas mimic LAMB, with an addition component on family grief support.

The LA HOPE instrument's 80 questions mainly were validated questions in MIHA, PRAMS, LAMB, and the National Fetal and Infant Mortality Home Interview instruments. Stakeholder and focus groups validated the cultural and linguistic appropriateness of the questions. The initial instrument was piloted in two LAC regions with high infant mortality rates—the AV and South Los Angeles. The final version also appeared in Spanish, and shares the LAMB's telephone translation service. The HOPE questionnaire was also approved by the DPH Institutional Review Board.

Survey Funding and Constraints of the Survey

LAMB is conducted every other year. LA HOPE is ongoing because the number of annual infant and fetal deaths is comparatively small. MCAH staff handled all components of survey administration. The initial cycles of LAMB required no external funding; subsequently, LAMB has been partially funded by external grants. LA HOPE relies solely on internal funds.

The result of supplementary subsidies to support project research has been the development of a survey now nationally recognized for its scientific merit and practical importance. While such an instrument must be relevant to current priorities, health trends also need to be assessed. The LAMB and LA HOPE surveys maintain the continuity of key questions in their respective main content areas while including pertinent new questions and removing those no longer relevant (see Table 9–1). The primary goal is always to collect the most actionable information with the greatest impact factors on the health of LAC women and babies.

TABLE 9–1 *Topic Areas, Los Angeles Mommy and Baby (LAMB) and Los Angeles Health Overview of a Pregnancy Event (LA HOPE) Projects, 2010*

	LAMB	LA HOPE
Socio-demographics	X	X
Preconception health experiences	X	X
Access to health care	X	X
Preconception planning	X	X
Folic acid use	X	X
Birth control and pregnancy intention	X	X
Prenatal Care	X	X
Access, content, and satisfaction	X	X
Prenatal care counseling	X	X
Maternal risk behavior during pregnancy	X	X
Alcohol, drug, and tobacco use	X	X
Intimate partner violence	X	X
Food insecurity	X	X
Maternal medical conditions and obstetrical history	X	X
Infant health care	X	X
Sleep position	X	X

(continued)

TABLE 9-1 *(Continued)*

	LAMB	LA HOPE
Breastfeeding	X	X
Well-baby checkup	X	X
Postpartum health	X	X
Postpartum checkup	X	X
Quality of care	X	X
Social determinants	X	X
Environmental exposures	X	X
Education	X	X
Neighborhood cohesiveness and characterization	X	X
Perceived racism	X	X
Stress, coping, and social support	X	X
Grief support		X
Offered or received bereavement material		X
Offered or attended support group or individual counseling		X
Self-identify a service or support that could have been helpful to the mother or her family		X

■ IMPLEMENTATION OF SOLUTIONS

Each project year, over 10,000 LAMB surveys are mailed three to seven months after eligible mothers deliver. A stratified random sample of birth certificates is selected quarterly based on race/ethnicity and place of residence. African American, Asian, and Native American women and women who deliver a low birth weight infant are overrepresented to ensure adequate samples for these smaller populations. Sampling at the census tract level was introduced to permit examination of individual factors and neighborhood effects on birth outcomes. LAMB data collection is similar to PRAMS. Potential respondents receive a survey packet. Non-respondents receive a reminder postcard, telephone follow-up, and reminder survey packet. A gift certificate goes to each person who completes the survey. The telephone follow-up improves response rates among those hardest to reach (see Figure 9-1).

Social marketing improves response rates, too. We have reached out to local faith-based organizations, WIC centers, and Black Infant Health programs. Staff attend fairs and other gatherings to conduct surveys, raise awareness of the project, and provide news on how people can use the findings to improve birth outcomes.

LA HOPE procedures are modeled after LAMB. LA HOPE samples are drawn three times each project year using state death record files. Participants are contacted within a year of suffering a fetal or infant loss. As with LAMB, LA HOPE is an ongoing, population-based survey and uses similar data collection methods. Survey primary content areas overlap and use many of the same questions, permitting comparison of the two groups of women. Given the smaller sample size and more sensitive LA HOPE survey, its protocol is somewhat modified from that of LAMB. LA HOPE mails letters to the hospitals to validate addresses and phone numbers.

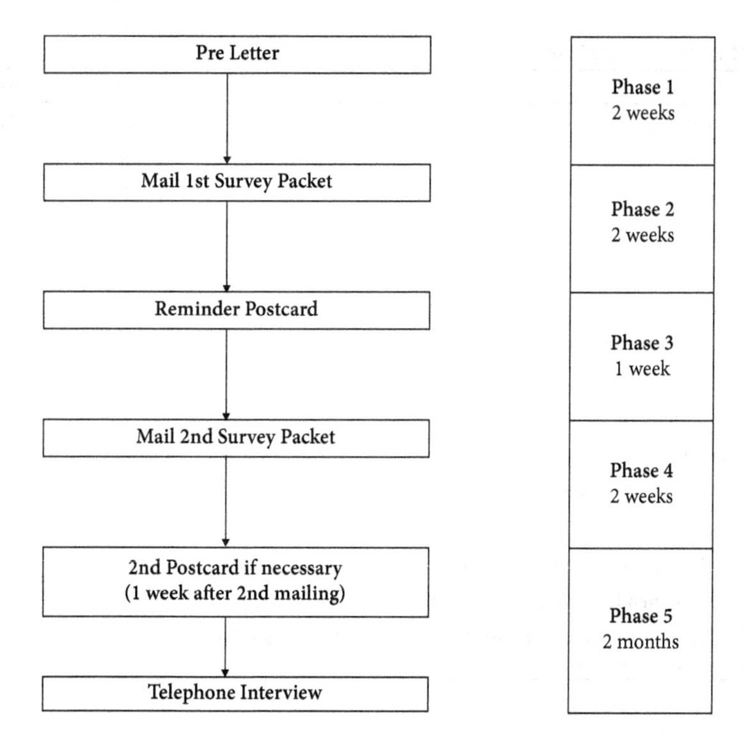

Figure 9–1 Los Angeles Mommy and Baby (LAMB) Survey Procedures.

An incentive accompanies initial survey packets. While both projects use telephone follow-up, LA HOPE completes a greater portion of surveys via phone interviews. A sympathetic and supportive voice often helps selected mothers to share their experiences and opinions.

■ EVALUATION

LAMB and LA HOPE allow the DPH to conduct ongoing perinatal health surveillance. Both help the DPH to identify factors associated with adverse birth outcomes. LAMB generates county-specific data for comparisons within county regions and national PRAMS sites.

As with all mail surveys, the sampling frame for LAMB and LA HOPE excludes the estimated 10% of county residents for whom there is a bad address. To reduce such bias, non-respondents receive telephone follow-up. Up to two survey mailings and eight call attempts are made to contact an eligible woman. Response rates for LAMB surveys range from 50% to 56%. Local LAMB results support national findings on key indicators; for example, the rate of LAC breastfed infants was 85% among those born in 2007, compared with 77% in 2005–2006 nationwide (8).

The average response rate for LA HOPE was 60%, ranging from 58% to 62%; a large portion of women who suffered a fetal or infant death were willing to share their experiences. LA HOPE has many additional advantages compared to the traditional

FIMR data collection process; it permits MCAH to go well beyond the FIMR analysis of medical records data by also collecting information on maternal perinatal behaviors to reveal underlying experiences, attitudes, and histories of pregnant and parenting women whose babies die. From a systems design perspective, the LA HOPE survey method required much less time per case for data collection and eliminated the need to review individual medical records and maternal interviews. In each survey year, LA HOPE sampled over 600 cases, netting some 300 respondents each year. In comparison, the conventional FIMR approach would have reviewed only 45 cases per year.

Many initial LAMB and LA HOPE respondents wrote positively about the survey that they answered. They appreciated being able to respond in their own language. They also expected that some follow-up actions would be based on survey findings. Typical statements were:

"[T]his survey is an EXCELLENT idea. Again, thanks for the opportunity to participate. Keep up the good work; we appreciate it."

"I hope that those surveys really count as a tool to come out with helpful programs to benefit women who really need support during their pregnancy."

Since LAMB and LA HOPE data are self-reported months after delivery (or loss), responses might reflect recall bias, which could vary among different populations and affect estimates of disparities. For example, women who experience pregnancy complications or who suffer a fetal or infant loss might recall events and feelings differently from those who deliver uncomplicated births. While the results of LAMB and LA HOPE are representative of LAC, they cannot be generalized to other counties or California as a whole.

■ IMPACT

With participants throughout LAC, LAMB allows the DPH to monitor trends and examine changes in maternal and child health indicators, including rates of unintended pregnancy, prenatal care, smoking and drinking during pregnancy, breastfeeding, well-baby checkups, infant illnesses, babies' sleep position, and exposure to secondhand smoke. LAMB complements information from birth certificates for planning state and local maternal, child, and infant health programs. Sampling refinements enable individual and neighborhood effects of socioeconomic factors and stressors on birth outcomes to be evaluated. LAMB has taken MCH population surveillance to a more refined level and provides a rich data set for research.

Before LAMB and LA HOPE, LAC struggled to describe health and demographic indicator trends or correlations pertaining to birth outcomes due to lack of perinatal health data. Since the projects began, findings from LAMB and LA HOPE have helped the LAC public health community to improve birth outcomes by focusing interventions on policy issues identified by the studies; these include preconception health, perinatal mental health, racism, and healthy weight for pregnant women. Ways that MCAH and community stakeholders use these data include:

- High infant mortality rates prompted the AV community to use LAMB data to prioritize activities to improve birth outcomes. The community used data to develop strategies to address infant mortality (see Chapter 33 for details).

- LAMB data identified 38% of women as overweight or obese. Additionally, 47% of African American and 43% of Latino women were overweight or obese before pregnancy. LA HOPE showed that 49.6% who experienced a fetal or infant loss were obese or overweight before pregnancy. These data helped the Healthy Weight for Women of Reproductive Age Action Learning Collaborative promote healthy weight before pregnancy. In 2008, MCAH developed health messages specific to African American and Latino women and developed tools to support worksite wellness programs.
- LAMB data shows that 43% of women took vitamin pills with folic acid or multivitamins before pregnancy and 9% smoked. LA HOPE findings were similar: 38% and 12%, respectively. LAMB and LA HOPE found that 40% of pregnancies were unplanned, highlighting the need to promote healthy lifestyles and access to reproductive health services (see Chapter 32).
- LAMB findings demonstrate that 34% of women report depressed mood during pregnancy and that Latino and African American women in Los Angeles are at increased risk for depression during pregnancy; 41% of LA HOPE respondents also reported depressed mood during pregnancy. Clinical depression during pregnancy increases a woman's risk of giving birth to a preterm or low birth weight infant (9). These critical findings supported formation of the Los Angeles Perinatal Mental Health Task Force (LAC PMHTF), which aims to improve the mental health of perinatal women. LAMB data helped the LAC PMHTF to secure a grant to address perinatal depression.
- LAMB findings show that half of new African American mothers experienced discrimination, more than any other racial or ethnic group. In late 2008, MCAH was selected from among six teams nationwide by three leading maternal-health agencies to form the LAC Partnership to Eliminate Disparities in Infant Mortality Action Learning Collaborative; its purpose is to address racial disparities in infant mortality.
- The high LA HOPE response rate and requests for bereavement support prompted MCAH to establish a peer parent grief support group, led by a public health nurse.
- LA HOPE also has changed the way in which MCAH Programs collect FIMR data. CDPH approved this and sees the new approach as providing more comprehensive information, suitable for large metropolitan areas, than traditional reviews of a few cases. San Diego and Sonoma counties are adopting LA HOPE methods for their FIMR programs.

CONCLUSION

The LAMB and LA HOPE projects allow MCAH to collect and disseminate more comprehensive risk factor data on fetal and infant deaths, low birth weight and preterm births, and resiliency factors that improve birth outcomes. Findings enable community stakeholders to identify effective intervention strategies to decrease fetal and infant morbidity and mortality in LAC's varied demographic and geographic groups. We have found that:

- Adverse birth outcomes are a major public health concern affecting LAC women and infants.

- LAMB and LA HOPE play significant roles in public health surveillance by monitoring and disseminateing information on maternal behavioral risk factors before and during pregnancy, as well as after delivery.
- LAMB and LA HOPE provide reliable maternal and infant health data for health professionals to use to evaluate and plan perinatal health programs and for policy decisions affecting the health of mothers and babies.
- LAMB and LA HOPE data both raise questions and suggest hypotheses about the associations between maternal behaviors and poor birth outcomes.
- Monitoring of adverse birth outcomes enables public health practitioners, community stakeholders, and researchers to learn more about the women who are at risk and to evaluate intervention and prevention efforts.
- Following established scientific methods can strengthen public health surveillance.
- The success of a surveillance system based on voluntary participation benefits from active community engagement and demonstration of the benefits to them.
- Availability of data from LAMB and LA HOPE has been essential to acquiring funding for programs and initiatives to improve birth outcomes in LAC.

REFERENCES

1. Los Angeles County Department of Public Health, Office of Health Assessment and Epidemiology. *Key Indicators of Health by Service Planning Area; June 2009*. Available from: http://publichealth.lacounty.gov/ha/docs/2007%20LACHS/Key_Indicator_2007/KIR_2009_FINALr1.pdf. (accessed June 15, 2012).
2. California Department of Public Health, Center for Health Statistics. OHIR vital statistics section, 1990–2007.
3. Pies C, Parthasarathy P, Kotelchuck M, Lu M. Making a paradigm shift in maternal and child health: A report on the national life course meeting. June 9–10, 2008. Available from: http://www.cchealth.org/groups/lifecourse/pdf/2009_10_meeting_report_final.pdf (accessed June 15, 2012).
4. Maternal and Infant Health Assessment (MIHA) Survey. Available from: http://www.cdph.ca.gov/data/surveys/Pages/MaternalandInfantHealthAssessment(MIHA)survey.aspx (accessed June 15, 2012).
5. Pregnancy Risk Assessment Monitoring System. U.S. Department of Health and Human Services, Centers for Disease Control and Prevention, National Center for Chronic Disease Prevention and Health Promotion, Division of Reproductive Health. *2002 PRAMS Surveillance Report: Appendix A. Detailed Methodology*. Available from: http://www.cdc.gov/prams/Methodology.htm (accessed June 20, 2012).
6. Department of Health Services, County of Los Angeles. *Cultural and Linguistic Competency Standards*. 2003. Available from: http://www.ladhs.org/wps/PA_1_QDN2DSD3005DD02DJ6VQC830C4/DhsSite/DiversityPrograms/pdf/dhsculturalstds.pdf (accessed June 15, 2012).
7. Los Angeles Unified School District, Office of Data and Accountability, School Information Branch. *R30 Language Census Report, Spring 2010*. Available from: http://www.lausd.k12.ca.us/lausd/offices/bulletins/r30r2009.pdf (accessed June 20, 2012).
8. McDowell MA, Wang C-Y, Kennedy-Stephenson J. *Breastfeeding in the United States: findings from the National Health and Nutrition Examination Surveys 1999–2006*. NCHS data briefs, no. 5, Hyattsville, MD: National Center for Health Statistics; 2008.
9. Grote NK, Bridge JA, Gavin AR, Melville JL, Iyengar S, Katon WJ. A meta-analysis of depression during pregnancy and the risk of preterm birth, low birth weight, and intrauterine growth restriction. *Arch Gen Psychiat*. 2010;67(10):1012–24.

■ PART TWO

Health Promotion

10 Underlying Determinants of Health

Putting Local Data to Work

MARGARET SHIH

THE NATURE OF THE PROBLEM

Los Angeles is characterized by tremendous racial and ethnic diversity, coupled with large, persistent health and socioeconomic disparities (see Chapter 1). To reduce disparities and improve Los Angeles County (LAC) residents' health and quality of life, the Department of Public Health (DPH) recognized the need for renewed emphasis on addressing underlying social and physical environmental determinants of health.

The department historically had done relatively little to engage the 88 cities within its boundaries on these issues. The DPH Director wanted to use the existing local government infrastructure to increase engagement and to mobilize efforts with cities, communities, and community groups, The county's cities and unincorporated communities were viewed as important partners in addressing health disparities and underlying determinants. Examining indicators at that level was viewed as an important first step in identifying and prioritizing issues, and attracting the attention of stakeholders to encourage active partnerships to address underlying health determinants.

CONTEXT

Over the past century, public health actions have dramatically reduced deaths from infectious diseases, injuries, and some chronic diseases, resulting in a 30-year increase in life expectancy. Much of this increase has resulted from improvements in sanitation, water treatment, and housing, as well as community education, along with improvements in clinical care. With the aging of the population and a related shift in disease burden to chronic diseases, there has been renewed interest in examining upstream health determinants and impacts across the life course. Today, there is increased emphasis not only on preventing mortality, but also on preventing disability and improving quality of life through policy and environmental change.

Creating healthy communities where residents live, work, learn, and play is a primary DPH objective. Community environments critically impact a person's health potential, longevity, and quality of life; the important effects of both physical and social environments on health across a person's lifespan are well recognized (1–3). Thus, communities are important partners for implementing interventions to maximize health and reduce disparities (see Figure 10–1).

Health determinants in the social environment include education, economic policy, employment, neighborhood safety, and social cohesion (4). These social and economic factors form the base of the Health Impact Pyramid, having the greatest

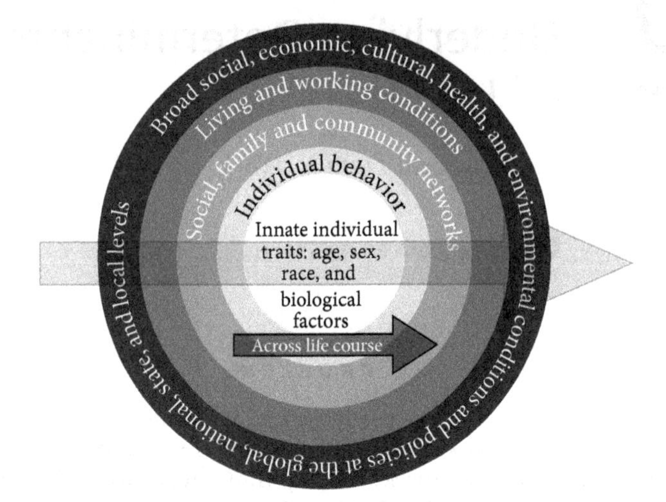

Figure 10–1 Ecologic Model of Health (Adapted from Healthy People 2020).

potential to improve population health (5, 6). However, changes in this realm have been difficult to effect because they require fundamental societal changes to sociocultural norms, and what some consider to be actions outside traditional public health roles, often in areas with little political consensus.

The physical environment includes the design of our cities and transportation systems, as well as exposures to environmental toxins and pollutants. Common land use and zoning decisions can either make it easier or more difficult for residents to be physically active and to eat nutritious foods, for example, by influencing whether residents have convenient access to affordable fresh fruits and vegetables, walking paths, or outdoor recreational areas.

These environmental factors interact to create communities that are either health promoting or health limiting. Demonstrating their health impacts by providing data at the local level is necessary to promote a common understanding of how the community-level physical and socioeconomic conditions influence health. Relevant data also help to engage cities, communities, and community-based private and not-for-profit organizations in policy-oriented prevention efforts.

■ APPROACH TO THE PROBLEM

Department leaders considered how policies in different sectors could impact the health of local populations and how best to use local data to engage community leaders, business leaders, city officials, city planners, and schools in discussions about environmental determinants of health. They decided to begin with a city/community-level health indicator report, possibly the first in a series, whose purpose would be to increase dialogue with local leaders and promote a common understanding of how the physical and social environments influence health. The idea was to help local leaders take action to improve the health of their communities.

The department formed a small team to conceptualize, design, and produce the report. The DPH did not have previous experience reporting data for small areas, so the initial step involved reviewing a range of local indicators and published data. An extensive discussion ensued regarding which health indicators and outcomes to include. The team considered the largest health problems facing LAC, the policy areas and sectors where the DPH was already engaged, the availability of local data, and what data city officials would find most useful. Potential population-level indicators and outcomes included leading causes of mortality, premature mortality, disease burden, general health status, and life expectancy. The consensus was to begin with mortality data, which were readily available, already geographically referenced, and easy to aggregate across multiple years if needed. Cardiovascular disease was chosen as the inaugural topic, since heart disease and stroke together accounted for 40% of all deaths in LAC. Since cardiovascular risk behaviors, including physical inactivity, poor diet, and smoking, can be influenced significantly via local land use and urban planning decisions, as well as local policies such as public smoking bans and food policies, this focus succeeded in engaging city leaders and planners in discussions of environment and health.

Finally, the geographic boundaries had to be defined for unincorporated communities within LAC. This was problematic since there were no standardized boundaries for such communities, which comprise about 10% of LAC's population. U.S. Census 2000 Incorporated Places and Census Designated Places were chosen to define boundaries for cities and communities, respectively; the City of Los Angeles was further broken down into its 15 city council districts due to its large size.

The California Endowment generously assisted with funding of the report design, production, and dissemination.

■ IMPLEMENTATION OF SOLUTIONS

The initial report was organized into several sections: a message from the DPH Director introduced and provided background on the health issue at hand; a brief description of the methods followed, along with a comprehensive table of results for each city and community; maps were used to show geographic patterns and disparities; and, finally, a menu of potential strategies that cities and communities could implement was outlined.

A key goal was to present useful and easily understandable information for a wide audience. The development team decided to present premature deaths (defined as any death before the age of 75 years) in the form of years of potential life lost due to heart disease and stroke. In order to produce reliable results for smaller communities, three years of mortality data were combined. Even using combined years, several communities had to be excluded because they reported fewer than 20 cardiovascular disease deaths during this period.

The development team also felt strongly that the report needed an overall socioeconomic indicator that could be compared across communities, since social determinants have the greatest impact on health. Possible measures included poverty, income, unemployment, high school completion rate, incarceration rates, housing, social cohesion, social capital, and the Townsend Index of deprivation. After reviewing these and others, the Intercity Economic Hardship measure developed by the Nelson A. Rockefeller Institute of Government (7–9) was chosen as the most robust single measure. The Hardship measure is a composite index of 6 indicators (crowded housing, poverty, unemployment, education, dependency, and income) that can be used to compare social and economic conditions among cities and communities. It has the advantage of being composed of data available from the U.S. Census at the census block level. While the Hardship measure is not as simple to describe as an individual measure might be and had not been previously applied specifically in relation to health, it includes important social determinants and provides a more complete picture of neighborhood socioeconomic conditions. It also facilitated easy-to-understand presentations of tables and maps analogous to the use of other well-known measures such as the gross national product or the consumer price index. People can easily grasp such measures conceptually without knowing the full details of how the measures are calculated (see Figures 10–2a and 10–2b).

An important consideration was whether to present the information as scores, grades, or rankings. While grades or rankings might garner more attention, local governments and/or the LAC Board of Supervisors, which provides oversight over LAC's large unincorporated areas, might object to an indicator report that directly compared very disparate communities. In addition, the small numbers for some communities lead to high variability in year-to-year estimates, resulting in large yearly shifts in community rankings. As a compromise, broader quartile groupings were included along with rankings to reduce the emphasis on numerical rankings (see Table 10–1).

As the report began to take shape, the development team solicited input on the report's comprehensibility and usefulness for engaging local stakeholders. Its format was widely vetted with stakeholders inside and outside the department. This lengthened the development process, but provided valuable feedback that shaped the report content, appearance, and overall utility. External input was particularly helpful for

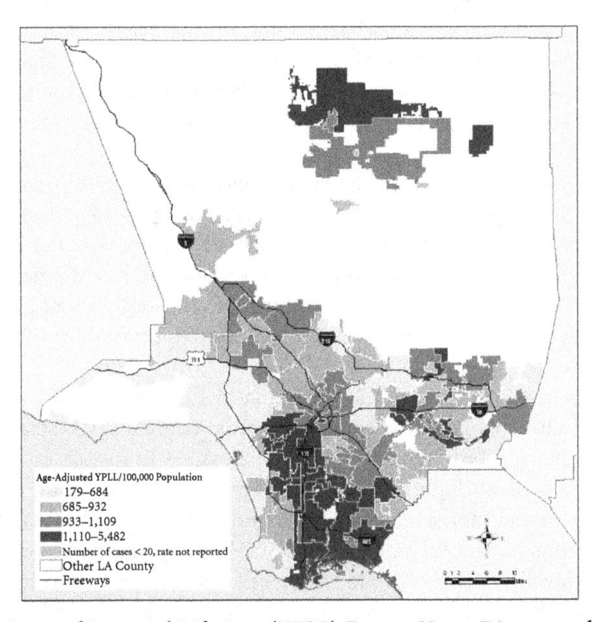

Figure 10–2a Years of Potential Life Lost (YPLL) Due to Heart Disease and Stroke, Los Angeles County, 2000–2002.

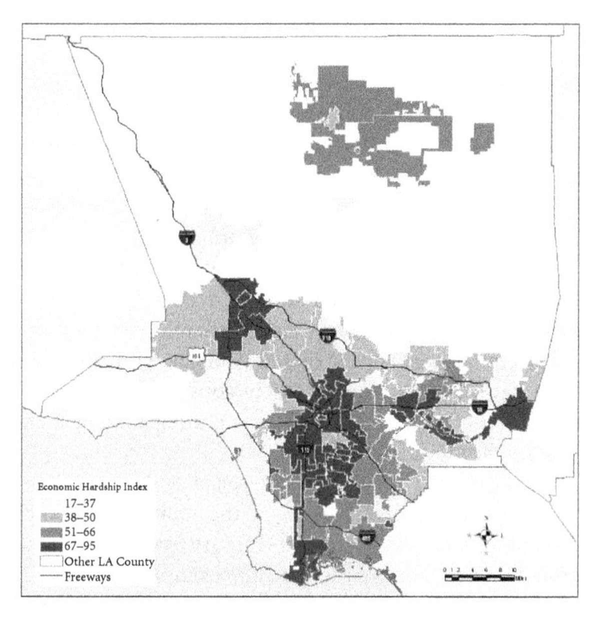

Figure 10-2b Economic Hardship in Cities and Communities, Los Angeles County, 2000 (10).

TABLE 10-1 *Example of Report Table (10)*

Premature Mortality from Heart Disease and Stroke, and
Economic Hardship by City and Community, Los Angeles County

City or Community	Heart Disease & Stroke (2000–2002)		Economic Hardship (2000)	
	Years of potential life lost per 100,000 population per year	Rank 1 = lowest loss 133 = highest loss	Index (1–100)	Rank 1 = least burden 133 = most burden
Los Angeles County, Overall	1,183	NA	NA	NA
◆ Agoura Hills	664	20	28.6	11
◆ Alhambra	736	22	50.9	67
Alondra Park	1,151	66	57.0	82
Altadena	1,241	84	41.0	41
◆ Arcadia	638	18	37.8	35
◆ Artesia	1,322	93	53.4	74
◆ Avalon	1,799	118	45.5	58
Avocado Heights	1,400	104	59.0	86
◆ Azusa	1,082	58	61.0	90
◆ Baldwin Park	1,278	88	71.3	108
◆ Bell	1,158	70	80.1	120
◆ Bellflower	1,764	115	56.0	81
◆ Bell Gardens	1,219	80	87.9	130
◆ Beverly Hills	406	7	31.3	20
◆ Burbank	894	41	41.5	47

= 1st quartile (rank 1–33) = 2nd quartile (rank 34–66) = 3rd quartile (rank 67–100) = 4th quartile (rank 101–133)

refining the section on strategies that cities could use to reduce the burden of heart disease and stroke. Cities provided useful feedback on what recommendations would or would not be feasible to implement, and programs helped align the recommendations with programmatic activities and goals.

The final published report was disseminated to city officials, city planners, community leaders, and public health leaders both electronically and in print (10). Shortly after its release, the department held its first Built Environment Workshop, convening nearly 200 city officials, planners, transportation engineers, public health staff, and nonprofit organization representatives. This was the first time that public health staff met with local leaders from so many different sectors to discuss common issues. Small group discussions during the workshop facilitated networking among representatives from different sectors and furthered dialogue with city planners and local leaders. The report became a key tool in discussions of how the built environment influences health and also what concrete actions participating agencies could begin to take to improve the health of communities.

A series of reports ensued on a range of social and physical determinants of health. With release of the second report, on the topic of childhood obesity, the department's Division of Chronic Disease and Injury Prevention's newly established Policies for Livable, Active Communities and Environments (PLACE) program (see Chapter 12) and a cadre of PH liaisons from the Community Health Services division used its findings in face-to-face meetings with city planners and city officials, particularly with the City of Los Angeles. Due to the high level of community interest in the problem of childhood obesity, DPH staff members were invited to attend city council meetings and to meet with city officials and community groups wanting to learn more about it and related health issues facing their communities. We also noted increasing recognition that the DPH could offer valuable information regarding land use, transportation planning, and the built environment. The report was also widely used to emphasize the relationship between health and neighborhood socioeconomic conditions by demonstrating the strong correlation between childhood obesity and economic hardship (see Table 11–1 in Chapter 11).

The PLACE program proactively contacted city planners, mayors, and city staff, to engage them in dialogue regarding built environment issues, emphasizing the need for implementing policy and environmental changes in their cities to promote active living and healthy eating. This directly translated into the creation of policies to promote active transportation (e.g., through creating city bike plans and transit-oriented districts), the incorporation of health elements into city and county general plans, community mobilization to create or improve parks and green spaces, and the broader incorporation of health considerations into other local planning decisions. This strengthened LAC ties with city planning agencies, and DPH input was increasingly sought regarding community development plans, city general plans, and other land use or transportation-related projects. Incorporating health elements into general plans was viewed as an important goal, since these are policies used to guide the current and long-term growth and land development of communities.

Subsequent reports have built on these relationships, helping establish the DPH as an important partner in many non-health sectors. In addition to economic hardship, other environmental determinants have been assessed, including park area in relation to childhood obesity, and motor vehicle crashes and violent crimes in relation to alcohol outlet density. Report topics have been chosen based on the availability of data for small areas, county disease burden, preventable burden, relevance to strategic departmental priorities, and the potential for partnering with cities and communities to effect changes at the community level. Over time, the focus of the reports has been shifting from determinants of health in the built environment to social determinants of health.

To date, this report series includes:

- Premature mortality from cardiovascular disease and stroke (10);
- Childhood obesity (11);
- Tobacco cessation (12);
- Life expectancy (13);
- Alcohol outlet density and alcohol-related harms (14).

A new report, currently under development, will be the first to focus on underlying social determinants. A social environment workgroup was formed within the department to increase awareness and engagement of DPH programs and of external partners in social environment work. The workgroup recommended creation of an indicator report to increase awareness of social environment determinants' impacts on health both within the department and with external collaborators. After reviewing a broad range of social indicators, an initial set of indicators from four key domains was selected: poverty, education, housing burden, and economic hardship. Indicators from other key domains such as employment, social cohesion, incarceration, and discrimination are planned for future reports.

By promoting broader awareness of underlying environmental determinants of health, by increasing dialogue and engagement between the DPH and different sectors, and by establishing and strengthening relationships, these reports have helped lay groundwork for a health-in-all-policies approach (15).

■ EVALUATION STRATEGY

Media coverage through print, internet, radio, and television was monitored to track the report's dissemination, use, and impact. As the department's first report in the series, the cardiovascular disease report received significant local media coverage, while the childhood obesity and life expectancy reports received even broader coverage in local, national, and international media. Although media coverage for the tobacco report was more limited, it generated intense local interest in several communities, and contributed to policy changes due to more strategic dissemination not only to city and state officials, but also to local community and advocacy groups (see examples below).

The DPH also tracked engagement with civic leaders by monitoring the number of communities initiating direct dialogue with the department. Events included invitations to participate in city council meetings, meetings to provide input on community development plans, meetings with city planners, and other meetings with representatives from non-traditional health sectors. Engagement has increased steadily, yielding frequent requests for additional data at the local level, but this has been difficult to quantify since so many programs are engaged in this work. The initial report was successful in opening communication channels; subsequent reports built on this by increasing engagement, such that public health is now viewed as an important partner in discussions of land use planning. For example, the tobacco cessation report has been widely used to provide information to cities considering bans on smoking in public areas. The City of West Hollywood, which has one of the highest smoking rates in the county, disseminated the report to staff having ongoing discussions about an outdoor smoking ban. In the City of Los Angeles Council Meeting, the report was frequently cited in support of a citywide comprehensive smoke-free ordinance. The report on life expectancy increased awareness among cities of the connection between social issues and health, and has been used in a proposal to incorporate health issues into the General Plan for the City of Los Angeles. Similarly, the childhood obesity report forced some city leaders to acknowledge childhood obesity as a previously unrecognized health issue for their communities. It has prompted cities to consider how land use decisions affect health and has encouraged policies to promote active transportation. One city was skeptical that the prevalence of childhood obesity in their city was higher than the county average. After investigating contributory factors, the city acknowledged that something about their environment was different from that of a neighboring city with a drastically lower prevalence. Another city already knew that childhood obesity was an important local issue and had been working on programs to address it, but when they saw the actual number printed in the report, they resolved to initiate a policy to promote their own active transportation opportunities. Another city mayor was keenly interested in comparing his city's profile with that of others; while he was not surprised by his city's relatively low life expectancy ranking, which he saw as related to the high crime rate, he was surprised by the high prevalence of childhood obesity in his as compared to other cities. These results provided motivation to work on a master bicycle plan.

■ IMPACT

This series of reports yielded several impacts. First, it facilitated increased engagement with local governments, planners, and other sectors such as schools, transportation, and the business community. Second, specific data and recommendations focused discussions, facilitated new partnerships, and increased recognition of the importance of the physical and social environments. Third, the reports raised awareness of the importance of a Health-in-All-Policies approach, and they changed traditional views of public health's role internally and externally. This resulted in increased awareness of the Public Health Department, and increased community engagement and mobilization (see Chapter 5). Fourth, rankings and comparisons among communities appeal to the general public. The reports received broad media coverage in local newspapers, radio stations, and local news channels. These raised public awareness about how underlying determinants affect a person's health. Finally, the reports helped the DPH to secure grant funds for other projects to implement recommendations for the prevention of childhood obesity and for smoking cessation.

Initial responses to these reports were not uniform among jurisdictions. Already engaged communities, which tend to be more affluent, were more likely to use the information. However, once specific policies or approaches were applied in one community, the examples encouraged others to implement them as well, creating a spillover effect. Then, too, some local leaders still view the scope of public health's purview as very narrow.

Using local data continues to be challenging (see web references in Box 10–1 on methodologic considerations). Small area estimation methods can be applied but are

BOX 10–1 ■ Methodologic Considerations in Analyzing and Presenting Data for Small Areas

1. **Limited availability of local data**. While demand for data at the local level to perform community-level assessments is high, community-level data resources are limited. However, several potential data sources include state and local surveys, birth and death records, hospital discharge data, the U.S. Census, and the American Community Survey. Additionally, data from multiple years can be aggregated in assessing very small jurisdictions.
   Examples of websites with local indicator data:
   U.S. Department of Health and Human Services Community Health Status Indicators website: http://www.communityhealth.hhs.gov.
   Federal government's health data portal: http://www.data.gov/health;
   CDC Chronic Disease Indicators website: http://apps.nccd.cdc.gov/cdi/;
   Website with indicators on the health and well-being of children in communities across California, sponsored by the Lucille Packard Foundation for Children's Health: http://www.kidsdata.org/.
2. **Defining geographic boundaries**. Choosing geographic boundaries can be challenging. Community boundaries are often non-discrete; Census Tracts often do not align with city and community boundaries; communities, community groups, and local agencies may all use different boundaries; and geographic boundaries—for example, zip codes, census tracts, and community definitions—change over time. Check with local city or county governments and/or planning departments for standardized boundary definitions. The U.S. Census has standard boundary definitions for cities and communities, but Census-defined community definitions may differ from local definitions.
3. **Choice of outcome measures**. Here are a few criteria for deciding which outcome measures to examine—importance to local leaders and community groups, overall and preventable burden, whether the outcome can be influenced through policy and environmental changes, and potential synergy with other efforts.
4. **Small area estimation methods**. Small area estimation approaches have become increasingly popular. Obtaining direct survey estimates for small areas is often cost prohibitive. Several small area estimation approaches include spatial smoothing techniques, creation of synthetic estimates, and regression-based estimates (16). While model-based approaches are becoming common, they typically require drawing on multiple data sources, assumptions, and time-intensive model building, which is difficult to systematize.

labor intensive, since the modeling process cannot be automated. Additionally, the year-to-year variability in some indicators can be quite high for communities due to small numbers of cases. Using quantiles can reduce the emphasis on numerical rankings.

CONCLUSIONS

Among the important lessons learned are that:

- Local elected officials and other leaders want data on their communities.
- The ability to compare results from one community to those from neighboring communities is highly motivational.

- Actively taking the data on social and physical determinants of health to policy makers can influence decisions in non-health sectors and can be a catalyst for policy changes.
- Data alone is usually insufficient to "sell" a case, but coupled with recommendations and expert consultation, can add value to efforts to change policy for improved health.
- Cities and communities vary in their levels of readiness to address different issues. It is usually easier to engage communities on an issue on which they are already active.
- One success story of healthy policy change can motivate other communities to take action.
- This approach involving targeted reports on key social and physical determinants of health in small areas can be replicated for broader use.
- While the content of these reports differs from that of disease- or risk factor-based reports typically published by public health departments, it has been effective. We have increased LAC DPH engagement with cities and other non-health partners; increased awareness of the societal determinants of health and reframed discussions around these determinants; provided motivation for cities and communities to act; and raised the profile of public health input as valuable in policy making for non-health sectors.

REFERENCES

1. Marmot M, Friel S, Bell R, et al. Closing the gap in a generation: health equity through action on the social determinants of health. *Lancet.* 2008;372:1661–9.
2. Fielding JE, Teutsch S, Breslow L. A framework for public health in the United States. *Public Health Rev.* 2011;32:174–189.
3. Barker DJP. Commentary: birthweight and coronary heart disease in a historical cohort. *Int J Epidemiol.* 2006;35:886–887.
4. Commission on Social Determinants of Health. *Closing the Gap in a Generation: Health Equity Through Action on the Social Determinants of Health.* Final Report of the Commission on Social Determinants of Health. Geneva, Switzerland: World Health Organization; 2008.
5. Frieden T. A framework for public health action: the health impact pyramid. *Am J Public Health.* 2010;100:590–595.
6. Galea S, Tracy M, Hoggett JK, et al. Estimated deaths attributable to social factors in the United States. *Am J Public Health.* 2011;101(8):1456–65.
7. Nathan RP, Adams CF Jr. Understanding central city hardship. *Polit Sci Quart.* 1976;91:47–62.
8. Nathan RP, Adams CF Jr. Four perspectives on urban hardship. *Polit Sci Quart.* 1989;104:483–508.
9. Montiel LM, Nathan RP, Wright DJ. *An Update on Urban Hardship.* Albany, NY: The Nelson A. Rockefeller Institute of Government; August 2004.
10. Los Angeles County Department of Health Services, Public Health. *Premature Death from Heart Disease and Stroke in Los Angeles County: A Cities and Communities Health Report.* January 2006. Available from: http://lapublichealth.org/epi/docs/CHR_CVH.pdf. (accessed June 15, 2012).
11. Los Angeles County Department of Public Health, Office of Health Assessment and Epidemiology. *Preventing Childhood Obesity: The Need to Create Healthy Places.*

A Cities and Communities Health Report. October 2007. Available from: http://lapublichealth.org/wwwfiles/ph/hae/epi/chr2-childhood_obesity.pdf (accessed June 15, 2012).

12. Los Angeles County Department of Public Health, Office of Health Assessment and Epidemiology. *Cigarette smoking in Los Angeles County: Local Data to Inform Tobacco Policy. A Cities and Communities Health Report.* June 2010. Available from: http://www.lapublichealth.org/ha/reports/habriefs/2007/Cigarette_Smoking_Cities_finalS.pdf (accessed June 15, 2012).
13. Los Angeles County Department of Public Health, Office of Health Assessment and Epidemiology. *Life Expectancy in Los Angeles County: How Long Do We Live and Why? A Cities and Communities Health Report.* July 2010. Available from: http://www.lapublichealth.org/epi/docs/Life%20Expectancy%20Final_web.pdf (accessed June 15, 2012).
14. Los Angeles County Department of Public Health, Office of Health Assessment and Epidemiology. *Reducing Alcohol-Related Harms in Los Angeles County: A Cities and Communities Report.* December 2011. Available from: http://www.lapublichealth.org/epi/docs/AOD%20final%20revised%20web%20ed.pdf (accessed June 15, 2012).
15. Sihto M, Ollila E, Koivusalo M. Principles and challenges of health in all policies. In: Ståhl T, Wismar M, Ollila E, et al., editors. *Health in All Policies: Prospects and Potentials.* Helsinki: Ministry of Social Affairs and Health; 2006, p. 3–20.
16. Rao JNK. Some recent advances in model-based small area estimation. *Survey Methodology.* 1999;25:175–86.

11 Tackling Toxic Food Environments

A Response to the Obesity Epidemic

PAUL SIMON AND SUZANNE BOGERT

THE PROBLEM

Poor nutrition contributes to a host of chronic diseases. It is a major cause of preventable mortality in the United States (1). Excess caloric intake as well as physical inactivity has fueled an epidemic of obesity among children and adults. In Los Angeles County (LAC), the prevalence of obesity (BMI > 30) among adults (18 years and older) increased from 14.3% in 1997 to 22.0% in 2007, a collective weight gain of 51 million pounds across the adult population in an 11-year period (2). Among the county's 5th, 7th, and 9th grade public school students, obesity prevalence increased from 18.9% in 1999 to 23.0% in 2008 (3). Among three- and four-year-olds receiving services in the Women, Infants, and Children (WIC) Program, a health and nutrition program serving more than half of the county's families with children under five years of age, obesity prevalence increased from16.8% in 2003 to 21.8% in 2009 (4).

The data also highlight marked disparities in the obesity epidemic among various populations and communities in LAC. Among 5th, 7th, and 9th graders, the obesity prevalence in 2008 was considerably higher among Latinos (27.5%) and African Americans (21.8%) than among whites (13.0%) and Asians (11.8%) (3). A geographic analysis of some 130 LAC cities and communities revealed even more striking disparities: here the obesity prevalence ranged from a low of 3.4% in the affluent coastal city of Manhattan Beach to a high of 38.7% in Walnut Park, a predominantly low-income community in south Los Angeles, less than 15 miles away. The factor most strongly correlated with a high rate of childhood obesity is neighborhood economic hardship, a composite measure that includes median household income (see Table 11–1), crowded housing, unemployment, lack of education, and dependency (percentage of the population under 18 or over 64 years of age) (see also Chapter 10 on social determinants).

These disparities and the link with economic hardship are consistent with studies documenting the important influence of physical and social environments on dietary practices and obesity risk (5). Low-income communities, in particular, are frequently characterized by "toxic" food environments with heavy concentrations of fast food restaurants and convenience stores offering super-sized portions of calorie-dense and nutrient-poor foods at low prices. These communities often offer limited access to supermarkets and grocery stores with fresh produce and other healthy options. Where produce is available, it is generally much more expensive than the less healthy packaged products, and is sometimes of inferior quality relative to produce sold in more affluent communities (6).

TABLE 11-1 *Cities/Communities with Lowest and Highest Childhood Obesity Prevalence and Associated Rank for Economic Hardship, Los Angeles County, 2008*

Top 10*		
City/Community Name	Obesity Prevalence (%)	Rank of Economic Hardship (1–128)
Manhattan Beach	3.4	2
Calabasas	5.0	8
Hermosa Beach	5.1	1
Agoura Hills	5.3	10
Beverly Hills	5.4	19
Malibu	5.9	4
Palos Verdes Estates	7.3	5
San Marino	7.8	15
Rolling Hills Estate	8.4	9
La Canada Flintridge	8.5	18
Average 10 lowest	6.2%	
Ave Median Household Income		$99,555
Bottom 10*		
City/Community Name	Obesity Prevalence (%)	Rank of Economic Hardship (1–128)
West Athens	30.6	94
South Gate	30.7	110
Florence-Graham	31.0	128
West Whittier-Los Nietos	31.1	81
West Carson	31.4	56
Vincent	32.2	69
East Los Angeles	32.9	117
Hawaiian Gardens	33.4	107
South El Monte	34.5	111
Walnut Park	38.7	113
Average 10 highest	32.7%	
Ave Median Household Income		$37,747

* Table excludes cities/communities where number of students with BMI data < 500.
Source: California Physical Fitness Testing Program, California Department of Education. Includes 5th, 7th, and 9th graders enrolled in LA County public schools; 2000 Census.

CONTEXT

Over the past decade, widespread media coverage of the national obesity epidemic raised public awareness of the problem and need for intervention (7). A recent survey in California found broad public support for government action to address the epidemic. This includes support for nutrition education and efforts to increase access to healthy food and beverage options, and reduce access to unhealthy options, particularly in school settings (8). Another California survey of local, state, and federal elected officials also found support for government action, though with less support for restrictive policies, such as placing limits on the density of fast food restaurants or restricting junk food advertising (8).

In LAC great community and political concern is voiced about obesity, particularly its impact on children. In 2002, the Los Angeles Unified School District (LAUSD), the second-largest district in the nation, became one of the first to remove soda from all K-12 school campuses, despite concern that the revenue loss from soft drink sales and donations from the beverage industry would adversely influence the cash-strapped district. But fears were overcome by a single Board member who championed the cause, using compelling data from the Department of Public Health (DPH) about the problem's severity. District action led to a progression of state legislation that strengthened and expanded school food and beverage nutrition standards.

In 2002, the County Board of Supervisors established a Task Force on Children and Youth Physical Fitness and charged it with preparing recommendations to address this epidemic. Its report included policy and program recommendations plus a public awareness campaign to promote healthy eating and physical activity (9). Not all recommendations are yet implemented, but the report has marshaled increased resources and has led to more organized efforts to address childhood obesity. These efforts were further advanced by the leadership and support of one county supervisor who publicly disclosed his own diagnosis of type 2 diabetes and has since championed the cause.

APPROACH TO THE PROBLEM

Public health efforts to promote nutrition and prevent obesity historically focus on educating the public at both individual and community levels. Since 1998, the DPH's nutrition promotion work has been funded by the U.S. Department of Agriculture's (USDA) Supplemental Nutrition Assistance Program Education Program (SNAP-ED). The USDA requires that the funding be used solely for education and promotion to increase fruit and vegetable consumption, physical activity, and enrollment of food stamp–eligible individuals and families into the program. Activities must be focused on low-income populations eligible for food stamps and not for policy or environmental change to improve food environments.

The importance of the food environment as a target of intervention is reflected in recent guidance from both the Centers for Disease Control and Prevention (CDC) and an Institute of Medicine report on community strategies that address the childhood obesity epidemic (10, 11). Many of these strategies focus on policy interventions to improve local food environments (e.g., policies that require or create incentives for healthy food retail sales, promote healthy food procurement, and establish nutrition standards for meals served in schools and institutional settings). The federal government and other funding sources embrace these environmental strategies in their recent calls for projects (12, 13), reflecting a growing awareness of the need to apply an ecologic framework in addressing the multiple influences on people's dietary habits (see Figure 11–1) (5).

However, the potential role of local public health departments in this enterprise is not clear. Unlike other areas of public health practice (e.g., communicable disease control and prevention) where the public health department is the lead authority

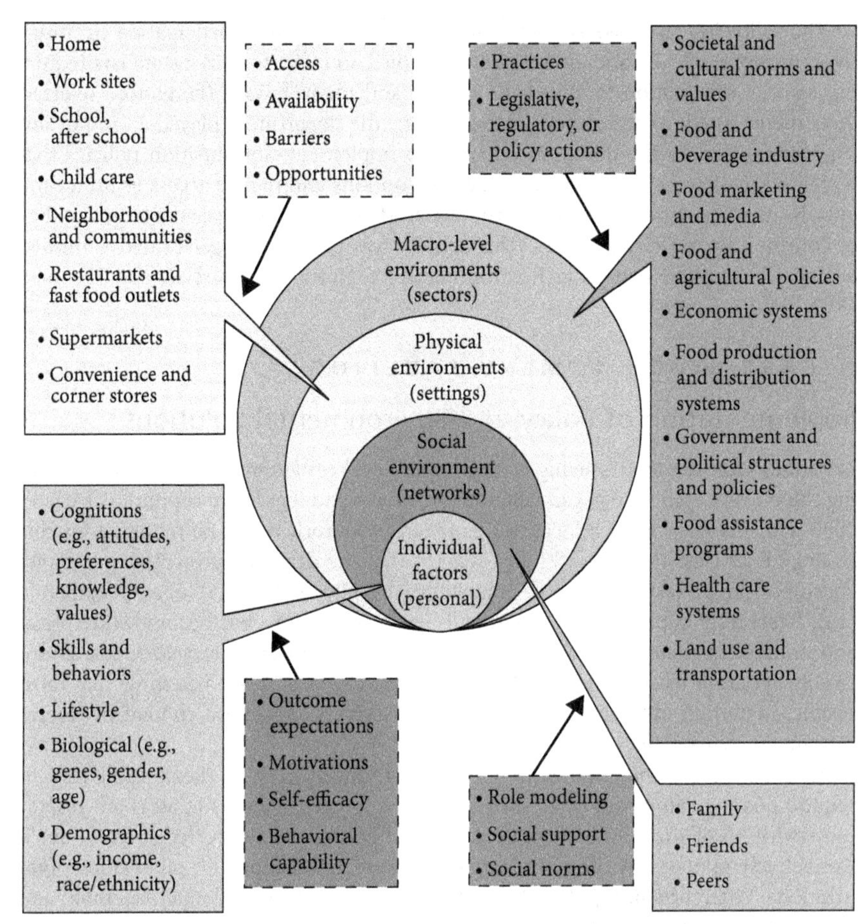

Figure 11–1 An Ecological Framework Depicting the Multiple Influences on What People Eat.
Source: Story M, et al., Creating healthy food and eating environments: policy and environmental approaches. Annu Rev Publ Health. 2008;29:253–272. Reproduced with permission of ANNUAL REVIEWS, INC. in the format Other book via Copyright Clearance Center.

and has regulatory oversight, obesity prevention and other areas of chronic disease prevention involve many stakeholders, some outside local government. Two of the county's major funders of community-based obesity prevention efforts are a nonprofit foundation (The California Endowment) and a large health care provider (Kaiser Permanente). Both have invested heavily in place-based strategies (i.e., interventions that address the broad determinants of health in a defined geographic area), including focus on the increased availability of healthy foods and community-based organizational leadership. The DPH provides information on evidence-based strategies; local health data for advocacy, planning, and evaluation; assistance in engaging community constituencies; and assistance in making the case to policy makers of the critical need for policies and practices that improve local food environments.

The following two case studies describe the department's participation in initiatives to improve LAC food environments. In one, an effort to pass a state law requiring calorie information to appear on menus and menu boards (heretofore referred to as menu labeling) at large chain restaurants, the department played an important supporting role. In the other, an initiative to implement city nutrition policies that increase access to healthy food and beverage options and reduce access to unhealthy options, the department was one of the two lead entities and engaged a large number of community and city partners. This activity was part of a larger initiative funded by the CDC called Renewing Environments for Nutrition, Exercise, and Wellness (RENEW LA County).

■ CASE STUDY 1: MENU LABELING

Implementation of Policy and Environmental Solutions

Laws that require menu labeling at large chain food restaurants as a means of reducing the obesity epidemic began generating interest and legislative support as early as 2006 with the passage of a local ordinance in New York City. The rationale for this strategy is at least threefold. Studies suggest that the dramatic growth in per capita consumption of restaurant food contributes heavily to the U.S. obesity epidemic (14). Restaurant super-sizing of food and beverage portions has become widespread and, unlike mandated calorie and nutrition information on packaged foods, is not readily apparent to customers at the point of purchase. And studies show that most people, including nutritionists, greatly underestimate the caloric content of restaurant menu items (15).

In California, a menu labeling bill was introduced in 2007 (Senate Bill 120) to require posting calorie information on menus and menu boards at all chain restaurants with 15 or more in-state outlets. The public broadly supported the bill, but it was actively opposed by the California Restaurant Association and other trade organizations. After bruising political debate, it was passed by the State Assembly and Senate but vetoed by the governor.

A similar bill (Senate Bill 1420) was introduced in 2008 but was limited to chain restaurants with 20 or more in-state venues. To inform the decision-making process on the bill, LAC DPH staff reviewed related research literature to assess the strategy's potential impact on obesity. Finding very limited direct information, the department initiated a health impact assessment (HIA) using small studies and assumptions to project the likely impact of a menu labeling law on obesity in LAC. It assumed that in response to calorie postings, 10% of restaurant patrons ordered reduced-calorie meals, resulting in an average reduction of 100 calories per meal. The analysis found that menu labeling would avert 40.6% of the 6.75 million pound average annual weight gain in the LAC population aged five years and older (16). A sensitivity analysis suggested that substantially larger impacts could be realized if more patrons ordered reduced-calorie meals, or if average per-meal calorie reductions increased.

The May 2008 report of the study came at the height of the public debate on the menu labeling bill, and garnered much media coverage. Several DPH staff testified before state legislative committees on the HIA findings and on the toll of the obesity epidemic. One sponsor of the bill reported that the HIA was instrumental in negotiations with legislators and the governor. In response to the report, the County Board of Supervisors voted to implement a county menu labeling ordinance if the state bill was not enacted. In response, the California Restaurant Association lowered its opposition, recognizing the advantages of a uniform statewide measure compared to this threat and similar action in other counties, enacting a patchwork of varying county ordinances. The bill was passed and signed into law by the governor. Two years later, a similar measure was approved at the national level as part of federal health care reform, preempting the California law.

Evaluation Strategy

Once the federal menu labeling law is implemented, the department's Environmental Health Division staff will assess compliance with posted calorie counts on menus at large chain restaurants as part of their routine restaurant inspections. If funding allows, Environmental Health staff also will collect food specimens from randomly sampled chain restaurants to check the accuracy of posted calorie information. Grants also will be sought to conduct pre- and post-implementation surveys of customers at chain restaurants to assess the law's impact on menu selections and calories consumed. The calorie content of restaurant offerings will be monitored before and after implementation of the law to determine if restaurant operators have modified recipes to reduce calorie content of menu items. Finally, the department will track the trajectory of the obesity epidemic, though the independent effect of the menu labeling law may be difficult to ascertain in the context of many complementary obesity prevention efforts.

Impact

Studies of the impact of menu labeling in New York City and Seattle have produced mixed results, some showing modest reductions in the caloric content of food purchases, others showing no effect (19–21). However, these short-term studies reflect consumer response relatively soon after menu labeling began, and it will be important to replicate them to see whether the impacts grow or diminish as customers become more familiar with the calorie information. Results may depend on the degree to which the intervention is accompanied by community education that promotes the use and interpretation of the calorie information.

Perhaps the most interesting early impact of menu labeling is the restaurant industry's response. Newspaper articles and industry trade publications and websites report that many chains are reformulating their menus, reducing the caloric content of standard items, or adding new low-calorie options. We are unaware of any formal assessment or quantification of this phenomenon, but the anecdotal reports suggest that the menu labeling policy may have additional benefits not measured in the department's HIA.

■ CASE STUDY 2: RENEW LA COUNTY, CITY NUTRITION POLICY

Implementation of Policy and Environmental Solutions

In March 2010 the DPH received a two-year CDC grant (part of the national Communities Putting Prevention to Work initiative) to improve nutrition, increase physical activity, and reduce obesity through "policy, systems, and environment change interventions." The initiative included a focus on improving local food environments through policy change at the city and county levels. With over 10 million people and encompassing 88 cities and a large unincorporated area, LAC is considered an ideal laboratory for local policy innovation. Cities and unincorporated communities were prioritized based on population size, need (as determined by child obesity rate, poverty level, and measures of the food environment), and political and community readiness to implement policy change. The policy interventions fell into three strategic areas: 1) food and beverage procurement and distribution (e.g., vending machines, cafeterias, community programs); 2) administrative and financial incentives for healthy food/beverage retail; and 3) regulation (e.g., zoning, taxation).

The department provided funding to the California Center for Public Health Advocacy, a nonpartisan, nonprofit organization that has expertise in nutrition policy, to conduct outreach and education to communities and cities on healthy food and beverage policies. A priority goal was to get cities to adopt policies that reduce access to soda and other sugar-sweetened beverages, given accumulating evidence of their key contribution to the obesity epidemic (17, 18). Department staff assisted in the efforts to inform communities and city officials about policy options. An important aspect of the initiative was its structured process. This included assessments of cities and their communities to determine readiness for policy change, community outreach and engagement to define a policy goal, development of a policy campaign strategy to build broad support for the initiative, implementation of the campaign, drafting of policy language, and securing approval of the policy (e.g., city council votes).

Early results suggest that the food/beverage procurement and distribution policy strategy is the most politically viable and offers solid opportunity to introduce a policy perspective and achieve relatively rapid wins. Within four months, five LAC cities adopted policies mandating healthy foods and beverages in vending machines on city property and in city programs serving youth.

Alternatively, the regulatory approach engendered heated debate on the appropriate role of government in addressing nutrition, including vocal opposition from those who oppose any government action and who believe that dietary choices are matters of personal responsibility best left solely to individuals. But this perspective does not recognize the influence of social, economic, and environmental conditions on food purchasing and consumption patterns. The debate has mobilized communities and has increased public awareness of the importance of the food environment but has made it difficult to achieve significant regulatory policy gains. One city council passed a moratorium on new fast food outlets, generating a flurry of newspaper articles and editorials, but six months later reversed its decision as it faced opposition from the business community and some members of the public.

Using fiscal or administrative incentives for healthy food retail sales has been less politically divisive but has still been challenging because of the cost and the need for changed administrative procedures to implement most incentives. A recent initiative, the California Fresh Works Fund, provides funds for loans and grants to supermarkets and grocery stores willing to locate in underserved communities or, if already present, to increase their refrigeration and shelf space for fresh produce and other healthy products.

Evaluation Strategy

To evaluate the city-level nutrition policy efforts, the RENEW LA County community action plan is tracked. This plan, approved by CDC, includes intermediate milestone activities toward policy adoption. Examples include systemic assessment of cities to identify those targets for outreach and education, preparation of fact sheets and a slide presentation for use in meetings with community and city representatives, establishment of a community coalition, identification of candidate policies to pursue, a strategic policy campaign, a city council vote on the policy, and an implementation plan once the policy is adopted.

The policy impact on dietary practices will be assessed using data from the LAC Health Survey, a biennial random-digit-dialed telephone survey of some 8,000 adults and parents of 6,000 children (see Chapter 2). These data will be supplemented with data from the California Health Interview Survey (CHIS), a survey that includes data on about 10,000 adults and 3,000 children in LAC. Both surveys include self-reported adult heights and weights to permit tracking of adult obesity prevalence. Data from the California Physical Fitness Testing Program includes measured heights and weights on public school 5th, 7th, and 9th graders, and will be used with data from the WIC program to assess impact on obesity trends in children.

Impact

The impact of this policy work remains unclear, given the short time over which it has been conducted. But progress in city policy adoption over the first half of 2011 suggests that it holds great promise. Definitive evidence of its impact on dietary practices and obesity rates among residents of the targeted cities will require data collection and analysis over the next several years.

■ CONCLUSIONS

- The obesity epidemic continues unabated in adults and children in LAC and is characterized by marked disparities among communities and demographic groups.
- In addition to educating the public on nutrition, efforts to address the epidemic must include policy and environmental change interventions to increase access to healthy food and beverage options and to reduce access to unhealthy options (i.e., making healthy choices easy choices).
- Local public health departments can play useful support and leadership roles in promoting policy and environmental change strategies to improve local food environments.
- Health impact assessments can be a vital tool to support policy development but must be carefully timed to maximize usefulness.
- The successful early policy efforts to create healthier food environments in K–12 school settings in LAC are now being replicated in cities.
- Despite this progress, these efforts are likely to face continued strong opposition, especially to policies that restrict or reduce access to unhealthy food and beverage options.
- More effective public messaging strategies can increase public awareness of the importance of environmental influences on dietary choices. They also can

counter the common belief that such choices are solely under an individual's control.

REFERENCES

1. Mokdad AH, Marks JS, Stroup DF, Gerberding JL. Actual causes of death in the United States, 2000. *JAMA*. 2004;291:1238–45.
2. Data from the LAC Health Survey, LAC Department of Public Health.
3. Data from the California Physical Fitness Testing Program, California Department of Education.
4. Data from the Public Health Foundation Enterprises' Women, Infants, and Children Program.
5. Story M, Kaphingst KM, Robinson-O'Brien R, Glanz K. Creating-healthy food and eating environments: policy and environmental approaches. *Annu Rev Publ Health*. 2008;29:253–272.
6. Sloane D, Nascimento L, Flynn G, et al. Assessing resource environments to target prevention interventions in community chronic disease control. *J Health Care Poor Underserved*. 2006;17 (2 Suppl):146–58.
7. Evans WD, Renaud JM, Finkelstein E. Kamerow DB, Brown DS. Changing perceptions of the childhood obesity epidemic. *Am J Health Behav*. 2006;30:167–176.
8. Presentation by Larry Bye, Field Research Corporation, 6th Biennial Childhood Obesity Conference, San Diego, California, June 30, 2011.
9. LAC Task Force on Children and Youth Physical Fitness. *Paving the Way for Physically Fit and Healthy Children: Findings and Recommendations*. August, 2002.
10. Centers for Disease Control and Prevention. Recommended community strategies and measurements to prevent obesity in the United States. *MMWR*. 2009;58(RR-7):1–30.
11. Parker L, Burns AC, Sanchez E, eds. *Local Government Actions to Prevent Childhood Obesity*. Washington, DC: The National Academies Press; 2009.
12. Centers for Disease Control and Prevention. *Funding Opportunity Announcement: American Recovery and Reinvestment Act (Recovery Act), Communities Putting Prevention to Work*. Available from: http://www.cdc.gov/nccdphp/recovery/faq.htm (accessed Mar. 15, 2011).
13. Samuels SE, Craypo L, Boyle M, Crawford PB, Yancey A, Flores G. The California Endowment's Healthy Eating, Active Communities program: a midpoint review. *Am J Public Health*. 2010 Nov;100(11):2114–23.
14. Kant AK, Graubard BI. Eating out in America, 1987–2000: trends and nutritional correlates. *Prev Med*. 2004;38:243–9.
15. Backstrand J, Wootan MG, Young LR, Hurley J. *Fat Chance*. Washington, DC: Center for Science in the Public Interest; 1997.
16. Kuo T, Jarosz CJ, Simon P, Fielding JE. Menu labeling as a potential strategy for combating the obesity epidemic: a health impact assessment. *Am J Public Health*. 2009;99:1680–1686.
17. Malik VS, Schulze MB, Hu FB. Intake of sugar-sweetened beverages and weight gain: a systematic review. *Am J Clin Nutr*. 2006;84:274–88.
18. Woodword-Lopez G, Kao J, Ritchie. To what extent have sweetened beverages contributed to the obesity epidemic? *Public Health Nutr*. 2010;14:499–509.
19. Bassett MT, Dumanovsky T, Huang C., et al. Purchasing behavior and calorie information at fast-food chains in New York City, 2007. *Am J Public Health*. 2008;98:1457–9.
20. Elbel B, Kersh R, Brescoll VL, Dixon LB. Calorie labeling and food choices: a first look at the effects on low-income people in New York City. *Health Aff*. 2009;28:w1110–21.
21. Finkelstein EA, Strombotne KL, Chan NL, Krieger J. Mandatory menu labeling in one fast-food chain in King County, Washington. *Am J Prev Med*. 2011;40:122–7.

12 Enticing People Out of Their Cars

Promoting Active Living

JEAN ARMBRUSTER, GAYLE HABERMAN, LOUISA FRANCO, AND MARGOT OCANAS

THE NATURE OF THE PROBLEM

Health statistics in Los Angeles County (LAC) paint a dismal picture. Between 1997 and 2007 obesity rates among adults rose from 14% to 22% (1), and between 1999 and 2008 among 5th, 7th, and 9th graders rose from 19% to 23% (2). This epidemic puts residents at risk for heart disease and stroke (the county's leading causes of death), as well as diabetes, cancer, and depression. Health behaviors contribute significantly to these outcomes: only 38% of children and 53% of adults in the county achieve recommended levels of physical activity (3).

Individual choices play a role, but the physical environments in which people live influence how physically active they can be. When communities are designed to encourage healthy lifestyles, people make healthier choices (4–8). For example, improving access to bike lanes and sidewalks increases opportunities for physical activity in daily life. In LAC, streets have been designed mainly for automobiles with little consideration of alternative travel modes. The LAC public transit system is improving but is still usually slower than car travel, and pedestrians and bicyclists are often overlooked. In this environment, public health has many opportunities to partner with local cities to improve health by designing and building streets and communities that encourage "active living" and "active transportation."

CONTEXT

As part of the Department of Public Health's (DPH) strategic planning (see Chapter 3), the Director tasked a cross-departmental workgroup with developing a plan for improving the physical environment to create safe places for increased physical activity. Members studied evidence-based built environment strategies that increase opportunities for physical activity and considered how to implement these (9–13). Interventions examined included city-level policies with the potential for increasing safety and accessibility for bicycling and walking ("policies" and "plans" are hereafter used interchangeably). These also included safe-routes-to-school plans to encourage children to walk and bicycle to schools. Given strong evidence that streets designed for walking and biking increase physical activity—and the knowledge that only 30 minutes of exercise a day significantly decrease the risk of chronic disease and obesity among adults—the workgroup recommended that the DPH begin working directly with cities to encourage policies that promote active living and other evidence-based strategies—a large undertaking.

The conclusions helped focus a newly established DPH program. Since chronic disease and injury prevention were severely underfunded in the DPH, the Director convinced the LAC Board of Supervisors, the county governing body, to allocate resources for chronic disease and injury prevention and to better align DPH resources with the actual burden of disease. The DPH used this funding to help launch a new program to implement the strategies identified in the physical environment action plan. The new program—Policies for Livable Active Community Environments (PLACE)—assists cities with policy change through: 1) Grant-making to cities and community partner organizations; and 2) DPH staff and technical support to cities without direct grants.

■ APPROACH TO THE PROBLEM

Most city governments have primary oversight over land use and community design—such as the continuity and safety of streets and sidewalks and the proximity of residential areas to stores, jobs and schools—and are thus empowered to create more walkable, bikeable streets. The DPH had related experience when the Tobacco Control and Prevention Program successfully used the Policy Adoption Model (PAM) to promote adoption of city-level tobacco policies restricting access to tobacco (see Chapter 13). The PAM uses an "outside/inside" approach: community coalitions advocate for change from "outside" city hall, then support the efforts of staff "inside" to draft policies adopted by city council. Alternatively, land use plans require an "inside/outside" emphasis. For these, city staff in planning, public works, and transportation must be involved from the beginning in the development, review, and approval of lengthy technical documents. Simultaneously, "outside" advocacy by community supporters is crucial for policy adoption and implementation. The new approach would entail funding cities directly to create policy change.

With little related practical experience, staff conducted extensive outreach to other funders and experts to identify entities using such models. This generated interest and advice and one excellent model: Active Living by Design (ALbD), a nonprofit funded by the Robert Wood Johnson Foundation, which provided funding and technical assistance to create environmental change supporting walkable and bikeable communities, using both "inside" and "outside" approaches. ALbD provided staff with generous technical assistance, and their model became a template for the new unit.

Staff then developed a request for proposals (RFP), inviting cities and community organizations to respond for a policy initiative to increase opportunities for physical activity (see logic model, Figure 12–1). This included a menu of evidence-based policies from which cities could choose (see Table 12–1). Cities and community organizations were required to partner on proposed activities, with city staff responsible for crafting the policy and ensuring internal buy-in. Community organizations were responsible for securing meaningful input and building a base of supporters to demonstrate to decision makers the community's desire for the policy. RFP selection criteria included evidence of political will and strategies for community engagement. PLACE then funded five cities and community organizations to create policy changes that would increase physical activity, and provided seed money to construct streetscape improvements to encourage biking and walking.

As awareness grew about the role of the environment in shaping the obesity epidemic, the Centers for Disease Control and Prevention (CDC) provided funding to reduce obesity through policy and environmental change, and the DPH received a

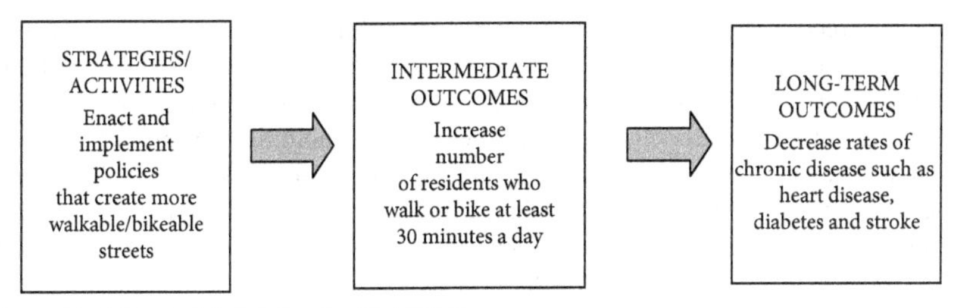

Figure 12–1 Logic Model for the PLACE Program.

two-year grant from the national Communities Putting Prevention to Work initiative. Our Renewing Environments for Nutrition, Exercise and Wellness (RENEW) program supported additional grants for environmental change that promoted active living and healthy eating.

After administering PLACE and RENEW grant cycles, the DPH realized that our grant-making model was not eliciting responses from many cities with the greatest need. Despite extensive efforts to encourage grant proposals from high-need/low-income cities, many simply did not have the resources to develop time-consuming grant applications. So, even though the RFP strongly prioritized need, low-income cities could not compete successfully against more highly resourced cities, some of which hired professional grant writers to develop their proposals.

So, the DPH targeted local cities with very high rates of childhood obesity and secured funding from the Kaiser Foundation and The California Endowment to implement a new approach called the Healthy Policies Initiative (HPI). In eleven cities with high rates of childhood obesity and economic hardship, DPH staff set up meetings with directors of public works and planning departments to assess interest in partnering with the DPH on creating policy change. Five cities accepted and currently receive technical assistance from expert consultants and DPH staff.

IMPLEMENTATION OF SOLUTIONS

Strategy 1: Make Grants for the Development of Healthy Plans and Policies

Through its grant programs, the DPH directly funds city and community organizations to develop bicycle and pedestrian master plans, safe routes to school plans,

TABLE 12–1 *Sample "Menu" of Policies and Plans in DPH Request for Proposals*

- Develop a health element of a general plan that promotes active transportation as well as access to parks and other health-related policies
- Create a pedestrian or bicycle master plan
- Develop "complete streets" initiatives to design streets for all users, not only cars
- Develop and implement safe routes to schools plans
- Develop joint-use agreements between school districts and cities to open school playgrounds after school hours so people can engage in physical activity
- Develop mixed-use and transit-oriented development policies that locate housing in close proximity to transit hubs and stores to encourage walking and bicycling

complete streets policies, and transit-oriented development plans. A first step that the DPH requires of grantees is to develop a time line that identifies the milestones of the initiative. Milestones include: researching similar policies from other cities; developing outreach materials to explain the initiative; holding community meetings to solicit ideas and concerns from stakeholders; recruiting new policy supporters; using local media to promote the policy; educating city commissions, city council, and other key community leaders about the policy; producing a draft policy for public review; and securing policy adoption by city council.

The policies adopted are key steps for cities; they guide city leaders and staff in future decision making, serve as a tool for community members to hold city officials accountable, and put cities at an advantage in applying for grant funds. For example, a city seeking subsidy for bike facilities has more funding options and a greater chance of success if it has an established bike master plan. One DPH grantee, Culver City, created its first bike and pedestrian master plan and had it approved by their city council. It then went on to develop its first safe-routes-to-school grant proposal, receiving an award of $450,000 to construct improved pedestrian intersections and bicycle facilities along key routes to an elementary school.

Strategy 2: Approach Land Use Planning Holistically to Avoid Unintended Consequences

When LAC residents voted for a ½ cent sales tax increase to fund 12 new rail projects in the region, an enormous opportunity arose to improve community health through transit oriented development (TOD) plans, that is, land use planning around transit stations. DPH responded by financing the City of Los Angeles' development of TOD plans for 10 transit stations in low-income areas, the goal being to design neighborhoods near stations where it would be safe, easy, and appealing to walk and bike to popular local destinations. TOD policies potentially increase the bikeabilty and walkability of streets, which in turn can increase physical activity, reduce bicycle/pedestrian injury, and improve air quality. This is an important opportunity for public health because transit lines are often located in dense, urban areas with large populations of low-income residents.

TOD planning also can lead to unintended consequences. Neighborhood revitalization often accompanies new transit investment and can raise property values, increasing rent for nearby housing and businesses. The loss of affordable housing and storefronts can displace low-income residents, who are forced to move to other areas where rents are lower (14). While each TOD differs and these issues may not apply everywhere, it is crucial that land use planning be conducted holistically, with sensitivity to its impact on vulnerable populations. Policies for TODs and transit corridors, for example, should prioritize equitable development that emphasizes preservation of existing and production of new affordable housing.

Strategy 3: Provide Seed Funds for the Construction of Physical Projects

The DPH also has provided "seed" funds for constructing physical projects related to policy initiatives. For example, if a policy being developed is a bicycle master plan, the aligned physical project might be paint-striping bicycle lanes, installing traffic calming measures, designing way-finding signage, or planting trees. The purpose of physical projects is to help grantees to start implementing their policies, and to help organize community members to advocate for change. Many times, the DPH's small investment has been leveraged by cities contributing significant additional amounts. The City of Glendale, collaborating with the Los Angeles County Bicycle Coalition, adopted a Safe and Healthy Streets plan spelling out bicycle and pedestrian engineering, encouragement, enforcement, and education policies for the city. The initiative's physical project—a model two-mile bicycle- and pedestrian-friendly corridor—features newly planted trees, traffic calming features, traffic signals, bicycle facilities, and way-finding signage. It generated great enthusiasm among residents and city officials, and even garnered additional city funding.

Strategy 4: Target Staff and Expert Resources to Cities with Very High Rates of Childhood Obesity

The Healthy Policies Initiative targets policy development resources to cities with very high rates of childhood obesity. Cities that commit to policy change processes are offered technical and DPH assistance to help develop their plans. Key steps of these policy initiatives are similar to those in cities that receive DPH grants. The City of Lynwood, for example, receives technical assistance from a transportation planning consultant to develop its first bicycle and pedestrian master plan, and is contributing its own funds to broaden their plan's scope.

Strategy 5: Organize "Game Changing" Events, Conferences, and Site Visits

Inspiring people with real life success stories influences policy change and shifts the way that people think. The DPH hosts conferences to foster solution-oriented thinking among leaders and advocates, recently partnering with the UCLA Luskin Center for Innovation to host a full-day Complete Streets conference to craft a new vision for Los Angeles County streets, that is, streets designed for users of all ages—pedestrians, bicyclists, transit users, and motorists. Participants included 250 political officials, researchers, and advocates from the fields of planning, public works, public health, and transportation. The DPH also encourages city staff and advocates to take high-level city officials on site visits to other cities for inspiration, to learn about their policy change successes, and to experience firsthand their innovative streetscape improvements.

Strategy 6: Provide Technical Assistance to Partner Cities

A key component of both DPH approaches to partnering with cities—grant-making and the Healthy Policies Initiative—is to contract with local transportation experts to provide technical assistance in support of policy and environmental change. These consultants have designed pedestrian networks and streetscape improvements for safe-routes-to-schools plans. Assistance has also featured inspirational speakers to build support among community members and city decision makers; transportation planners to lead workshops; facilitators to lead community meetings; and graphic designers to create way-finding signage, renderings of proposed improvements, and maps.

Strategy 7: Require Community Engagement and Advocacy in Policy Initiatives

Involving and mobilizing community members in policy initiatives is important for several reasons: 1) outreach builds support among ordinary residents; 2) advocacy is usually needed to get bold policies passed by city council; and 3) overcoming significant community opposition requires education, information, and time. Most cities are accustomed to conducting basic outreach to invite residents to public meetings to solicit their concerns and ideas regarding proposed policies. However, many DPH grantees create additional approaches for building support. The City of Long Beach branded their initiative "Bike Long Beach"; promoted "Bike-to-Work Fridays" for everyone working in the city; organized weekly bike rides with the city's mobility coordinator; and sponsored an annual bike festival. Pacoima Beautiful, a nonprofit organization, presented plans to over 20 local groups and organized volunteer community clean-up days to build support for their initiative to turn the Pacoima wash flood control channel into a recreational greenway. The City of El Monte enlisted their school district partner to use their automatic-dialing system to call all parents to attend community meetings at nearby schools.

Community advocacy is key to creating bold and ambitious policy change; without advocacy, policies may be watered down or forgotten. Or, policies may not get passed at all if strong opposition emerges. Community supporters play instrumental roles in meeting one-on-one with elected officials to educate them about the need for the policy. New policies can be controversial, and initiatives must take the time to address stakeholders' concerns if significant opposition arises.

For example, despite expected increases in traffic from new bike and pedestrian facilities, business owners sometimes fear that removing car travel lanes or parking spaces to accommodate walkers and bicyclists could detrimentally affect their businesses in reducing customers coming by car. When the City of Long Beach encountered this problem, it gathered data to convince business owners that proposed streetscape changes would not adversely affect sales. The city used sales tax data to evaluate the impact of a unique bike lane on retail performance. This showed that the bicycle facilities in one business district did not negatively impact retail sales growth there, and that sales at adjacent restaurants and grocery stores were higher than sales in control neighborhoods. Thus, targeted outreach to concerned stakeholders—whether businesses, residents or other groups—converted policy opponents to supporters.

Strategy 8: Create Innovative Procedural Change Within Local Jurisdictions

Creating new *procedures* within a city can also promote health. The City of Los Angeles is developing a demonstration program called Streets for People (S4P), to allow city staff and residents to quickly and inexpensively repurpose underused street rights of way for short-term, low-cost, pedestrian "plazas," including improvements such as planters, tables, and chairs. Supporting S4P, the City of Los Angeles passed a motion that requires an interagency task force to develop the program with an expedited permit process for community members seeking to improve their streets. Another example of procedural change is a Model Street Design Manual for LAC, which provides detailed guidance for designing safer streets for walking and biking. The manual was developed by over 50 street design experts nationwide and will be made freely available in an editable format so that any city or county can modify it to meet its needs. The City of Baldwin Park, for example, is customizing the manual for their city.

■ EVALUATION STRATEGY

The DPH's evaluation of its policy work with cities to increase opportunities for physical activity—grant-making and the Healthy Policies Initiative—includes tracking processes in the short term and health outcomes in the long term. In the short term, the DPH documents cities' progress made toward achieving their milestones (see discussion of milestones in "Implementation" section). One such—passage of a policy by the city council—is a key short-term indicator of success. Over time, as policies are implemented, DPH hopes to see health outcomes in these cities such as reduced rates of heart disease and diabetes and lower levels of childhood obesity. Of course, any reduction in chronic disease rates cannot be attributed solely to the policies of DPH grantees since multiple population-based and community interventions also are underway. While it is difficult to demonstrate progress toward better health over the term of a grant, the DPH monitors health outcomes through the LAC Health Survey (see Chapter 2), analyzing data and assessing trends at the local jurisdiction level (15).

Until specific health data are available, assessing behavioral outcomes—such as levels of physical activity—are important measures of success. As part of grant deliverables, for example, grantees conduct bike and pedestrian counts to evaluate the numbers of users and assess whether their efforts result in increases over time. These counts are executed yearly or biannually, at the same intersections and same time of day. In addition to providing valuable health data, such counts also help cities seeking funding for infrastructure projects by providing evidence of demand for street-designed active living. Early results are encouraging. In Long Beach, counts indicate that bicyclists riding at identified locations increased 12% over one year. In addition to improved health and behavioral outcomes, other public health benefits of policy initiatives are greater community cohesion and resiliency when residents advocate collectively to meet common needs.

■ IMPACT

The policies adopted by city councils and implemented by city staff—including the built physical projects—give tangible evidence of DPH success (see Table 12–2). There are less tangible impacts, too. The *process* of developing a new policy creates enthusiasm and momentum among city staff, residents, and elected officials. In a survey of the DPH's first round of grantees, 70% of staff from city and partner organizations felt that their elected officials were more committed to making changes to promote active living. As an illustration, El Monte's approval of a health element led quickly to passage also of a healthy food procurement policy and efforts to develop a tobacco retail licensing policy—policies also prioritized in the health element.

The process of developing these policies increases city interdepartmental coordination. Grantees describe how DPH grants required them to work more closely

TABLE 12-2 *Examples of City Council Policies Adopted via DPH Grant-Making Program*

- Culver City—Bicycle and Pedestrian Master Plan
- Glendale—Safe and Healthy Streets Plan
- Long Beach—Active Living Principles Integrated into City General Plan
- El Monte—Health and Wellness Element for City General Plan
- Baldwin Park—Complete Streets Policy

with other city departments than previously and that increased cross-department collaboration aids policy implementation. Further, 92% of city staff reported personally becoming stronger supporters of health-related policy change, and 76% stated that their city colleagues in general were more committed to health-related policy change. One planner mused, "This has been one of the greatest projects I've worked on. It has taken me in a new direction...the active living agenda wasn't even on my radar and now it's shifted my way of thinking about my work."

A critical success factor is that DPH staff pushed city staff to make their policies bold and ambitious in order to prompt real impact on health outcomes. The DPH often gave detailed public health feedback on draft plan language; strongly suggested that each policy include an aggressive action plan with time frames for implementation once adopted by city council; and continually ensured that grantees were on track for success.

KEY LESSONS LEARNED

- The funder role has enabled the DPH to develop strong relationships with grantee cities. The DPH has now positioned itself as a legitimate partner in decision-making processes regarding land use and community design.
- Public health can contribute by funding cities to develop bicycle and pedestrian plans. Few funders provide grants for bicycle and pedestrian master plans, yet many require cities to have a plan before seeking support.
- Political will and community support are important criteria for evaluating the potential success of policy initiatives. Given higher rates of chronic disease in lower-income communities, equity should also be a driving force in selecting cities and communities for policy efforts.
- Public health should remain vigilant about the impact of land use planning on low-income communities to avoid unintended consequences such as the loss of affordable housing and affordable storefronts, or subsequent displacement that can occur during neighborhood revitalization.
- Requiring and funding a physical project—such as planting trees, creating way-finding signage, building walking circuits, and paint-striping bike lanes—serves as a catalyst for garnering other funds and generates community support and excitement.
- Land use policies are controversial. Cities and community partners should expect opposition to policy change and should take time to build sufficient community and political support to address it effectively.
- Two years is sufficient for a city to pass a land use policy such as a bike and pedestrian master plan; the third and/or fourth year of a grant should be used

to fund policy implementation. A two-year time frame allows elected officials to become champions of the policy during their tenure.

NOTE

More information about the policies and plans described in this chapter may be accessed at: www.ph.lacounty.gov/place.

REFERENCES

1. Data from the Los Angeles County Health Survey, Los Angeles County Department of Public Health.
2. Data from the California Physical Fitness Testing Program, California Department of Education.
3. Los Angeles County Department of Public Health, Key Indicators of Health, 2009.
4. Ewing R,Dumbaugh E. The built environment and traffic safety: A review of empirical evidence. *J Plan Lit.* 2009;23:347–67.
5. Pucher J, Buehler R, Bassett DR,Dannenberg AL. Walking and cycling to health: A comparative analysis of city, state, and international data. *Am J Public Health.* 2010;100(10):1986–92.
6. Davison KK, Werder JL, Lawson CT. Children's active commuting to school: Current knowledge and future directions. *Prev Chronic Dis.* 2008;5(3). Available from: http://www.cdc.gov/pcd/issues/2008/jul/07_0075.htm (accessed Aug. 3, 2011).
7. Frank LD, Winter M, Patterson B, Craig CL, and The Vancouver Foundation. *Promoting Physical Activity Through Healthy Community Design: The Active Transportation Collaboratory.* Available from: http://health-design.spph.ubc.ca/files/2011/07/VanFdnStudy.pdf (accessed June 16, 2012).
8. Sallis J, Bowles H, et al. Neighborhood environments and physical activity among adults in 11 countries. *Am J Prev Med.* 2009 (6);484–90.
9. Kettel Khan LK, Sobush K, Keener D, et al. Recommended strategies and measurements to prevent obesity in the United States. Centers for Disease Control and Prevention. *MMWR Rec & Reports.* 2009;58(RR07):1–26.
10. Guide to Community Preventive Service. *Promoting Physical Activity: Environmental Policy Approaches.* Available from: www.thecommunityguide.org/pa/environmental-policy/index.html (accessed June 19, 2012).
11. Centers for Disease Control and Prevention. *CDC Recommendations for Improving Health Through Transportation Policy.* 2010. Available from: http://www.cdc.gov/transportation/docs/FINAL%20CDC%20Transportation%20Recommendations-4-28-2010.pdf (accessed Aug. 3, 2011).
12. Institute of Medicine and National Research Council. *Local Government Actions to Prevent Childhood Obesity.* Washington, DC: The National Academies Press; 2009.
13. Robert Wood Johnson Foundation. *Action Strategies Toolkit: A Guide for Local and State Leaders Working to Create Healthy Communities and Prevent Childhood Obesity.* 2011. Available from: http://www.leadershipforhealthycommunities.org/index.php?option=com_content&task=view&id=352&Itemid=154 (accessed Aug. 3, 2011).
14. Pollack S, Bluestone B, Gartsman A. *Maintaining Diversity in America's Transit-Rich Neighborhoods: Tools for Equitable Change.* Boston: Dukakis Center for Urban and Regional Policy; October 2010.
15. Los Angeles County Department of Public Health, Office of Health Assessment and Epidemiology. *Life Expectancy in Los Angeles County: How Long Do We Live and Why? A Cities and Communities Health Report.* July 2010.

13 From Health Education to Health Policy

A Paradigm Shift in Tobacco Control

MARK D. WEBER AND
LINDA M. ARAGON

THE PROBLEM

Cigarette smoking remains the leading cause of preventable morbidity and mortality in the United States, resulting each year in an estimated 443,000 premature deaths and $193 billion in direct health care expenditures and productivity losses (1). After decades of declines in smoking prevalence, progress appeared to have stalled nationally and in California (2, 3). Yet more recently, smoking prevalence in California again decreased for youths and adults, leading to expectations that the downward smoking trends might be resuming. California's adult smoking prevalence (11.9%) achieved the Healthy People 2020 target of 12% (Utah is the only other state achieving this milestone) (3). In Los Angeles County (LAC), cigarette smoking remains the leading cause of preventable illness and death, causing one in every seven deaths (4) and costing $4.3 billion dollars ($2.3 billion in direct health care and $2.0 billion in lost productivity) annually (5). Significant progress has reduced smoking prevalence in California's general population to among the nation's lowest—14.3% (6) of adults and 10.6% (7) of youth—but marked disparities among subgroups persist. Smoking prevalence in 2007 was significantly higher among African American males (32.1%) than among white (16.2%), Latino (17.7%), and Asian/Pacific Islander (20.5%) males (8). Smoking prevalence strongly relates to geography, socioeconomic status, and race/ethnicity. In LAC's South Service Planning Area, smoking prevalence among African American males and females was 39.0% and 24.5%, respectively, increasing to 54.3% and 32.5% among those living below 100% of the federal poverty level (8).

Exposure to secondhand smoke (SHS) remains a significant public health problem in LAC where 585,000 (10.1%) non-smoking adults were exposed to SHS (9) and exposure was higher among Latinos (14.0%) and African Americans (10.8%) than among whites (6.1%) and Asian/Pacific Islanders (5.7%) (9). Among LAC households with children, 13.2% (some 336,000 children) were exposed to SHS at home (9), the highest exposure found among households of African Americans (18.2%), followed by Latinos (14.3%), whites (9.3%), and Asian/Pacific Islanders (8.1%) (9). Latinos accounted for 66.2% and 72.0% of all adult and child household SHS exposures, in part due to their large population size (9).

Disparities in smoking prevalence and SHS exposure generally correspond to smoking-related chronic diseases. Age-adjusted smoking-attributable mortality rates among males and females were highest for African Americans (425/100,000 and

215/100,000), followed by whites (304/100,000 and 179/100,000), Asians (185/100,000 and 37/100,000), and Latinos (170/100,000 and 49/100,000) (4).

CONTEXT

In 1988, Proposition 99 (Prop 99), a tobacco tax, was passed and led to the creation of the California Tobacco Control Program (CTCP). Through Prop 99 funding, CTCP coordinates the efforts of 61 state public health departments, including the LAC Department of Public Health's (DPH) Tobacco Control and Prevention Program (TCPP). CTCP adopted a comprehensive strategy based on a community-focused social norm change model positing that "the thoughts, values, morals and actions of individuals are tempered by their community" and that "durable social norm change occurs through shifts in the social environment of local communities, at the grass roots level" (10). CTCP's strategy included policy change, media campaigns, raising tobacco taxes, preventing youth tobacco use initiation, and cessation services.

Following this strategy, TCPP worked with community-based organizations (CBOs) to spearhead local tobacco control activities. However, the lack of experience in health policy among TCPP and CBO staff limited TCPP's pursuit of the CTCP mandate for regulatory policy change. Instead, tobacco control efforts focused on health education and voluntary policy adoption. The lack of systematic and sustained policy efforts backed by staff trained to conduct regulatory tobacco control policy (hereafter referred to as "tobacco control policy") campaigns at the local level produced limited policy adoption.

APPROACH TO THE PROBLEM

In 2004, TCPP appraised its program goals, organization, and capacity. The revised goals emphasized the primacy of adopting and implementing tobacco control policies, which in turn led to a concerted planning effort. TCPP's ready access to many resources on planning and implementing tobacco control policies included "best practices" publications from the Centers for Disease Control and Prevention (CDC) and CTCP (10, 11); expertise from the CDC, CTCP, and CTCP-funded statewide projects (e.g., The Center for Tobacco Policy and Organizing [The Center] and the Technical Assistance Legal Center [TALC]); as well as the field-tested experience of 60 Prop 99–funded local health departments. TCPP's restructuring efforts also expanded access to and use of smoking cessation services, but a description is beyond the scope of this chapter.

IMPLEMENTATION OF SOLUTIONS

Following TCPP's appraisal of program goals, organization, and capacity, a new framework was developed to advance local tobacco control policies. Key components eliminated gaps exposed in previous tobacco control efforts.

Organizational Changes and Team Approach

A new Policy and Planning Unit provided leadership, analysis, and coordination of tobacco policy efforts, including technical assistance to CBOs charged with spearheading local campaigns. The existing Contract Management Unit was reoriented to play an active role in implementing policy campaigns, including a system for incentivizing CBOs to conduct policy work, continuously monitoring the type and number of campaign activities, and providing feedback on progress. Similarly, the Research and Evaluation Unit was reorganized to focus on policy support functions, including the rapid collection, analysis, and dissemination of qualitative and quantitative data (e.g., focus groups/key informant interviews, public opinion surveys, population-based surveys) specific to tobacco control policies under consideration. A team approach involved all TCPP units to support a consistent strategy for the CBO policy campaigns and jointly promote them. Further, staff from TCPP and the CBOs met regularly during the campaigns to resolve issues and revise strategies in response to unfolding events.

Establishing Key Partnerships for Technical Assistance and Training

CTCP provided leadership and critical infrastructure to support TCPP's policy efforts. Most important were the availability of tobacco policy training for organizing campaigns, legal analysis of potential policies, and ongoing technical assistance from policy experts throughout the campaigns. TCPP proactively engaged CTCP-funded organizations to create strong partnerships, "leveraging" policy expertise and an array of training not available within TCPP.

Embracing a Structured Model for Policy Change

TCPP collaborated with The Center to develop a step-by-step approach for planning and implementing tobacco policy campaigns called the Policy Adoption and Implementation Model (PAIM) (see Figure 13–1). This model separates the policy

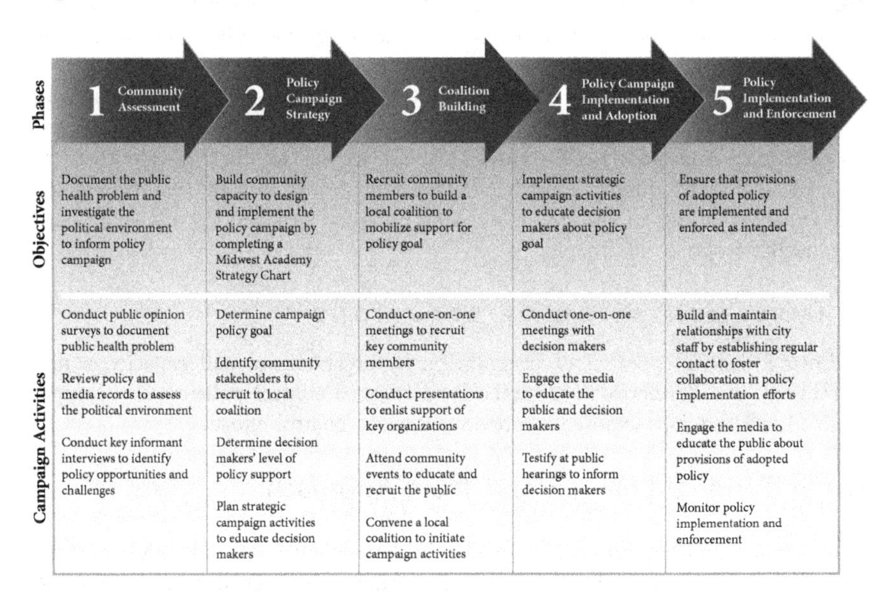

Figure 13–1 The Policy Adoption and Implementation Model.

adoption and implementation process into five phases: community assessment (phase 1); policy campaign strategy (phase 2); coalition building (phase 3); implementation of policy campaign and adoption of the policy (phase 4); and policy implementation and enforcement (phase 5). A heuristic tool, the Midwest Academy Strategy Chart, was adopted for planning policy campaign activities during phase 2 (12). The strategy chart has five components: 1) developing campaign goals; 2) assessing organizational resources; 3) identifying constituents, allies, and opponents; 4) selecting appropriate policy/decision makers; and 5) choosing campaign tactics. These five components yield a blueprint for conducting a policy campaign.

Community Mobilization

To increase public support and mobilize communities, TCPP and partnering CBOs established a local community coalition in each city for the specific tobacco control policy under consideration. Coalitions included local residents interested in tobacco issues, health advocacy groups, business owners, and ethnic/religious/cultural organizations. TCPP, CBOs, and local coalitions collaboratively planned and implemented each campaign.

Capacity Building

Intensive training of TCPP and CBO staff on each phase of the PAIM was critical to the success of TCPP's restructuring. This included comprehensive all-day trainings, webinars, small group workshops, and ongoing one-on-one technical assistance led by TCPP staff and The Center. CBOs also received training in data collection methods to ensure the reliability and validity of data provided to stakeholders.

Aligning the Incentives

Despite intensive training on the PAIM, CBO staff were initially reluctant to implement the model's phase-specific campaign activities. This barrier was overcome by fiscal incentives linking the completion of each phase-specific activity to financial reimbursement. The CBOs submitted monthly invoices describing the activity type, number completed, and supporting documentation in order to receive payment. This incentive-based approach also allowed CBO staff flexibility in responding to campaign developments by changing the type and timing of activities.

Increasing Program Funding

Since 1988, California dropped from 1st to 30th in both tax and programmatic spending on tobacco (13). Its per capita budget spending ($2.19) is well below the CDC's recommended $12.12 for an effective tobacco control program in California (14). Because TCPP obtained nearly all funding through Prop 99, it was directly affected by the state budgetary constraints. Additional funding sources were secured from:

- L.A. Care Health Plan to increase access to and use of cessation services by low-income uninsured and Medi-Cal populations;

- The Master Settlement Agreement to increase smoking cessation services among mental health and substance use patients;
- Communities Putting Prevention to Work (CPPW) to partner with community coalitions, cities, school districts, community leaders and technical consultants to reduce smoking prevalence and decrease exposure to secondhand smoke, especially in disadvantaged communities;
- Peer-Mentoring Consultative Services and Training Initiative to collaborate with the CDC, national organizations, technical experts, and other funded mentoring communities on training, technical assistance, and mentoring services to other CPPW grantees;
- Multi-Unit Housing (MUH) Cohort Study to evaluate the health and social impact, and cost-effectiveness of smoke-free MUH policies in LAC in conjunction with Healthy Housing Solutions, Inc.;
- Community Transformation Grant to reduce chronic diseases and underlying risk factors, especially among vulnerable populations bearing the highest disease burden.

Promoting Visibility and Recognition of TCPP

TCPP's initial tobacco control efforts lacked a strong policy focus; hence few policies were adopted. Yet, evidence-based practice recommendations from the CDC and CTCP were available. Thus discrepancies between state and national policy and TCPP's efforts hindered establishing strong partnerships for change.

In restructuring, the number of policy adoptions steadily increased and recognition of TCPP's tobacco control achievements and expertise grew. Today, TCPP is a nationally recognized leader, and its visibility provides tangible benefits. TCPP regularly publishes in peer-reviewed journals, gives presentations at state and national tobacco conferences, and receives funding opportunities for its demonstrated expertise. TCPP was one of only five awardees of a CDC peer-mentoring grant to provide tobacco control policy training across the nation.

Implementation Challenges

Organizational changes are now well established, the policy campaign organizing capacity of TCPP and CBO staff is vastly improved, and over 100 tobacco control policies have been adopted and implemented in LAC cities. Yet the transition from a primarily health education and voluntary policy approach to a health policy focus faced early challenges. Some staff were reluctant to relinquish their health education orientation; others resisted shifting from voluntary to regulatory control policies. The regulatory policy approach required staff to acquire knowledge and experience with legislative procedures and to develop keen understandings of political decision-making processes, to develop tobacco policy expertise, and to learn how to plan and implement tobacco control policy campaigns; in effect, TCPP and CBO staff had to become policy campaign strategists.

Initial efforts by the CBO staff in using new organizing tools, such as the PAIM, were somewhat mechanical. The model's five individual phases and associated activities were viewed as discreet, unrelated activities. However, as they gained field experience, CBO staff could view the five phases and corresponding activities as a continuous, dynamic campaign process that optimized likelihood for policy adoption and implementation. The transition period between initiation of the organizational changes, capacity building, and the possession of high-quality policy organizing skills took about two years.

Another challenge was high CBO staff turnover during a policy campaign, which typically lasts two years. Responding, TCPP created a policy training unit, developed training materials, and trained CBO's replacement staff in all aspects of planning and implementing a tobacco control policy campaign. Together, these efforts minimized potential campaign disruptions.

Some CBOs challenged the highly structured and prescriptive policy campaign approach. TCPP's extensive array of training, policy campaign activities, and ongoing campaign oversight differed dramatically from the independence to which CBOs were accustomed. This was addressed by establishing fiscal incentives for the funded CBOs to conduct activities identified in the PAIM. TCPP and CBO staff also had to adhere to requirements not to lobby for regulatory tobacco policies while conducting educational activities. To minimize the potential for problems, TALC's legal experts trained TCPP and CBO staff on lobbying laws.

■ EVALUATION STRATEGY

Standard evaluation practice includes roughly equal efforts for the collection and analysis of process and outcome measures. However, given the overarching evaluation goal of TCPP's restructuring efforts—to demonstrate reductions in smoking-related chronic diseases and underlying risk factors—evaluation emphasized outcome over process evaluation.

To successfully complete outcome evaluation goals, both baseline (pre-) and follow-up (post-policy) short-, intermediate-, and long-term outcome measures are collected. And as feasible, data collection also measured relevant covariates and confounders for use in stratified and multivariate analyses, and evaluation designs that yield greater internal validity (e.g., quasi-experimental rather than one-group pre-/post-test). These evaluation strategies strengthen the ability to make casual inferences about impact of TCPP's efforts.

To date, short-term pre-/post-test outcome evaluation measures (e.g., number of tobacco policies adopted and implemented), intermediate-term (e.g., prevalence of cigarette smoking, SHS exposure) pre-test measures, and long-term pre-test measures (e.g., number of child and adult asthma and adult acute myocardial infarctions) have been collected. Post-test long-term outcomes will soon become available.

Although process data collection activities are not central to the evaluation, they do provide important information for quality assurance, quality improvement, and for understanding the context of lessons learned. Such activities guide strategic development, document the intervention process, identify facilitators of and barriers to campaign strategy implementation, and collect tracking measures of tobacco policy campaign activities. These methods were adapted to each policy campaign, including public opinion surveys, key informant interviews, focus groups, education/participant surveys, media/policy record reviews, and youth purchase surveys (i.e., youth decoy or "sting" operations). Evaluation goals include:

- Contributing evidence for community-based tobacco control by identifying strategies with broad reach, high impact, and sustainability;

- Documenting lessons learned and the comparative effectiveness of tobacco control strategies implemented in LAC;
- Documentation, including peer-reviewed publications, to support replication of evidence-based tobacco control strategies or best practices in other communities.

EVALUATION METHODS FOR EXAMINING IMPACT OF POLICY ADOPTION AND IMPLEMENTATION

Data analysis procedures were performed appropriate to the type of data and evaluation question. For example, qualitative analysis procedures such as content analysis were used for key informant interviews and focus groups. The overall analytic strategy for quantitative data (e.g., population surveys, mortality data) employed a "stepwise" approach starting with univariate analyses (e.g., descriptive statistics such as frequencies and percentages), followed by bivariate (e.g., two-way cross-tabulations, correlations), stratified analyses (e.g., three-way cross-tabulations using confounder or control variable), and multivariate procedures (e.g., logistic regression, multilevel modeling). Advanced modeling of the potential health impacts using health impact assessment methodology or forecasting analyses are under consideration.

IMPACT

Through coordinated efforts of TCPP and its community partners, 79 local tobacco control policies were adopted in 43 LAC cities and unincorporated areas from 2004 to 2010; 18 additional policies were passed without TCPP assistance. The adopted policies cover 77% of LAC's 10.4 million population and include these ordinances: 29 tobacco retail licensing, 18 smoke-free parks, 11 smoke-free beaches, 7 comprehensive smoke-free outdoor areas, 5 smoke-free outdoor dining, 5 smoke-free multi-unit housing, and 4 other policy type variations. In comparison, only 15 smoke-free ordinances were adopted from 1998–2003 (see Table 13–1). This represents a 427% increase in policy adoption.

TABLE 13-1 *Number of Tobacco Control Policies Adopted in Los Angeles County, 1998–2010*

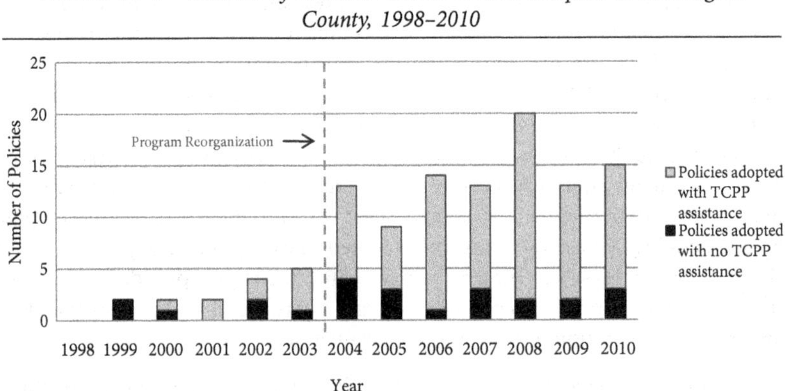

Although LAC cities dramatically increased tobacco control policy adoptions in the six years following TCPP restructuring, the lack of a control study condition (e.g., matched cities without TCPP's highly structured tobacco control policy approach) precludes making strong causal inferences about program restructuring effects. However, the 427% increase in policy adoption grew in spite of 58% and 43% decreases in TCPP funding and CTCP media funding targeting LAC, respectively, during 2004–2010 as compared to 1998–2003. No other systematically coordinated, well-funded tobacco policy efforts targeted LAC cities from 2004–2010, during which time over 80% of policies were adopted with TCPP's assistance. But evaluation of intermediate- and long-term outcomes awaits additional data.

■ CONCLUSIONS

TCPP improved its capacity for adopting and implementing local tobacco control policies. Key elements of TCPP's restructuring framework included: 1) creating a fully staffed and trained Policy and Planning Unit; 2) partnering with state-funded tobacco control organizations to provide high-quality training and ongoing technical assistance; 3) implementing a highly structured policy adoption approach; 4) expanding the CBOs' capacity to plan and implement tobacco control policy campaigns; 5) establishing local coalitions to mobilize communities; 6) establishing fiscal incentives for the funded CBOs to conduct the activities of the PAIM; 7) increasing TCPP's funding to expand the reach and impact of tobacco control efforts; and 8) promoting the visibility and recognition of TCPP.

Seven years of field-based tobacco control policy campaign experience provides a solid foundation for promulgating key lessons learned. Among them:

- Intangibles such as commitment, passion, enthusiasm, and tenacity were critical to achieving TCPP's goal to advance LAC local tobacco control policies.
- Transitioning from a health education and voluntary policy approach to a regulatory policy focus required extensive organizational changes and capacity-building efforts but led to substantially more tobacco control policy adoptions and implementations.
- A team approach, including collaboration with CBOs to jointly promote and strategize about specific policy campaigns, is considered essential to achieving the policy successes.
- Creating and strengthening collaborations and partnerships with organizations funded to provide technical expertise "leveraged" resources and built TCPP and CBO staff capacities.
- Use of campaign organizing tools (e.g., the PAIM, Midwest Academy Strategy Chart), coupled with ongoing technical support, contributed greatly to tobacco control policy adoption and implementation.
- Establishing fiscal incentives for the funded CBOs to conduct the PAIM activities was instrumental to their adherence, and consequently, achieving policy successes.
- TCPP's experience in LAC suggests that policy adoption readiness can be developed relatively quickly, but benefits from highly structured processes, strong community partnerships, and a robust technical assistance and capacity-building infrastructure.

- The successful restructuring of TCPP provides a model for other communities and health departments transitioning to a tobacco control policy adoption and implementation focus.

■ REFERENCES

1. Centers for Disease Control and Prevention. Smoking-attributable mortality, years of potential life lost, and productivity losses—United States, 2000–2004. *MMWR* 2008;57:1226–8.
2. Centers for Disease Control and Prevention. Ten great public health achievements—United States, 2001–2010. *MMWR* 2011;60:619–23.
3. Press Release, July 13, 2011. California adult smoking rate reaches historic low. California Department of Public Health.
4. Weber MD, Wong J, Casil J, Sklyar L. *Human Cost of Smoking in Los Angeles County.* Tobacco Control & Prevention Program, Los Angeles County Department of Public Health, 2011.
5. Max W, Rice DP, Zhang X, Sung H-Y, Miller L. *The Cost of Smoking in California, 1999.* Sacramento, CA: California Department of Health Services; 2002.
6. Los Angeles County Health Survey, Office of Health Assessment & Epidemiology, Los Angeles County Department of Public Health. 2007.
7. Centers for Disease Control and Prevention. *Youth Risk Behavior Surveillance Survey.* Los Angeles Unified School District. Los Angeles County CPPW Initiative, 2010, unpublished data.
8. Weber MD, Sze D, Simon P. Tobacco-related disparities among African Americans living in Los Angeles County: The case for change. Poster accepted for presentation at the 137th Annual Meeting of the American Public Health Association, Philadelphia, PA, 2009.
9. Weber MD, Sze D, Wong J, Sklyar L. Tobacco control & prevention program report for the County Public Health Commission, 2008–2010. Tobacco Control & Prevention Program, Los Angeles County Department of Public Health, 2010.
10. California Department of Health Services. Tobacco Control Section. A model for change: The California experience in tobacco control. October 1998.
11. Centers for Disease Control and Prevention. *Best Practices for Comprehensive Tobacco Control Programs—August 1999.* Atlanta, GA: U.S. Department of Health and Human Services, Centers for Disease Control and Prevention, National Center for Chronic Disease Prevention and Health Promotion, Office on Smoking and Health, August 1999.
12. Bobo KA, Kendal J, Max S. *Organizing for Social Change: Midwest Academy Manual for Activists,* 3rd edition. Santa Ana, CA: Seven Locks Press; 2001.
13. Tobacco Education and Research Oversight Committee. *Endangered Investment: Toward a Tobacco-free California 2009-2011—Master Plan.* Sacramento, CA: Tobacco Education and Research Oversight Committee; 2009.
14. Centers for Disease Control and Prevention. *Best Practices for Comprehensive Tobacco Control Programs—2007.* Atlanta, GA: U.S. Department of Health and Human Services, Centers for Disease Control and Prevention, National Center for Chronic Disease Prevention and Health Promotion, Office on Smoking and Health; October 2007.

14 Reaching Underserved Populations

Influenza Vaccination in the African American Community

JULIA HEINZERLING, MICHELLE T. PARRA, STEPHANIE N. CALDWELL, AND KIM HARRISON EOWAN

THE NATURE OF THE PROBLEM

In April 2009, the first H1NI influenza case in the United States was detected in a 10-year-old child in Southern California. By summer, the U.S. government had declared a public health emergency, the World Health Organization had declared a global pandemic, and the Los Angeles County (LAC) Department of Public Health (DPH) had mobilized a large-scale response that continued well into 2010.

Through its response, the LAC DPH promoted H1N1 vaccinations and vaccinated those without access through regular health care providers. African Americans (AA) had not benefited equitably from these efforts and were significantly less likely to be vaccinated than other racial/ethnic groups. With encouragement from an LAC supervisor who represents historically AA neighborhoods, the LAC Board of Supervisors instructed the DPH to develop a "more comprehensive, aggressive, innovative and strategic outreach campaign" to inform AAs about H1N1 vaccination (1) and to increase their vaccination rates. In this environment, the African American Engagement Project (AAEP) was designed and launched.

CONTEXT

Likelihood of Vaccination among African Americans

From the pandemic's onset, the DPH provided no-cost vaccinations to diverse individuals without health insurance or a regular health care provider at its health centers, large-scale points of distribution(POD), sites and smaller scale neighborhood clinics (see Chapter 27). The DPH vaccinated nearly 200,000 individuals, but AAs, who comprise 9.1% of LAC's population, received just 3.0% of doses at PODS; they were half as likely to be vaccinated against H1N1 as whites. Asians and Hispanics were more likely than whites to receive vaccine at PODs (2).

AAs were also more likely to experience H1N1 complications and be hospitalized than other racial/ethnic groups (3) perhaps because of limited access to and use of medical care, as well as elevated underlying health conditions that increase the risk for flu, such as asthma and diabetes.

■ THE SCALE OF RESPONSE

The disparity in H1N1 vaccination rates was not unexpected. Survey data suggest that in 2007, only 30% of AA adults in LAC received seasonal flu vaccinations, compared to 35% of Asian Americans and 38% of whites (4). Similar disparities were found for other vaccinations recommended for children, teens, and adults. Likely reasons include negative beliefs; access to care; perceived discrimination; misconceptions that the vaccine causes flu or serious side effects (5); and limited trust in government agencies, researchers, and health care providers (6). For over a decade, the DPH sought to understand and address these disparities through qualitative research, targeted media, a quality improvement project, community partnerships, and a community-led peer education intervention.

Anticipating possible disparities in H1N1 vaccine uptake, the DPH scheduled clinics in locations convenient for AA families and used targeted outreach to promote vaccination. However, the enormity of responding to the pandemic, the "unknowns" of H1N1's scale and severity, unpredictable vaccine supply, early vaccine demand that outstretched supply, and the fast pace of daily response limited the DPH's capacity to develop a comprehensive approach to reach under-vaccinated communities.

As the H1N1 response continued, concern about low vaccine uptake among AAs spurred a media campaign, a review of clinic sites and promotional strategies, and AA neighborhood walks to educate and build trust. The Board of Supervisors' "call to action" prompted the development of the African American Engagement Project, which offered an opportunity, albeit a late one, to address the disparity. The Board's request was covered by local media, and the DPH presented its plan within one week, signaling the issue's urgency.

■ APPROACH TO THE PROBLEM

A Focus on Short- and Long-term Gains

A small DPH workgroup developed a comprehensive plan that acknowledged the challenge of improving vaccination rates among AAs. H1N1 had proven milder than feared, cases were declining, and media and public interest in H1N1 had waned, posing barriers to improving uptake in any population, let alone a population where interest had initially been low. Even intensive promotional efforts might yield modest increases in vaccinations. Hence, while the primary project goal was to increase H1N1 vaccination coverage levels for AAs, a secondary, but important, goal was to test strategies and build partnerships for future campaigns.

The DPH developed a multilevel approach to address H1N1 vaccination barriers and concerns, improve access, and build confidence in the vaccine in two areas with historically large AA populations: the South and South Bay regions (7). Key components of the approach were to engage trusted community leaders and ethnic media sources; address common concerns about flu vaccination; use tailored educational materials, peer health educators, and targeted outreach; and improve access to vaccines in convenient community settings. Throughout implementation, strategies, messages, and materials were refined based on partner input (see Figure 14–1).

To meet goals, dedicated resources were required. Federal Public Health Emergency Response (PHER) funds went to the AAEP to support materials development, media buys, and contracts with local agencies to promote and offer vaccinations.

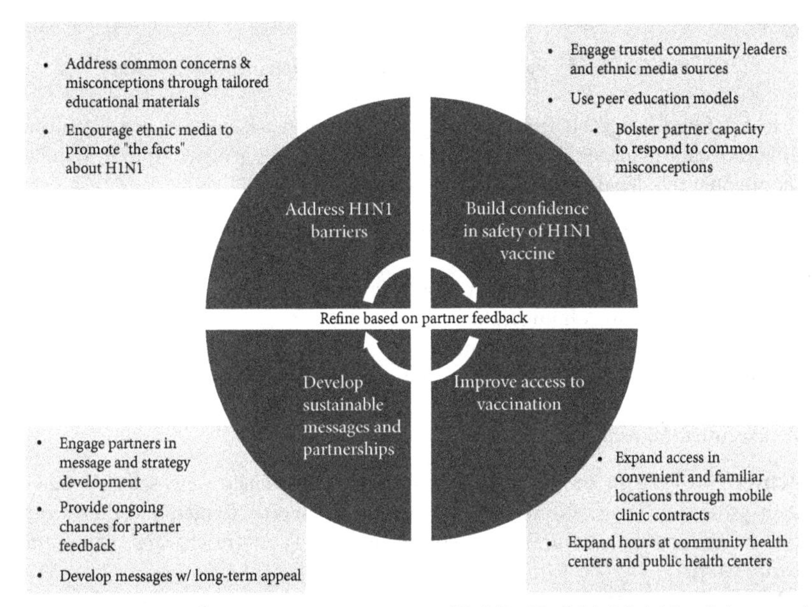

Figure 14–1 Los Angeles County Department of Public Health's Multi-level Approach to Promoting H1N1 Vaccination in the African American Community.

■ IMPLEMENTATION OF SOLUTIONS

Outreach and Partnerships

Mistrust of government can be a barrier (6), so strong community support was critical. The best intended plans can fail without the explicit support of community organizations that have worked with a target population, so the DPH drew up contracts with community-based organizations to conduct outreach and vaccination activities. Eighteen agencies that served large numbers of AAs, were well-regarded professionally, and were trusted by the community were invited to support the project. Six declined due to project timing and staff limits. Six agreed to handle outreach and vaccination promotion: a chemical dependency agency, two Black Infant Health Programs, an agency that conducts health insurance enrollments, and two receiving federal funding to implement community-based disparities campaigns. Three community health centers contracted to provide H1N1 vaccinations at fixed clinic sites, and two hospitals contracted to provide H1N1 vaccination at mobile sites. One public relations (PR) agency would provide targeted media outreach. Given LAC's diversity, partners were encouraged to target energies to AAs but to engage all residents. The DPH provided technical assistance, training, and financial resources to strengthen partner capacity (see Box 14–1).

Continuation of Outreach and Development of Resources

The DPH worked with partners to develop scopes of work that built on their respective areas of expertise (e.g., one-on-one consultations, group classes, and

BOX 14–1 ■ Public Health's Internal Implementation Team

A team of knowledgeable frontline and management representatives was established to launch and manage the H1N1 African American Engagement Project. Members represented the department's:

- Emergency Preparedness and Response Program
- Immunization Program
- Maternal, Child and Adolescent Health Program
- Health Education Administration
- External Relations and Communications
- Community Health Services (manages public health centers and flu vaccination clinics)
- Executive Administration.

Actively involved in the H1N1 response, these individuals were selected due to their professional roles in the DPH's routine vaccination activities, and their expertise in vaccination, cultural competency, messaging, outreach, and community partnership.

Community partners were not represented on the implementation team but served in a consultative role to the team, sharing input and feedback throughout the implementation period.

community promotion campaigns). This process capitalized on partner strengths, but took time—over a month for some agencies. Although prioritized as H1N1 response contracts, it took several weeks to process contracts. Thus, project implementation was delayed until March.

During contracting, the DPH continued its own targeted outreach, scheduling vaccination clinics in AA neighborhoods, placing billboards and radio messages, and enlisting two volunteer community health centers to provide H1N1 vaccinations at two events well attended by AAs, including a Martin Luther King Jr. Day parade and a Southern California Leadership prayer breakfast. The DPH also developed tailored materials to address concerns and common misconceptions in the AA community.

All contracts were executed by March, and each agency attended a mandatory orientation (see Box 14–2). Agencies received an electronic tool kit with H1N1 flyers; brochures; posters; presentations; presentation evaluations; flyer, agenda, e-mail, and newsletter templates; talking points; a resource guide; and a list of H1N1 vaccination sites. Partners also prompted DPH to develop a suite of narrow-cast materials to reach groups at special risk—persons with diabetes, pregnant women, and young children—since partners believed that community members felt that H1N1 was "not a big deal."

■ ACTIVITIES INITIATED BY PARTNERS

Media Messaging: Getting the Word Out

The PR partner encouraged ethnic media outlets to support key messages and used advertisements in local newspapers, radio spots featuring a local African

BOX 14-2 ■ Partner Orientation Conference

Partners were required to attend a half-day orientation conference upon final execution of their contract. To accommodate partner schedules and differing contract start dates, two sessions were held. The conference was designed to build agency capacity to address misconceptions, promote vaccination, and strengthen relationships. Objectives were to:

- Establish relationships among all agencies;
- Discuss project expectations;
- Increase partner knowledge and self-efficacy for educating the public about H1N1 and responding to common vaccination misconceptions;
- Promote effective outreach strategies;
- Identify mechanisms for cross-agency coordination; and
- Obtain feedback on the H1N1 educational materials.

Agency staff learned about H1N1, received the H1N1 tool kit, learned how to order free materials, shared methods to coordinate activities, and identified additional support needed from the DPH. Conference evaluations indicated that the session increased partner ability to address vaccine concerns and built confidence in H1N1 vaccinations among staff, some of whom questioned the safety and effectiveness of the vaccine. Learning about H1N1 and flu myths was reported to be the most helpful aspect.

American physician, billboards, and bus ads in AA neighborholds to promote vaccination. Nearly 700 local TV spots also ran on national stations, including Black Entertainment Television. These efforts were supplemented by vignettes on YouTube, Transit TV, and local access stations. AA leaders were encouraged to promote H1N1 vaccination in their community. This strategy was based on the principle that when leaders model a behavior, innovations may diffuse more quickly.

The PR partner supplemented these efforts by distributing H1N1 materials and promotional cards at job/health fairs, hair salons, barber shops, the oldest church in LAC founded by AAs, and Los Angeles' largest street festival. President Obama was also shown receiving his vaccine at a school.

Reaching Families Through Peer-to-Peer Education

Peer health educators offered a promising approach for this project. They have been used widely to promote healthy behaviors in communities of color because they provide trusted culturally relevant information to individuals who may not otherwise have access to health information and services. They have improved health-related knowledge, behaviors, and/or self-efficacy with AAs (8–10). Community partners used lay health educators to conduct outreach in schools, churches, and Women, Infants, and Children (WIC) centers. They also educated community members through one-on-one consults, support groups, newsletters, websites, and e-blasts.

Meanwhile, DPH staff gave over 200 H1N1 presentations in a variety of venues, including schools, faith-based sites, day care, senior, community and WIC centers, and health fairs.

Improving Access to Vaccinations

LAC DPH had offered vaccinations at no charge through its PODs and outreach sites. The AAEP clinical partners coordinated with community outreach partners to expand access in health centers and mobile clinics. Enhanced efforts continued through the end of the flu vaccination season.

By the end of April, flu hospitalizations had returned to expected levels, and by the end of May, California no longer reported widespread flu activity (11). Thus, at the end of May, the DPH ended the AAEP and H1N1 vaccination activities.

■ EVALUATION

Tracking Progress and Impact

The DPH's evaluation identified best practices; tracked vaccine doses received by AAs; and assessed campaign reach. Findings enabled real-time changes to strategies, messages, and materials and will inform strategies for future emergency responses and reducing disparities.

Agencies were reluctant to enter into contracts requiring intense reporting given the short contract period, so the DPH selected simple mechanisms, including a monthly report. For each outreach activity, outreach partners were asked to record the event name, location, number of materials distributed, number of contacts (by race), and other relevant details. Clinical partners provided their H1N1 vaccine clinic schedules, reported vaccine doses, and approximated the percent of doses administered to AAs. To minimize administrative burden, vaccination records were captured in the electronic California Immunization Registry (CAIR). Contractors were encouraged, but not required, to enter patients' race/ethnicity and zip code, which, in retrospect, led to these data being captured inconsistently.

Qualitative data from staff discussion groups and a closing conference helped identify best practices and recommended strategies to enhance outreach to underserved communities. The conference acknowledged partner contributions, and solicited partner recommendations to improve future campaigns. Recommendations included the following suggestions: convene partnerships and initiate interventions early in the flu season; hold vaccination clinics in small, non-clinical sites; engage trusted community members as media spokespeople; expand outreach to include ethnic and social media; respond immediately and directly to misconceptions and false reports; and build more consistent, diverse, and deep community partnerships.

Education and Referrals

Through outreach and educational efforts, the campaign reached families, service providers, and AA leaders. With 100 outreach activities reported during the project period, the six outreach partners exceeded the project goal of participating in at least 10 outreach events each. Partners provided information and/or referrals to free- or low-cost H1N1 vaccine providers to over 5,600 individuals. While this number is modest, the project covered only three months at the time when interest in vaccination was lowest yet reached individuals who would not have otherwise been reached due to lack of engagement and trust in the medical system and government organizations.

Through intensified outreach, the DPH vaccinated over 40,000 individuals at small vaccination clinics in school and community settings. Earlier, PODS had vaccinated nearly five times more individuals but the smaller-scale events reached a higher proportion of AAs than the PODS—3.5% versus 3.0%. Still, the disparity remained stark since AAs represented 9.1% of the LAC population.

AAEP's 35 small-scale clinics provided 857 doses of H1N1 vaccine, an average of only 25 vaccines per event. However, a larger proportion of AAs were vaccinated. Though race/ethnicity was not recorded for nearly half of doses, approximately 11% of those recorded were given to individuals who self-identified as black/AA. About 32% and 15% of residents in the targeted South and South Bay communities, respectively, were AA (7).

■ IMPACTS

Long-term Gains

Strengthened Partnerships

Existing relationships with community-based organizations helped the DPH quickly mobilize partners, and the AAEP increased the ease with which future DPH collaborations will be realized. A solid group of dependable partners is now identified, and the DPH already has benefited as several partners became media spokespeople for a 2011 immunization campaign.

Renewed Commitment to Intra-division Cooperation

The AAEP afforded the DPH opportunities to engage in unparalleled intra-departmental partnerships and establish new networks of expertise. Cross-collaboration has been sustained by work on subsequent joint preventive health campaigns.

Sustainable Materials

New tool kit materials and messages demonstrated long-term utility. The DPH has adapted educational texts and templates for its seasonal flu vaccination campaign and has integrated key messages into subsequent PSA scripts and flyers.

Building for the Future

The project had only modest impact on the number of vaccinations given to AAs but appears to have slightly reduced the magnitude of disparity. It also yielded long-term benefits such as enduring messages, increased intra-departmental collaboration, and enhanced community engagement strategies. The recommendations below can help public health departments and others develop effective emergency response, influenza, and disparities campaigns.

CONCLUSIONS

Internal Collaboration and Coordination

- Intradepartmental coordination succeeded due to diversity in the implementation team, clearly defined strength based roles, shared decision making, open communication, flexibility, and recognition of contributions.
- Streamlined administrative processes are critical to effective emergency response. Contracting protocols need to be streamlined to expedite processing and payment. To help partners avoid delays, pre-negotiated contractor relationships should be established.

Community Partnerships

- External partnerships laid the groundwork for future collaborations on topics ranging from maternal, child, and adolescent health to chronic disease prevention.
- Community partners may help public health departments connect with hard-to-reach communities. External agencies can help overcome community mistrust of government; identify outreach venues; and promote awareness, knowledge and vaccination using culturally appropriate approaches.
- Depending on project aims, public health departments should carefully consider the best role for partners. If the goal is high-volume vaccination clinics, small neighborhood clinics may not be the best choice, but could be enlisted to co-sponsor an event, or to conduct targeted event promotion. Through small-scale neighborhood events, individuals who are not connected to the medical system or who distrust government can be vaccinated.

Message Development and Dissemination

- Partner involvement can enhance message relevance and acceptance. Partners should engage early in developing strategies, messages, and materials and meet face-to-face to build relationships and open communication.
- Working from diffusion-of-innovation and popular-opinion-leader principles, the project enlisted key opinion leaders to accept and model healthy behaviors. Such opinion leaders are central to educational efforts to address common misconceptions.
- Immunization registries facilitate timely data capture for evaluation. Data can be entered in real time, so reports can be generated frequently to ascertain whether target groups are being reached, identify coverage and programmatic gaps, and evaluate performance of contracted entities. Data entry requirements should be built into contracts, especially if partners are expected to collect data elements such as race/ethnicity that they are not accustomed to collecting.

Mobilizing to Address Persistent Disparities

- Launching a targeted campaign to reach under-vaccinated groups requires careful planning. Such planning during the heat of a large-scale emergency response can divert resources, confuse and delay implementation, and result in suboptimal outcomes due to delayed responses. Public health organizations should anticipate the need for targeted campaigns, identify potential partners, understand promising messages and strategies for the community of interest, and assure resources. Flu and other vaccination campaigns provide chances to strengthen partnerships, test messages and materials, and vet promising strategies for reaching under-vaccinated communities.

- Despite significant efforts and resources, H1N1 vaccine uptake in the AA community remained modest due to fading interest in vaccination when the campaign launched, and underscores the importance of starting promotional campaigns early each flu season. Low uptake also highlights the significant challenges to eliminating disparities. Long-term partnerships, educational efforts, and systemic changes are required to address entrenched beliefs, practices, and access issues that contribute to persistent disparities.

■ REFERENCES

1. Hennessy-Fiske M. L.A. County opens up distribution of H1N1 flu vaccine to the public. *Los Angeles Times*. December 15, 2009. Available from: http://latimesblogs.latimes.com/lanow/2009/12/la-opens-up-distribution-of-h1n1-flu-vaccine-to-the-general-public.html (accessed July 15, 2011).
2. Plough A, Bristow B, Fielding J, Caldwell S, Khan S. Pandemics and health equity: Lessons learned from the H1N1 response in Los Angeles County. *J Public Health Management Practice.* 2011;17(1):20–7.
3. Centers for Disease Control and Prevention. *Information on 2009 H1N1 Impact by Race and Ethnicity.* February 24, 2010. Available from: http://www.cdc.gov/h1n1flu/race_ethnicity_qa.htm (accessed July 15, 2011).
4. California Health Interview Survey. CHIS 2007 Adult Public Use File. [computer file]. Los Angeles, CA: UCLA Center for Health Policy Research; January 2007. (accessed July 27, 2011).
5. Hebert PL, Frick KD, Kane RL, McBean AM. The causes of racial and ethnic differences in influenza vaccination rates among elderly Medicare beneficiaries. *Health Serv Res.* 2005;40(2):517–37.
6. Boulware LE, Cooper LA, Ratner LE, LaVeist TA, Powe NR. Race and trust in the health care system. *Public Health Rep.* 2003;118:358–65.
7. Los Angeles County Department of Public Health, Office of Health Assessment and Epidemiology. *Key Indicators of Health by Service Planning Area; June 2009.*
8. Mickens AD, Modeste N, Montgomery S, Taylor M. Peer support and breastfeeding intentions among black WIC participants. *Hum Lact.* 2009;25(2):157–62.
9. Heisler M, Spencer M, Forman J, Robinson C, Shultz C, Palmisano G, Graddy-Dansby G, Kieffer E. Participants' assessments of the effects of a community health worker intervention on their diabetes self-management and interactions with healthcare providers. *Am J Prev Med.* 2009;37(6 Suppl 1):S270–9.
10. Allicock M, Campbell MK, Valle CG, Barlow JN, Carr C, Meier A, Gizlice Z. Evaluating the implementation of peer counseling in a church-based dietary intervention for African Americans. *Patient Educ Couns.* 2010;81(1):37–42.
11. Centers for Disease Control and Prevention. Information 2009 H1N1 flu: Situation update. June 18, 2010. Available from: http://www.cdc.gov/H1n1flu/update.htm (accessed July 15, 2011).

15 The Asthma Coalition

Effective Prevention and Control Through Collaboration

ROBERT A. GILCHICK, JANET M. SCULLY, AND CYNTHIA HARDING

THE NATURE OF THE PROBLEM

Asthma is a common chronic respiratory condition characterized by inflammation and hyper-reactivity of the smaller airways. When poorly controlled, acute bouts of airway obstruction with resulting shortness of breath and low levels of oxygen in the blood may become frequent and severe. Some individuals require emergency treatment and repeated hospitalizations. However, asthma can be effectively controlled by minimizing exposure to environmental triggers and by appropriate clinical management to maintain stable airway functions and to prevent acute exacerbations. Poor outdoor and indoor air quality with reduced access to health care services, and sub-optimal clinical management can cause significant excess costs, including greater morbidity and reduced well-being of affected individuals and increased health care spending and missed school and work days (1).

Although asthma occurs in persons of all ages, the highest prevalence of active asthma occurs in children and youth. In Los Angeles County (LAC), the prevalence of active childhood asthma is 9.0%, while the lifetime prevalence of asthma in children younger than 18 years is 13.8% (2). These are similar to national rates. In 2008, nearly 19,000 children visited emergency departments for asthma, of whom 3,000 were hospitalized; the average charge per hospitalization was about $17,000 (2). Among those who missed school days because of their asthma, the average was 5.1 missed days. In LAC, asthma displays marked racial and ethnic disparities. Asthma is more than twice as prevalent in African American children compared to white children (4) (see Figure 15–1), African Americans with asthma were nearly four times more likely to visit emergency departments, and were more than three times as likely to be hospitalized (2).

CONTEXT

In recent decades, the nationwide prevalence of asthma has risen, particularly among children. This trend, along with the high rates and costs of hospitalizations and emergency department visits in Los Angeles, poor air quality, and significant disparities in asthma burden among race/ethnicity and socioeconomic strata, mobilized community nonprofit, nongovernmental organizations to focus on strategies to decrease the overall prevalence of asthma, improve asthma management, and reduce the marked disparities. This resulted in the formation of the Asthma Coalition of LAC (ACLAC).

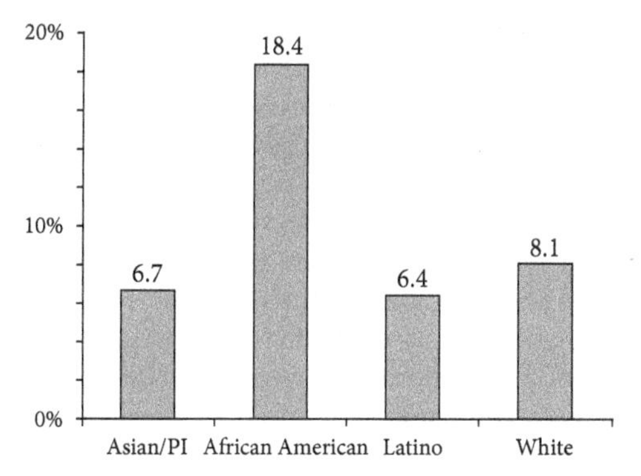

Figure 15–1 Lifetime Prevalence of Asthma in Children by Race/Ethnicity.
Source: LA Health Survey: Childhood Asthma, 2007.

Separate organizations independently addressing a problem affecting a particular community is neither efficient nor cost-effective. With asthma, as with many health problems, there were many advantages to working collaboratively as a coalition. With its county-wide recognition as an authority on health-related issues, the LAC Department of Public Health (DPH) was uniquely positioned to convene organizations committed to addressing the asthma problem.

■ APPROACH TO THE PROBLEM

Although few evidence-based community interventions existed to address asthma in large populations when ACLAC was formed, epidemiologic studies had shown a strong association between environmental triggers and asthma prevalence and severity (1).

Air pollution is of particular concern in LAC. California has the highest level of air pollution in the nation, and Los Angeles is among the worst in the state. Exposure to increased levels of air pollution correlates with asthma symptoms. Proximity to traffic also correlates with asthma severity; children living near busy roads are more likely to have symptoms. Similarly, indoor environmental triggers such as tobacco smoke, dust mites, cockroaches, and mold increase the frequency of asthma symptoms. Improving indoor and outdoor air quality requires strong advocacy to support policies and legislation regarding transportation, smoking, healthy homes, schools, and workplaces. Since public health initiatives alone do not have a strong enough presence in all of these areas, partnerships are needed to create sufficient synergy among the members of ACLAC so that its influence can exceed the impact of the sum of the individual members' impacts.

Clinically, appropriate asthma management can decrease the frequency and severity of asthma attacks. One evidence-based tool to improve asthma management is the recommendation for multi-component approaches to reduce indoor asthma triggers (5). Furthermore, training health care providers increases adherence to the National Asthma Education and Prevention program guidelines and decreases emergency room visits and hospitalizations (1). However, increasing the scale of limited pilots or research studies to a population the size of LAC requires health care system-level alterations that far exceed the ability of the DPH or any other single entity to achieve. ACLAC therefore convened health care–related entities from across LAC to develop a cohesive strategy. Its approach to asthma prevention and control is represented in a logic model (see Figure 15–2).

In response to the growing asthma problem and recognition that a community-level approach was needed, several LAC community organizations began to take action independently. An early collaboration of three community-based organizations (6) interested in addressing asthma, especially in minorities and lower-income families, came to the attention of The California Endowment (TCE), a private health foundation that makes grants to community organizations throughout the state. TCE had formed the Community Action to Fight Asthma (CAFA) initiative in 2002, targeting the reduction of asthma disparities through a comprehensive, place-based approach that addressed the impaired environments of children. This early three-member collaborative was contacted by TCE to gain insight into how the collaborative was addressing asthma. Following this assessment, TCE released a statewide request for proposals to fund local coalition grants. The local collaborative was awarded funds to expand its asthma work and became known as the CAFA Collaborative.

Simultaneously, the DPH was in the process of convening ACLAC. Recruitment of a diverse group of stakeholders reduced the "silo" effect, opened functional lines of communication between and among organizations, and alleviated duplication of effort. Not long after the formation of ACLAC, the CAFA Collaborative was contacted, and the two collaboratives combined forces to create a more robust ACLAC.

IMPLEMENTATION OF SOLUTIONS

Once membership and governance of ACLAC was formalized, a steering committee formed, and bylaws adopted (7), ACLAC recruited additional members who shared its mission to prevent, minimize, and manage the burden of asthma. Currently more than 60 diverse organizations have joined (8). The DPH coordinates all general membership, steering committee, and workgroup activities, providing in-kind staff support for this purpose. One of the private nonprofit members acts as the fiscal agent.

ACLAC's first substantial project was publication of a 2006 report, *Controlling Asthma in Los Angeles County: A Call to Action*, which described the asthma problem and proffered six general recommendations for solutions, each with numerous potential interventions (1) (see Figure 15–3). Four of the recommendations became basic goals within ACLAC's strategic plan. Two other recommendations address disparities and strengthening research, each with crosscutting priorities emphasized throughout the coalition's work. The Coalition functions largely through its four workgroups (see Table 15–1).

The successful publication of *A Call to Action* was followed by a formal strategic planning process designed to operationalize and prioritize the report's recommendations, potential policies, and interventions. With the help of an external consultant, the process began with a membership assessment of how the coalition should function. Most strikingly the assessment found that all respondents agreed that ACLAC should be involved in policy and advocacy. Following the self-assessment, each workgroup carefully examined strategic priorities from the *Strategic Plan for Asthma in*

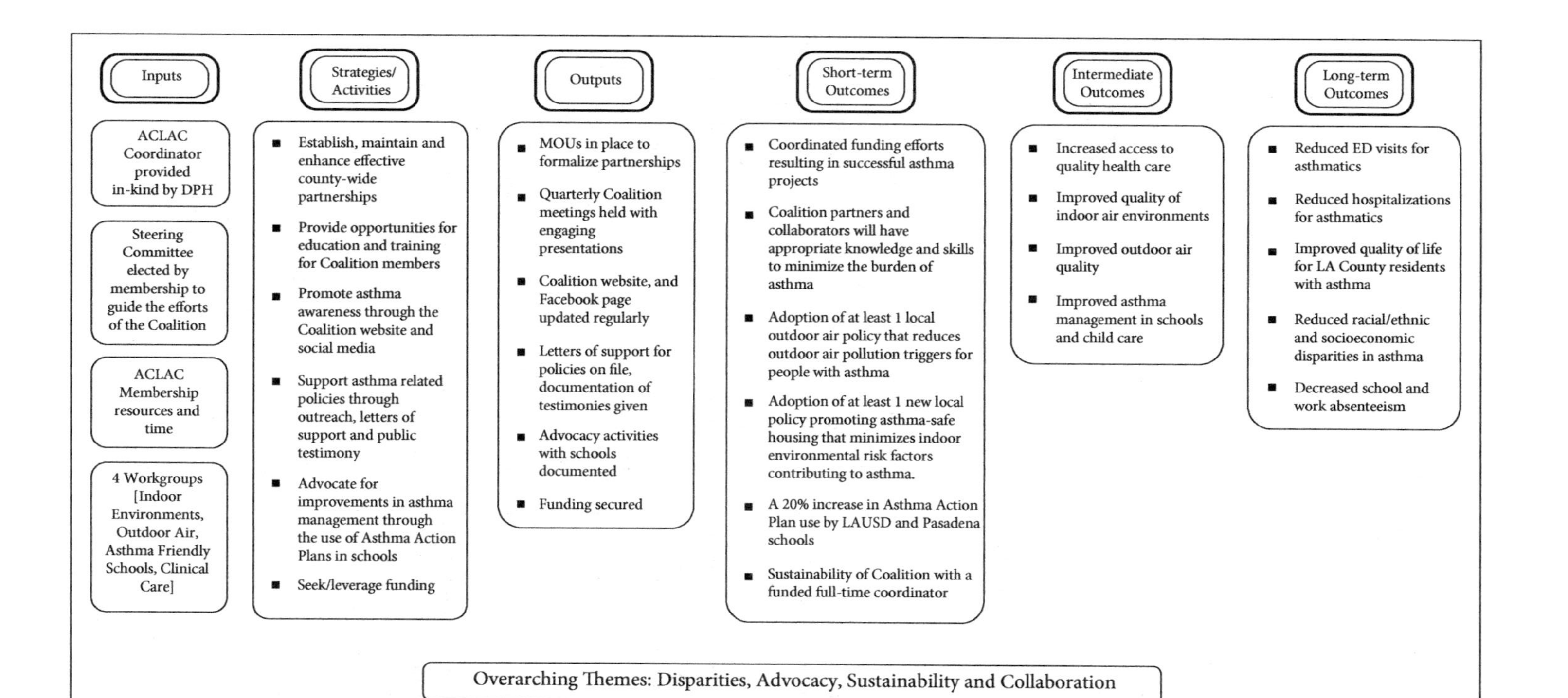

Figure 15–2 ACLAC Logic Model.

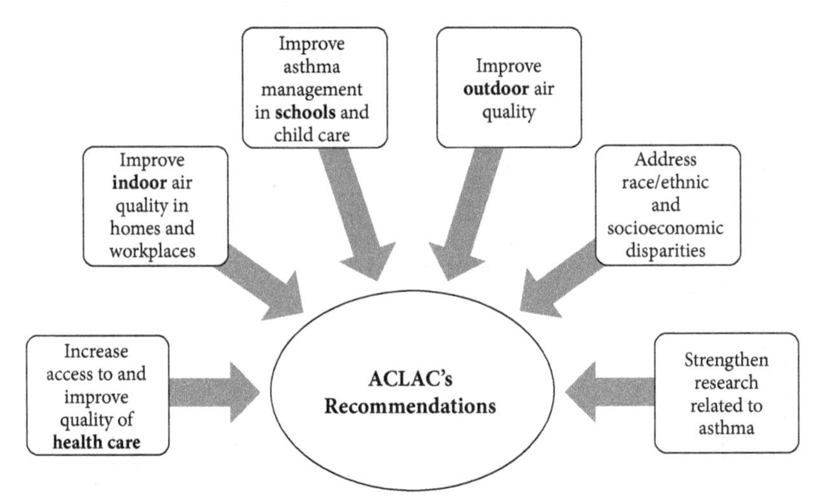

Figure 15-3 ACLAC Recommendations.

California (9) and *Controlling Asthma in LAC: A Call to Action* to ensure that workgroup priorities aligned with both documents. Ultimately, each workgroup selected one or more policy and advocacy priorities for its focus. The Health Care, Clinical Setting Workgroup chose to help expand medical access through the Breathmobile Program (mobile asthma clinic). The Indoor Environments Workgroup chose to promote indoor air quality and asthma-friendly housing systems and policies. The Asthma Friendly Schools Workgroup decided to advocate for adoption of a universal asthma action plan by all schools in the county. Finally, the Outdoor Environment Workgroup chose to emphasize smoke-free outdoor environments (e.g., dining areas, parks, and beaches) and Clean Trucks Programs that strengthen emission regulations.

As all members agreed on the importance of policy and advocacy, early general meetings of the Coalition included training and discussion on effective advocacy techniques. Individual member organizations were encouraged to provide letters and testimony on proposed ordinances, regulations, and legislation with an impact on ACLAC priorities, while ACLAC also provided letters representing the united coalition.

The steering committee remains the Coalition's most active body and provides ongoing direction to ACLAC activities via monthly meetings. The four individual workgroups meet bimonthly and have responsibility for most of the specific activities aimed at achieving strategic priorities. The four workgroups have not all progressed at

TABLE 15-1 *The Coalition's Four Workgroups*

Workgroup	Goal
• Health Care, Clinical Setting	Increase access to and improve quality health care
• Indoor Environments	Improve indoor air quality in homes and workplaces
• Asthma Friendly Schools	Improve asthma management in schools, child care centers, and child care homes
• Outdoor Environments	Improve outdoor air quality

the same pace or with the same level of success—a reflection of the available time of individual workgroup members and the frequency of workgroup meetings. Although the DPH continues to provide coordination of steering committee and general membership meeting activities, resource limitations make it difficult to do the same for the four workgroups.

Due to limited funding, ACLAC relies on donations collected directly from members at the general meetings and seeks opportunities for external funding. The Coalition would benefit enormously from a full-time coordinator to complement the in-kind support of DPH staff. As a short-term solution, ACLAC held a fund-raising event that raised several thousand dollars, which has supported the Coalition's asthma prevention work.

Another challenge faced by the Coalition is achieving consensus when there are strong opposing positions. One example is the disagreement that ACLAC members had over the issue of smoke-free multi-unit housing ordinances. Although all members of the coalition recognize exposure to tobacco smoke as a significant asthma trigger, and all agree that smoke-free homes is an important goal, there has been substantial disagreement about the most appropriate way to effect that change. Many strongly support expanded adoption of local ordinances mandating smoke-free housing units, but other members are concerned over social justice implications, concerned that ordinances may lead to the displacement from their homes of smokers having difficulty with cessation from a highly addictive substance. This is a particular problem for low-income individuals who depend on subsidized public housing and have few other housing options. As this particular policy issue remains contentious among ACLAC members, it demonstrates the ability of the Coalition to compartmentalize its priorities and continue to be effective in the many areas where consensus clearly exists. For now, ACLAC members "agree to disagree" on this issue, while progress on other objectives continues apace and brings ACLAC closer to achieving its overarching goals.

■ EVALUATION STRATEGY

ACLAC's Logic Model lays out a set of short-term, intermediate, and long-term outcomes (see Figure 15–2). Long-term outcomes refer to health and health care use metrics. Note that the ACLAC logic model does not include asthma prevalence per se as a long-term outcome. Although there is some evidence to suggest that environmental improvement may prevent the incidence of asthma, our understanding of the actual etiology of asthma remains incomplete, nor is there any recognized cure for the condition; thus it is difficult to predict what effect these interventions would have on prevalence (10). ACLAC is more focused on controlling existing asthma. Long-term outcomes include asthma-related decreases in emergency department visits and hospitalizations, decreases in school and work absenteeism, and a reduction in the significant racial/ethnic and socioeconomic disparities. With numerous cooperative and independent local, state, and federal efforts to address asthma, improvements in long-term health outcomes cannot be attributed directly to the activities of ACLAC. The logic model demonstrates the causal connections between ACLAC activities and outcomes, but dissecting the relative contribution of all the other influences and interventions cannot be done. Thus, we focus on shorter term process outcomes as a more direct measure of ACLAC's impact.

Each workgroup adopted at least one measurable objective to meet during the five-year strategic plan. For example, the Outdoor and Indoor Air Workgroups each agreed on an objective to adopt at least one local air policy (ordinance) to reduce outdoor air pollution asthma triggers, and one local policy related to asthma-safe housing that minimizes asthma risk factors at home. The Asthma Safe Schools Workgroup chose a 20% increase in use of asthma action plans over initial baselines in two large LAC school district partners as its target. SMART (11) objectives allows precise assessment at a later date as to the degree that ACLAC meets its targets.

In addition to asthma-specific objectives, ACLAC also set organizational objectives. Since the ability to continue its mission depends on continued funding and human resources, ACLAC included secured funding and dedicated staffing among its short-term outcomes.

■ IMPACT

ACLAC has achieved a number of its specific objectives and continues to collaborate successfully toward completion of the remainder. The Coalition advocated successfully for the recently adopted ordinance banning outdoor smoking at restaurants in the city of Los Angeles, thereby achieving the objective of the Outdoor Air Workgroup. The Asthma-Friendly Schools Workgroup also met its objective in achieving increasing use of asthma action plans in schools from partnering school districts, including Los Angeles Unified School District, which is the second-largest school district in the United States and serves approximately 40% of LAC students (12). A subset of ACLAC members, including the DPH, temporarily formed an Asthma Clinical Partnership, which developed a Pediatric Asthma Provider Toolkit that was distributed to over 1,000 pediatric primary care clinicians across the county.

Despite challenges in securing continued funding and staff support, ACLAC's successes demonstrate that numerous diverse organizations from various sectors (e.g., health care, education, research/academia, and community advocacy) can effectively collaborate as long as common goals are shared by all members, and participants are willing to share information and resources. In addition, the Coalition believes that its achievements require collaboration, and that its initiatives would not have been successful if the effort had been undertaken by any single member. ACLAC presents a model for collaboration that could be applied to other chronic disease or public health problems, for example, obesity, diabetes, mental health, violence and injury prevention.

It is worth noting the favorable trends in health outcomes and health care use (see Figure 15–4). While these gains cannot be attributed exclusively to ACLAC, the trends in asthma emergency department visits, and hospitalizations are consistent with ACLAC's logic model (Figure 15–2). Unfortunately, despite successes in the general population, closing the gaps in the health disparities affecting the more vulnerable populations remains a challenge (Figure 15–1).

■ CONCLUSIONS

Experience with the ACLAC yields these insights:

- Diverse organizations from the public and private sectors can effectively collaborate on achieving common population health goals by sharing

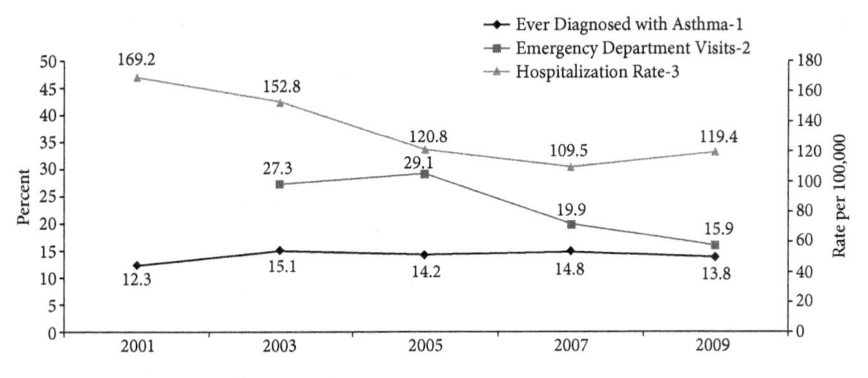

Figure 15–4 Trends in Childhood Asthma.
Sources: California Health Interview Survey (CHIS) and Office of Statewide Health Planning and Development (OSHPD).

networks and resources. The coalition can accomplish objectives that no single organization could achieve independently.

- Members need not agree on all strategies in order for a coalition to be effective, as long as all respect the right of others to disagree and are willing to focus on areas where there is consensus.
- The ACLAC is a successful model that can be applied to other chronic disease or public health issues.
- In the case of childhood asthma, ACLAC has contributed to significant decreases in emergency department visits and hospitalizations, suggesting improved control of existing asthma.
- Despite improvement in general population measures, significant asthma disparities remain, with higher disease burden in low-income communities of color. More innovative approaches, such as place-based initiatives targeting specific neighborhoods, may be required.

REFERENCES

1. Controlling asthma in Los Angeles County: A call to action. Available from: http://publichealth.lacounty.gov/mch/AsthmaCoalition/docs/CallToAction.pdf (accessed June 16, 2012).
2. California breathing—Los Angeles County asthma profile, May 2011. Available from: http://www.californiabreathing.org/asthma-data/county-asthma-profiles/los-angeles-county-asthma-profile# (accessed June 16, 2012).
3. California Health Interview Survey, 2009. Available from: http://www.chis.ucla.edu/.
4. Los Angeles County Department of Public Health, Office of Health Assessment and Epidemiology, 2007, Los Angeles County Health Survey.
5. The Community Guide. Asthma control: Home-based multi-trigger, multi-component environmental interventions. Available from: http://www.thecommunityguide.org/asthma/multicomponent.html (accessed June 16, 2012).

6. Esperanza Community Housing Corporation, St. John's Well Child and Family Center and Strategic Action for a Just Economy (SAJE).
7. ACLAC organizational guidelines. Available from: http://publichealth.lacounty.gov/mch/AsthmaCoalition/docs/CoalitionByLaws_draft_5_09.pdf (accessed June 16, 2012).
8. ACLAC member roster. Available from: http://publichealth.lacounty.gov/mch/AsthmaCoalition/docs/AsthmaCoalitionAgencyList.pdf (accessed June 16, 2012).
9. Strategic plan for asthma in California. Available from: http://www.cdph.ca.gov/programs/caphi/Documents/AsthmaStrategicPlan.5-5-08.pdf (accessed June 16, 2012).
10. Davis A, Herman E. Considerations and challenges for planning a public health approach to asthma. *J Urban Health*. 2011;88(Suppl 1):16–29.
11. Specific, measurable, achievable, realistic, time-limited.
12. Los Angeles Unified School District website. Available from: http://notebook.lausd.net/portal/page?_pageid=33,48254&_dad=ptl&_schema=PTL_EP (accessed June 16, 2012).

PART THREE
Health Protection

16 101 Deadly Days

Listeria monocytogenes Associated with Mexican-Style Cheese

LAURENE MASCOLA AND
S. BENSON WERNER

BACKGROUND

Los Angeles County (LAC) Department of Health Services' (DHS) involvement with the rare and unusual bacteria *Listeria monocytogenes* (LM) began in April 1985. The Epidemic Intelligence Service Officer (EISO) in the LAC Department of Acute Communicable Disease Control Program (ACDC) on telephone duty received notification from a local infection control practitioner (ICP) that cases of listeriosis among pregnant women and their offspring were being identified at an alarming rate in their hospital. The large volume of deliveries at this county hospital (approximately 50 deliveries/day, or 18,000 deliveries/year) provided staff an opportunity to notice an increase in this usually rare disease. While reports of *Listeria* infections were not reportable in 1985, the ICP had background incident data from the hospital, and one of the obstetricians had research interest in the disease. The ICP reported that 12 cases of listeriosis had occurred in mothers and their newborns in 1985 through the end of April, whereas there had been only 6 cases during the same time period in 1984 and 8 cases in 1983. Besides reporting an increased incidence, the ICP called to determine if other hospitals in LAC were experiencing an increased incidence in cases; and so "the investigation of a lifetime" began.

NATURE OF THE PROBLEM/CONTEXT

Listeria monocytogenes (LM) is a gram positive bacterium that was first isolated from rabbits that became ill in a laboratory epidemic in 1926, from a human in 1929, and in 1936 was found to cause disease in neonates. This organism is ubiquitous in the environment, in multiple ecological sites, and throughout the food chain. Humans become infected by inadvertently ingesting soil-contaminated foods and by ingesting products from animals that are infected commonly by soil-contaminated foods. Fortunately, although most humans are probably routinely exposed to small quantities of the organism (and indeed, this organism can be recovered from the stool of a small percent of perfectly healthy persons, i.e., healthy carriers), LM primarily causes disease in persons with immune-system dysfunction (due to chemotherapy, radiation, old age, or pregnancy). There are also rare outbreaks of LM gastroenteritis in otherwise healthy persons who acquire their infection from heavily contaminated food items. Seven species of *Listeria* exist, and LM is the principal pathogen in humans and animals. There are at least 16 different serotypes or serovars; yet, despite this diversity, only three serotypes are responsible for more than 90% of human disease (1). Therefore, serotyping organism is of limited epidemiologic use. In 1985, bacteriophage testing was the commonly used method to distinguish *Listeria* serotypes.

Stimulated by the 1985 LAC outbreak of LM, the largest in North America, the incidence of infections due to LM has decreased dramatically in the twenty-first century, largely due to a higher concern among food manufacturers and regulatory agencies. In 1996 a multistate, laboratory-based active surveillance program found the annual incidence of listeriosis to be 42 cases/100,000. Prevention efforts by the U.S. food industry and government regulatory agencies were probably responsible for most of this decline (see Figure 16–1) (2). In 2010, the nation came close to achieving its 2010 goal of 0.24 cases of listeriosis/100,000 population (3). Prevention of this disease remains a priority. In LAC in 2010, there were 4 perinatal cases (annual incidence of 3.23/100,000) and 14 non-perinatal cases of listeriosis (annual incidence of 0.14/100,000).

■ APPROACH TO THE PROBLEM

The Investigation

Epidemiologists use routine procedures to identify whether an outbreak is occurring (see Box 16–1). As the diagnosis of listeriosis is usually made by recovering LM from cultures of normally sterile sites, this part of the investigation was relatively easy. On the other hand, listeriosis was not a reportable condition in 1985. Therefore, ACDC sent letters to over 160 area hospitals with more than 100 beds, asking for the number of listeriosis cases seen in 1985, compared with cases found in 1984 and 1983. ACDC developed case definitions, namely that a pregnant/neonatal case of listeriosis had LM recovered from a normally sterile site in a mother, infant, or both, and a non-perinatal case of listeriosis was defined as the isolation of LM from a normally sterile body site in an individual neither pregnant nor in utero

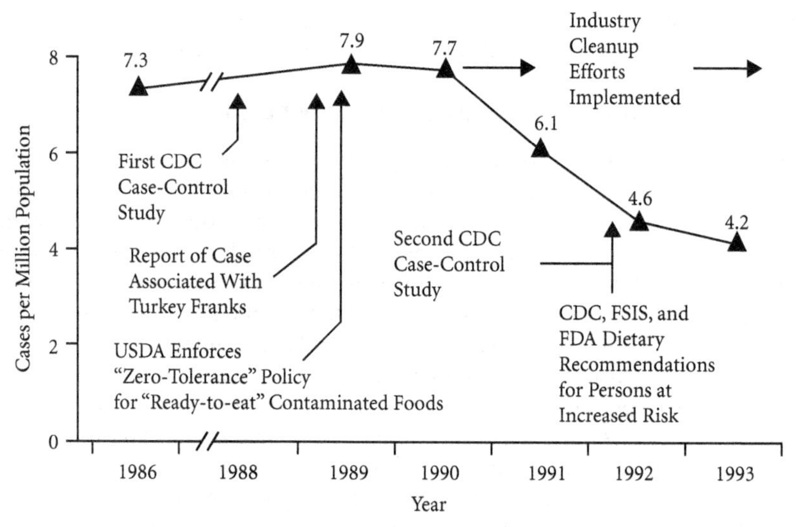

Figure 16–1 Incidence of Listeriosis Based on Data from all Nine Active Surveillance Areas in the United States, 1986 and 1989–1993.
CDC indicates Centers for Disease Control and Prevention; USDA: U.S. Department of Agriculture; FSIS: Food Safety and Inspection Service; FDA: Food and Drug Administration.

Box 16–1 ■ Outbreak Investigation Steps

- Verify the diagnosis.
- Determine whether the number of cases identified exceeds the expected number.
- Search for additional cases.
- Describe the cases with respect to person, time, and place.
- Formulate and test hypotheses.
- Analyze the data.
- Take action to prevent further cases if the outbreak is ongoing and make recommendations to prevent a recurrence.

nor within the first month of life. ACDC also queried the LAC public health laboratory, which mainly serves as a reference laboratory for the county for cases, and the lab reported 5 positive cultures for LM from March to May of 1985, whereas in the previous one and half years there had been none. ACDC also did some "fingertip epidemiology" by calling select larger county hospitals (one of us—Dr. S. Werner—has called personal communication by telephone the "epidemiologist's stethoscope"), and working with their ICPs and laboratorians to ascertain if they were experiencing an increase in listeriosis cases; it appeared that the other hospitals were, too. Inasmuch as listeriosis cases tend to be hospitalized, we concentrated on ICPs for case finding. We were later criticized by independent reviewers, charged by the Board of Supervisors to evaluate our investigation (see below), because the obstetrical community at that time was not contacted. In addition to the fact that there was no readily accessible list of current obstetricians, a belief existed that the diagnosis of listeriosis was straightforward, usually resulted in hospitalization, and standardized treatment for listeriosis existed. Citizens were exposed to daily media updates on the outbreak and its primary effect on pregnant women and their offspring.

In addition to dedicated ACDC staff, two additional "free physicians" began assisting in the investigation. One was a preventive medicine resident; the other was a visiting physician from France. When she returned to France, working in their public health department, she became and continues to be the leading expert in *Listeria* infections in that country.

By May, ACDC officially reported a county-wide outbreak of listeriosis, with over 60 listeriosis cases, and more than 25 deaths, reported by more than 30 hospitals. Only 40 listeriosis cases had been identified in those same hospitals throughout 1984. This had become a deadly epidemic. In May, the Centers for Disease Control and Prevention (CDC) sent two medical epidemiologists (EISOs) to assist in the investigation. Upon their arrival, meetings were held with various groups within DHS and LAC/USC medical center. An investigation plan was agreed upon.

■ IMPLEMENTATION

From Outbreak to Epidemic: Describing Epidemic Cases

Initially, early cases were viewed by zip code to determine if there was any central clustering; there was not. In addition, neighboring counties and states were contacted. Orange County had 9 cases of listeriosis in pregnant Hispanic women, while San Diego and adjoining states had none. At this point, a contaminated food product was suspected to have been widely distributed throughout LAC and Orange County and to be the source of the outbreak. As LM cases continued to be reported, the contaminated foods were likely still available for consumption by the public.

Historically, listeriosis primarily affects two groups of people: pregnant women and other immunocompromised adults. The striking point about the LAC pregnancy-related cases was that all, but one, were Hispanic. Accordingly, a decision was made to focus the investigation on pregnancy-associated cases and on those food items that might be common among Hispanic women. Prior to this outbreak, only one other North American outbreak of LM had occurred (in Nova Scotia, Canada, in 1981) (4). That outbreak was the first to conclusively document food-borne transmission of LM (via contaminated coleslaw), and a later outbreak of LM was associated with pasteurized milk (4, 5). ACDC investigators went to five of the initial cases' households to look at food items in their refrigerators, obtain samples for subsequent bacterial analysis and conduct open-ended interviews. In one household, Jalisco brand *queso fresco* (Mexican-style cheese) was found and sent to the CDC. Extensive, fact-finding questionnaires lasting over an hour were used to elicit food preferences that might yield possible sources of *Listeria*. Serendipitously, in June 1985, *Sunset Magazine* published a special section on the diversity of Mexican-style cheeses (some of which were hard, some soft, some semi-liquid) and helped our mostly non-Hispanic epidemiology group to develop a culturally appropriate questionnaire. After the interviews and a review of Hispanic food consumption practices, ACDC investigators collaborated with the Women, Infants and Children (WIC) nutritionists, consulted with the Nutrition Departments at the LAC Department of Public Health and the UCLA School of Public Health, talked to local *curanderos* about nostrums and herbal remedies, visited the LAC Mercado Central and local Pioneer Grocery Markets in cases' neighborhoods, and began formulating hypotheses and designing a final food-borne illness questionnaire. Informal discussions occurred at this time with the California Department of Health Services (CADHS) and the CDC.

■ THE ANALYTIC CASE-CONTROL STUDY: WAS IT THE CHEESE?

A number of questions were asked about underlying disease, prescription medications, home remedies, contact with animals, and other food items that have been historically linked to food-borne outbreaks of listeriosis. Of course, in LAC's affected population, special attention was directed to ethnic products, such as Mexican-style cheeses and Mexican raw fruits and vegetables (including jicama and cilantro). In sum, the first case control study evaluated the association of a variety of environmental factors, behaviors, and more than 60 food items for possible association with disease.

The case control study started with 66 cases, 40 of which were mother-newborn pairs. Two controls were chosen per case from the case's hospital, which amounted to performing nearly 200 interviews. For neonatal controls, one control was matched by race and age of the mother and the other control was matched only temporally. For non-neonatal cases, one control was matched by age, race, and underlying condition and the other control only by underlying condition. Food consumption histories can be different in chronically ill patients and in Hispanic pregnant women, and that is why matching was so important. This case control study was extremely laborious and difficult to perform. As many of the interviews were conducted three to four months after the onset of disease in cases, their addresses (as listed on the birth certificates of many of the perinatal cases) were no longer valid. We relied on the support of the public health investigators and public health nurses to walk street corners and perform real "shoe leather" epidemiology to find cases and controls for interviews. Non-neonatal controls were particularly difficult to obtain from hospital records, so occasionally we had to contact private physician offices to find similarly immunosuppressed patients for controls, a time-consuming and difficult task. Forty percent of all interviews were compiled in the field; weekend work was necessary. Three attempts were made to find each case and control; searches were made through welfare and WIC rolls, along with police logs, in an attempt to find people. To assist in this task, another medical epidemiologist from the CDC and a state EISO arrived to help find cases and controls and conduct interviews.

This was an extremely complicated investigation, conducted in an era before e-mail and incident command structure. One co-lead investigator from the CDC held morning conference calls with outside partners, while the other held morning meetings with all LAC staff to discuss objectives for that day. After these meetings, the co-lead investigators met to share findings, and at the end of each day a planning meeting was held with key staff for the next day.

▪ EVALUATION

What the Data Did or Did Not Tell Us

In June, a preliminary analysis of the case-control study was performed with 39 cases and their controls. McNemar matched analysis revealed that Hispanic mothers with listeriosis were much more likely to consume Mexican-style cheeses than age-matched Hispanic controls; the odds ratio was 5.5 with 95% confidence interval limits of 1.2–29.8. The biologic plausibility of this epidemiologic association was strong because: (a) milk had been implicated in earlier listeriosis outbreaks, and cheese is made from milk; (b) Mexican-style cheese has a long shelf life in the refrigerator; and (c) LM is a psychrophilic organism, meaning that it can survive and even multiply at refrigerator temperatures, so that an initially small amount of LM contamination in a cheese product could result in an extraordinarily large dose and pose a significant health hazard.

There were over 60 food items listed on the questionnaire, and often interviews were performed months after the cases' exposures. As brand name information for most products was spotty on the original questionnaire, ACDC faced a daunting decision. Should information be released to the public immediately, announcing that Mexican-style cheese products seem implicated as the source of the *Listeria* epidemic? At that time, there were 4 different Mexican-style cheese manufacturers in LAC. By releasing broadly stated information, DHS would interfere with the commerce of all brands of a normally safe, relatively affordable protein and dairy source for Hispanic pregnant women. There were also considerations and concerns that the attendant publicity would preclude ACDC from ever identifying the specific cheese manufacturer that caused the outbreak, preclude discovery of how this outbreak occurred, and preclude ACDC from learning enough to prevent the same problem from occurring in the same, as well as other, cheese manufacturers. The alternate option was to re-interview cases and controls and identify, where possible, specific brand information. By taking this route, one would have to realize that some LM cases might occur during a second case control study. Cases and controls were to be asked a few questions specifically about Mexican-style cheeses and to identify brands bought months earlier (subject to recall bias) or to look in their refrigerators and name the current brand in the hope of identifying brand loyalty.

ACDC, after consultation with the LAC Director of Disease Control Programs and the LAC Director of Department of Health Services, the CDC, the CADHS, and the California Department of Food and Agriculture decided to try to identify the responsible cheese manufacturer. Moreover, in addition to embarking on a second case control study (which focused on brands and types of foods implicated in the first study), a team of investigators from ACDC, the CDC, and the California Department of Food and Agriculture visited all Mexican-style cheese manufacturers located in LAC, obtained samples of the cheese and raw milk products for testing, and looked for any obvious breaches in safe food handling that might cause us to focus our attention on specific manufacturers. Only one of the four Mexican-style cheese manufacturers, Jalisco, was not fully automated. A memo was sent to members of the Board of Supervisors, and a letter was sent to all practicing LAC obstetricians informing them of the plan. After Mexican-style cheese was implicated through the case-control study, the investigators went to local grocery stores near recent cases' households and bought 20–30 packages of unopened Mexican cheeses of all brands and sent those to the CDC. All of these activities occurred concurrently. Teams composed of public health nurses and public health investigators went "into the field" to interview cases and controls for the second set of questions; environmental health teams visited the Mexican-style cheese processors and grocery stores; laboratorians cultured food products; and epidemiologists analyzed data and information as fast as they came in. It was a race against time to find the contaminated product.

Fortuitous timing supports investigations in strange ways. The biology and epidemiologic analysis of the outbreak led us to believe that Mexican-style cheese was the cause of the outbreak. These data were confirmed and discussed through daily team meetings and conference calls with external partners. However, in 1985, laboratory detection of *Listeria* in raw foods was a difficult and time-consuming process (taking up to 3–4 weeks for processing), so definitive laboratory confirmation of the presumptive explanation for the outbreak was still unavailable. While all these investigations (epidemiology, laboratory studies, investigation of Mexican-style cheese manufacturers) were progressing, the CDC reported that an opened food product (Jalisco Mexican-style cheese) that came from the household of one of the first listeriosis cases (visited in mid-May as part of initial investigation) grew LM serotype 4b, the same serotype found in our human cases. One can never prove that an opened package of a product is the source of an outbreak, as that product could just as well have been contaminated by a case. However, the analysis of our second case control study showed on June 12, 1985, that consumption of cheese from the same manufacturer, Jalisco, was associated with disease. Using 39 matched cases and controls, the odds ratio was 8.5, with 95% confidence intervals of 2.4–26.2 (6). The odds ratios were low and not significant with the other cheese manufacturer. Additionally, on June 12, 1985, an unopened package of Jalisco brand cheese purchased from a local grocery store was found to have LM serotype 4b. Now the implicated food product had been identified through both laboratory and epidemiologic investigations although, as per the *Los Angeles Herald Examiner*, this occurred after "101 deadly days" (7).

Unfortunately, the human toll in this outbreak was severe. By the end of the epidemic, which extended from January through August 1985, 142 listeriosis cases occurred, of which 93 were perinatal and 49 were non-perinatal cases, causing 48 deaths (34% case fatality ratio) involving 30 fetuses/newborn infants, and 18 non-perinatal cases. The incubation period for listeriosis can be as long as 90 days, explaining why cases had disease onset long after the cheese was removed from commerce. Of the *Listeria* isolates available for study, 82% (86 of 105) were serotype 4b, of which 63 (73%) were the same phage type. We called this the epidemic strain.

■ IMPACT

How We Made Decisions about the Analytical Results

With results of the second case control study and laboratory in hand, on June 13, 1985, the LAC Department of Public Health (DPH), in collaboration with the California Department of Food and Agriculture and the United States Department of Agriculture, advised the public to stop eating products made by the Jalisco Mexican Style Cheese Company and to discard any such products that were still in their refrigerators. The LAC Environmental Health Program was tasked with requesting retail environments to remove from sale any Jalisco products, and with performing spot checks in restaurants and small food markets throughout LAC (see Chapter 20). Identifying the implicated cheese product and preventing disease by removal of contaminated product from commerce were responsibilities of the LAC DPH.

Questions remained that needed to be answered, such as: How did this cheese get contaminated with *Listeria,* and why this particular cheese manufacturer? A team of engineers, bacteriologists, food scientists, and attorneys from the FDA, the California Department of Food and Agriculture, and the office of the Los Angeles District Attorney inspected the cheese manufacturer's factory. The team reviewed the operation of the pasteurizer, time and temperature records, cheese manufacturing processes, and general plant operations. Records of deliveries and shipments were reviewed, and plant personnel were interviewed for proprietary information. The pasteurizer was found to be operating properly, although the FDA investigators noted that it was possible to bypass the pasteurizer. They also documented delivery on several occasions of 10% more milk than could be pasteurized, given the capacity of the pasteurizer. Environmental samples from drains and condensates were taken at the Jalisco plant and tested positive for the epidemic phage type. An investigator hypothesized that raw milk was likely added to the pasteurized product and that the raw milk was contaminated with *Listeria*. Then, another medical investigator from the CDC came to assist the team with another investigation—to discover which dairy herds were contaminated with LM.

After the cheese manufacturer was closed, dairy herds supplying milk to the cheese plant and control herds were visited. Owners of these herds were extremely cooperative due to the positive relationship between the California Department of Food and Agriculture and the dairy industry. Epidemiologists, veterinarians, and regulators were also involved in this investigation. Noting that in cows as well as humans, LM also can cause an increase in spontaneous stillbirths, veterinarians at those dairy farms denied knowledge of clinical cases of listeriosis in the herds. The 27 dairy farms that supplied raw milk to the cheese plant were large (mean of 869 Holstein cows, median 650). They were modern, dry lot (feedlot) operations that typically used hay and grain for feed. Raw milk from the central collection tanks was collected five times between mid-June and the end of July of 1985. Epidemiologists from another LAC unit were reassigned and tasked with collecting the milk and placing the milk samples in freezers—not usual epidemiology practice! During the last week of June, milk-line filters and pooled milk samples from groups of 50 cows (subsequently pooled to 200-cow composite samples) were collected and cultured. No *Listeria* organisms were found in the samples obtained from the herds of dairies supplying the cheese factory in late June, two weeks after the cheese factory was closed. But, *Listeria* of the epidemic phage type was recovered from products produced at a separate plant that shared the same source of raw milk as the Jalisco manufacturer (6). Political lobbying from this manufacturer and lack of epidemiologic evidence implicating this plant prevented follow-up of this finding.

One particular offshoot of this 1985 outbreak was the intense attention of the media to the outbreak that mandated daily counts of cases and deaths, and the increased pressure for ACDC to explain its evolving and ever-expanding responses to the outbreak. Questions were raised as to the timeliness of the announcement to the public about the dangers in eating Jalisco brand cheese and the subsequent removal of Jalisco's cheese from the markets. Due to concerns about the department's response to the outbreak, the LAC Board of Supervisors demanded a chronology of major steps in the Jalisco cheese recall. And the Director of Health Services initiated an internal evaluation of all of the department's activities relating to the investigation and response by outside experts. In the end, these experts commended ACDC's work, despite inadequate staffing for such an extensive outbreak investigation. Their one criticism was that the obstetrical community should have been notified earlier in a more direct manner about the ongoing outbreak and its predilection for pregnant Hispanic women. The reviewers noted that two other important outbreaks, involving salmonellosis and hepatitis, were occurring concurrently with the listeriosis outbreak. These needed to be investigated as well, thereby demonstrating inadequate ACDC staffing. Because of these findings and recommendations, ACDC was authorized to augment its staffing with a physician and four epidemiology positions. This provided one of the authors her first appointment with the department.

In addition, an evaluation of the LM investigation showed that external communication with the Board of Supervisors, news media, and medical community might not have been as timely as it could have been and that there appeared to be a reluctance on the part of ACDC management to routinely inform upper management in an ongoing fashion of investigative findings. This reluctance was based on ACDC management's concern about a potential leak to the media of information that might derail the investigation, and a period of some mistrust among colleagues in the administrative chain and concern that the information would not be handled appropriately.

The Big Picture

As a result of this outbreak and to learn more about the epidemiology of the disease, in June 1985, the CADHS instituted mandatory reporting of listeriosis by clinical laboratories. Prompted by LAC's large outbreak, the FDA began monitoring dairy products for *L. monocytogenes* (2). To aid in the detection of other outbreaks or clusters of listeriosis, the Council of State and Territorial Epidemiologists recommended in 1986 that laboratory-based surveillance be conducted for cases of listeriosis to allow an ongoing assessment of the magnitude of this infection (8). From 1989–1993, *Listeria* became reportable in only five active CDC Emerging Infections Program's surveillance sites. But, in 1999, the Council of State and Territorial Epidemiologist made the condition reportable nationally.

Other studies prompted by the 1985 outbreak included two major studies that were performed by the CDC in 1988 (8, 9) to describe dietary risk factors for sporadic listeriosis. These studies showed that the consumption of undercooked poultry and non-reheated hot dogs posed a risk for sporadic listeriosis. Another study in 1992 (10) identified an association between the consumption of soft cheeses and delicatessen counter foods with sporadic listeriosis. And a complementary microbiological investigation of food specimens obtained from the refrigerators of case patients led to publication of dietary recommendations from the CDC, USDA's Food Safety and Inspection Service, and the FDA for preventing food-borne listeriosis, which remain relevant today (11). Additionally, the LAC outbreak eventually led to an FDA review from 1987–1989 that yielded a quantitative risk assessment on *L. monocytogenes* in ready-to-eat foods and a decision on whether the United States should establish a zero tolerance level for *Listeria* (2). The FDA eventually did recommend the enforcement of a "zero-tolerance policy" of LM in ready-to-eat foods. The industry implemented its own measures to reduce the risk of contamination by *Listeria*. And, over the years, the incidence rates of listeriosis have fallen. But there is still room for improvement. The latest food-borne illness summary for 2010 (12) showed that while the incidence of *E. coli* dropped 25% compared to the 2006–2008 period, there was little change in the incidence of listeriosis during that same period. Since illegal cheese is commonly smuggled into the United States from Mexico, continued vigilance is warranted.

CONCLUSIONS

The key lessons learned from this outbreak investigation are:

- Local health departments need to be agile in order to adapt to crises and, if needed, mobilize staff from other units. This outbreak occurred before the establishment of the Incident Command System and was managed creatively with internal cooperation between and among LAC public health departments. However, it consumed many resources, additional staff from the state and the CDC, and put substantial pressure on existing staff.
- Local health departments face many practical problems in trying to be transparent with data and in sharing information with the public, but, in doing so, not impugn an entire industry. In this case study, ACDC realized relatively early that Mexican-style cheeses were a risk factor for listeriosis but chose not to publicize that information until a specific brand could be implicated.
- Problems were identified in internal communication systems, particularly reluctance by middle management to routinely notify upper management. No apparent administrative processes existed, then, for emergency notifications. Also, the need to transmit information in a timely and effective manner

to individuals and organizations external to the department was identified. These problems resulted in comprehensive new notification processes.

- It is important to have extra-agency contacts in the field. In this case study, the ICP was a personal friend of the EISO, who had previously lectured at the ICP's hospital, and that contact facilitated the initial call for advice on evidence suspected to represent an outbreak.
- Do not underestimate the influence of the media on how the public perceives your work product or service. Informing the media in a regular, responsive, and respectful manner is vital to establishing a position of trust.
- Despite how well your program communicates with the public or general medical community, there is always room for improvement.
- Educating the public and officials about the stages and difficulties of performing outbreak investigations is critical for preventing unnecessary criticism. Keep in mind, and do not underestimate, the power of politicians. By providing preliminary communications and ongoing discussions with them about an outbreak, they can be forceful advocates instead of adversaries.
- Be open to volunteers, if they can be vetted and well trained.
- Do not underestimate the impact a local outbreak can have on national and international policy with regard to disease surveillance and regulatory control.

■ REFERENCES

1. Gellin BG, Broome CV. Listeriosis. *JAMA*. 1989;261:9:1313–20.
2. Tappero JW, Schuchat A, Deaver KA, et al. Reduction in the incidence of human Listeriosis in the United States: Effectiveness of prevention efforts? *JAMA*. 1995;273:14:1118–1122.
3. Centers for Disease Control and Prevention. Preliminary FoodNet data on the incidence of infection with pathogens transmitted commonly through food—10 States, 2009. *MMWR*. 2010;59:14:418–22.
4. Schlech WF III, Lavigne PM, Bortolussi RA, et al. Epidemic Listeriosis: Evidence for transmission by food. *N Eng J Med*. 1983;308:4:203–6.
5. Fleming DW, Cochi SL, MacDonald KL, et al. Pasteurized milk as a vehicle of infection in an outbreak of Listeriosis. *N Engl J Med*. 1985;312:7:404–7.
6. Linnan MJ, Mascola L, Lou DX, et al. Epidemic listeriosis associated with Mexican-style cheese. *N Engl J Med*. 1988;319:13:823–8.
7. The listeriosis chronology: 101 deadly days. *Los Angeles Herald Examiner*. Friday, June 21, 1985. A10.
8. Gellin BG, Broome CV, Bibb WF, et al. The epidemiology of Listeriosis in the United States—1986. *AJE*. 1986;133:4:392–401.
9. Schuchat A, Deaver KA, Wenger JD, et al. Role of foods in sporadic Listeriosis. I. Case-control study of dietary risk factors. *JAMA*. 1992;267:15:2041–5.
10. Pinner RW, Schuchat A, Swaminathan B, et al. Role of foods in sporadic Listeriosis. II. Microbiologic and epidemiologic investigation. *JAMA*. 1992;267:15:2046–50.
11. Update: Foodborne Listeriosis—United States, 1988–1990. *MMWR*. 1992;41:15: 251–8.
12. Robert Roos. CDC: E. coli down, most other foodborne illensses level. Available from: http://www.cidrap.umn.edu/cidrap/content/fs/food/news/apr1510foodnet.html (accessed June 19, 2012).

17 Infection Control

Public Health Outreach to Hospitals

DAVID E. DASSEY, SHARON SAKAMOTO, AND DAWN TERASHITA

THE PROBLEM

A previously unknown severe respiratory illness was first detected in southeastern China in the fall and winter of 2002–2003. Initial reports to the outside world were sketchy, and there was little impression that the problem had the potential to spread internationally. However, an ill Chinese physician traveled to Hong Kong in February 2003 and infected 10 other guests in his hotel. The world soon learned of the problem when many of these secondary cases carried the infection back to their home countries, two of them igniting outbreaks in Singapore and Canada. Severe acute respiratory syndrome (SARS), caused by a newly identified coronavirus (SARS coronavirus, SCoV), became the first global epidemic of the twenty-first century, infecting over 8,500 people in approximately 30 countries, with a mortality rate of 9% (1). What distinguished this illness was the fact that approximately half of the victims were health care workers, infected while caring for patients with recognized or unrecognized SARS (2).

CONTEXT

Although historically other disease outbreaks have required extraordinary public health response, the SARS outbreak was unique, characterized by its concentration in health care settings and infecting a large number of health care workers. Hospitals were rapidly burdened with its sudden emergence owing to its highly contagious epidemic transmission. Transmission of SCoV was shown to be mostly through droplet spread from contact with infectious respiratory secretions; however, there was also evidence of airborne spread in both health care institutions and residential settings. Cases were infectious for a longer period than with other respiratory pathogens, the highest risk occurring during the second week of illness. This meant that there were likely to be more minor breaches in personal protection while patients were infectious, which increased workers' risk of infection (3). Thus health care workers were at much higher risk than the public at large. Approximately half of the cases worldwide were associated with transmission in health care settings to other patients, visitors, and health care workers. Chaos, fear, and distress rose to extreme levels (4). Enhanced communication and collaboration became a crucial factor among infection preventionists, other hospital personnel, and the Los Angeles County (LAC) Department of Public Health (DPH), and the county's 102 hospitals and 72 fully staffed emergency departments, should cases be introduced into the county.

APPROACH TO THE PROBLEM

The SARS epidemic changed the paradigm of public health's interactions with hospitals (5). Surveillance was established worldwide, following guidance issued by the World Health Organization (WHO) and the U.S. Centers for Disease Control and Prevention (CDC). The LAC DPH, like many other local health departments, quickly promulgated procedures for surveillance, testing, isolation, and quarantine. To render appropriate and timely treatment, and containment, the DPH asked emergency departments and hospitals to conduct case surveillance based on patients' travel histories, signs, and symptoms. Although proper infection control practices and barriers can prevent spread, considerable consultation, education, and training on the use of personal protective equipment and other restrictions were needed.

In November 2003, the DPH invited public health officials from Toronto, Canada, for two days of presentations and discussions on SARS. There was one salient message—improving communication among public health entities and every hospital was critical to controlling SARS. To that end, authorities in Toronto placed a public health nurse (PHN) in every hospital to track reports of SARS cases, suspects, and contacts, and to relay orders from local and provincial government agencies directly to hospital administration (6). Despite media coverage, federal guidelines, and information in medical journals, what guided Toronto hospital officials was face to face discussions of their operational plans with their Canadian public health colleagues. It was clear—it would be necessary to establish a hospital liaison program in Los Angeles.

The DPH has provided communicable disease control and epidemiology services to hospitals for decades. Historically, a Hospital Outbreak team consisting of a medical epidemiologist, an epidemiologist, and a public health nurse (PHN) responded to reports of possible outbreaks in hospitals. There was no formal outreach or active engagement of infection control professionals, hospital-based providers, emergency departments, or laboratories. The nature of outbreaks in hospitals has changed in important ways since the early years of the Hospital Outbreak team.

In the 1980s and 1990s, the majority of outbreaks were caused by either scabies, *Staphylococcus aureus* (including methicillin sensitive and methicillin resistant [MRSA] strains), and vancomycin resistant Enterococcus species. However, over the last decade, the causative agents are more likely to be other multidrug resistant pathogens such as the Gram-negative bacilli (e.g., *Escherichia, Pseudomonas, Acinetobacter, Serratia,* and *Klebsiella*) and community-associated MRSA. Increasing numbers of patients are immunosuppressed by disease or age; more patients are undergoing dialysis or mechanical ventilation and thus are prone to infections that previously were rarely seen, but dealing with such agents did not prepare us to manage a SARS-like incident. Neither was our traditional outbreak response sufficient to address a potential bioterrorist incident on a county-wide level.

A new paradigm was needed to raise awareness of public health initiatives among health care facilities and of DPH resources. Effective and clear channels of communication, coordination, and collaboration with hospitals were needed to improve surveillance and provide up-to-date training and guidance for infection control, testing, prevention, and treatment. The department therefore established the Hospital Outreach Unit (HOU), a new liaison program in the Acute Communicable Disease Control Program as part of departmental emergency preparedness efforts; funding was derived mostly from the CDC Public Health Emergency Preparedness grant.

The HOU's mission is to enhance emerging infectious disease preparedness and response efforts and to improve disease reporting and outbreak detection by hospitals through strengthened communications, collaboration, and consolidation of resources. The HOU's goals are to strengthen communication and collaboration among public health and medical, nursing, and clinical staff, administrators, emergency departments, and employee health laboratories, in essence becoming the face of public health for each institution.

The principal point of contact at each hospital is the infection preventionist (IP) in the office of infection control. Hospital infection control services are mandated by law in many states and are also required by national accrediting agencies such as The Joint Commission (7) (TJC, formerly the Joint Commission on Accreditation of Healthcare Organizations [JCAHO]) and the Centers for Medicare and Medicaid Services (CMS) (8). The history of hospital infection control dates back to the 1960s, when U.S. hospitals established infection control programs to conduct surveillance, develop control measures, and enact and implement infection control policies. In 1976, JCAHO added the presence of an infection surveillance and control program for hospitals to its accreditation standards.

Infection preventionists are specially trained health care professionals, most often nurses, who oversee infection control programs. According to the Association for Professionals in Infection Control (APIC), infection preventionists identify and isolate sources of infection. They also educate to reduce the spread of infection, and devise strategies to prevent future outbreaks. They serve as consultants and educators to physicians, nurses, and other health professionals, applying their expertise in infection prevention to protect patients, visitors, and staff. Over the past decade, the role of the IP has expanded to include broader public health issues, such as response to bioterrorism agents, epidemics such as pandemic influenza, and preparedness and disaster management.

IMPLEMENTATION OF SOLUTIONS

Today, the HOU team consists of five PHNs and a supervising PHN, who report to a medical epidemiologist who also supervises the HOU. These PHNs serve as liaisons between the DPH, infection preventionists, and other health care professionals in over 100 acute care hospitals in Los Angeles County. Each liaison PHN (LPHN) conducts site visits once or twice a year, and to ensure quick and timely communication when needed, maintains a database of all key positions in each hospital, including the chief executive officer and director of nursing, emergency services, employee health, pharmacy, laboratory, infectious disease physician, and the infection preventionist. The database includes a hospital profile providing basic hospital information, such as the type of hospital and range of services (e.g., emergency department, trauma center, pediatric, obstetric, intensive care, transplant services) and its emergency preparedness and response plans. Also included are such detailed variables as the number of available hospital beds, negative pressure rooms, high-efficiency particulate air (HEPA) filters, and ventilators. In the event of a significant public health event, the capability that the HOU database provides can be critical to the management of a crisis.

This HOU has proved valuable in assisting hospitals and health care providers in planning for public health crises, such as health care–associated infections, pandemic influenza, and other novel pathogens and agents of bioterrorism. For example, when a new state law was enacted in 2006 mandating that all hospitals maintain a pandemic influenza plan and collaborate with their local public health department, the HOU provided assistance and recommendations to improve those pandemic response plans. Another example is the implementation of state and national initiatives for reporting and control of health care–associated infections. The National Healthcare Safety Network (NHSN) is a national surveillance system coordinated by the CDC and supported by CMS to track an array of process and outcome variables among hospitalized patients (9). In California, NHSN was selected to be the tool that all hospitals must use to comply with several state laws intended to improve hospital safety and reduce infections. A team comprised of a state worker and a LPHN visited every hospital to orient and assist with the NHSN web-based applications. The HOU assists with data validation studies and can generate reports that identify infection rates and gaps in practice, in an effort to improve hospital performance and patient outcomes.

- The HOU also has been involved in many DPH special projects to improve surveillance extending beyond the reporting of confirmed communicable disease cases. The HOU unit facilitates detection of reportable disease cases and outbreaks in the community through data obtained from electronic laboratory reporting and syndromic surveillance. Syndromic surveillance is an early disease detection system that uses chief complaint data from emergency room patient visits. If these data suggest a cluster or outbreak being treated at a particular hospital, the HOU LPHN facilitates the collection of patient data from the hospital to help determine if the event is of public health importance.
- Coroner case surveillance is overseen by a LPHN who performs a daily case-by-case analysis of coroner's data to identify and follow up suspicious and infectious disease-related deaths. The LPHN obtains medical records for hospitalized coroner cases, coordinates special testing provided by the Public Health Laboratory, and distributes notices of these deaths to the appropriate units within the DPH, such as the Tuberculosis Control Program and Toxics Epidemiology Program.
- A Web-based Confidential Morbidity Report (WebCMR) is based on an advanced electronic reporting system used by hospital infection preventionists and other providers to file state-mandated disease case reports and laboratory results. WebCMR is offered to all LAC hospitals to improve timely reporting, increase standardization and accuracy of reported CMR information, and to create a secure, user-friendly site that will encourage health professionals to comply with state regulations on reporting communicable diseases. LPHNs educate and train health care providers on initiating and using the WebCMR system, and offer web-based communication and training resources, assist with the collection of information on reportable cases, and promote its continual use.

Surveillance is the cornerstone for rapid detection of emerging or reemerging infections so that effective control measures can be implemented. In the hospital setting, the SARS epidemic illustrated that surveillance must focus on the detection of clusters of illness among health care workers (HCW) to ensure a timely containment strategy. In the Canadian outbreak, fever surveillance among HCWs proved vital to rapidly identify potential cases (unfortunately, this process was difficult to implement in many institutions due to concerns for worker privacy). Close relationships between DPH and the infection preventionist is key to ensuring quick detection of unusual patterns of illness among HCWs, visitors, and patients with the goal of implementing isolation and quarantine measures.

The HOU LPHN regularly attends infection control committee meetings in many of their assigned hospitals. They provide a variety of public health educational and promotional material in support of hospitals, provide training to infection preventionists and hospital staff when needed, and assist in numerous hospital outbreak investigations by reviewing and abstracting data from medical records. They interview and obtain epidemiologic data from cases, family members, and health care providers. The LPHN also assists in providing consultation and guidance on proper infection control practice.

Over time, additional health care facilities have been added to the scope of the HOU. These include large outpatient centers, university student health services, jail medical services, psychiatric hospitals, and ambulatory surgical centers. With additional resources, the HOU staff could expand their outreach to other levels of health care units to include skilled nursing facilities

■ EVALUATION STRATEGY

Currently, the HOU LPHNs conduct annual site visits and maintain statistics of over 200 health care facilities and service providers. These include all 102 hospitals in LAC, several comprehensive health centers, large physician groups, jail medical services, and psychiatric hospitals. The LPHNs assess use of WebCMR and follows up with all hospitals not utilizing the reporting tool. An overview of the system is reviewed, along with a hands-on demonstration of the WebCMR community reporting module, discussion of the Health Insurance Portability and Accountability Act (HIPAA) laws and compliance, and LAC DPH reportable diseases and conditions as outlined in California regulations. The LPHNs also train new staff to use WebCMR and are always available to assist with questions or problems. The security process for each user must be replaced every six months, and the LPHNs deliver this component as well.

The HOU tallies all the reportable diseases and conditions filed annually in the county, and follows up with low reporting sites to determine whether technical issues may be inhibiting use of the reporting module. A similar tally of disease outbreaks in hospitals is also assessed annually. Hospitals are contacted six months after an outbreak by the LPHN to insure adherence to the DPH's recommendations. One notable outcome in the first years of operation was an increase in consultation calls from IPs seeking advice and assistance on problematic findings. This suggests that IPs see LACDPH more as a resource than a regulator. Situations that might otherwise have festered and become an outbreak now are being addressed earlier.

A survey of all emergency department syndromic surveillance users is completed by the LPHNs annually and follow-up is initiated for all hospitals of non-user status during the site visit. Infection preventionists and hospital staff are encouraged to use the system for early detection of emerging infectious diseases. By increasing the numbers of hospitals participating in the system, representation of the health status of the community is improved.

The HOU LPHN conducts an annual assessment of users of the California Health Alert Network (CAHAN), and an overview and enrollment packet is distributed to potential non-users of the system on the annual site visit. CAHAN is used both by the California Department of Public Health and the DPH, and users may receive health alerts from both entities. In LAC, the CAHAN system is a key component of preparedness and response to significant public health incidents or threats, and works to protect the public's health. Health alerts and notifications that reflect local guidance and resources are distributed.

Annually, ACDC monitors all activities completed by the HOU LPHNs. This includes numbers of visits made, reasons for visits, number of communications such as phone calls, e-mails, and faxes to and from hospitals, number of syndromic clusters followed, number of outbreaks, number of presentations conducted, educational materials delivered, and so on. Periodic conference calls and annual meetings are now held with hospital IPs during which the HOU LPHN provides updates on public health issues, orientation to new surveillance system features, and infection prevention and control guidance.

IMPACT

Most hospitals and their IP lack a formal relationship with public health providers. Prior to the establishment of the HOU in LAC, the two seldom interacted, with the exception of investigation of hospital-based outbreaks. For the seven years prior to the establishment of the HOU, there were 146 outbreaks investigated by the Hospital Outbreak team (mean 21, range 8–31). In the following seven years since establishment of the HOU, from 2004 to 2010, the number of outbreaks investigated rose to 201 (mean 29, range 16–35). While more and more emerging infectious diseases pose increasing threats to the public's health, serious delays in reporting may lead to the spread of disease. Delays also may lead to ineffective interventions and delayed recognition of a potential public health emergency. Stronger relationships breed trust and earlier reporting and follow-up by public health. With hospitals likely to be the first point of contact for those affected, the LPHN serves as a key component of the public health link to hospital IPs to facilitate and strengthen communication, improve reporting, and enhance early detection and preparedness efforts, while protecting the health and safety of LAC residents and visitors. The HOU's services, annual site visits, and hospital profile assessments demonstrate the value of joint collaborative efforts. Providers see the LPHNs as the local face of the DPH and a source of information, referral, and resources. HOU LPHNs now attend infection control committee meetings of over 30 acute care hospitals, providing access to hospital staff from the laboratory, pharmacy, food services, housekeeping and environmental services, and offering the LPHN opportunities to further strengthen links and raise the DPH's stature among hospital providers. The invitation to participate in these committees indicates intent by hospitals for collaboration and transparency with public health.

Hospital staff involvement and commitment to public health initiatives are essential in our efforts to reduce the risk of emerging infectious disease, including multidrug resistant infections and health care–associated infections. Public health engagement of the IP and key hospital staff encourages commitment and fosters trusting and collegial relationships that ensure sustainability. The Hospital Outreach Unit and its

LPHNs are an integral component of a new public health paradigm that promotes collaboration with hospitals and IPs that best serve the public's health in rapid detection and effective containment of infectious disease threats.

CONCLUSIONS

A dedicated hospital liaison unit has proved invaluable to the LAC DPH. The unit has:

- Given a face to public health, and educated hospital staff on our role and mission;
- Enhanced communication and collaboration between hospitals and public health agencies, leading to increased and prompt reporting;
- Strengthened the surveillance infrastructure to enhance detection of severe and emerging infectious diseases;
- Enabled rapid implementation of effective control measures;
- Increased awareness of planning and emergency preparedness for infectious disease control;
- Enhanced infection prevention and control strategies through education and training efforts on behalf of state and federal control efforts;
- Increased awareness among hospital and other health care providers of the importance of infection prevention and control;
- Educated hospital infection preventionists on emerging diseases, health care associated infections, changes in DPH policies, and available resources from local, state and federal programs.

REFERENCES

1. Christian MD, Poutanen SM, Loutfy MR, Muller MP, Low DE. Severe acute respiratory syndrome. *Clin Infect Dis.* 2004 May 15;38(10):1420–7.
2. Wenzel RP, Bearman G, Edmond MB. Lessons from severe acute respiratory syndrome (SARS): Implications for infection control. *Arch Med Res.* 2005 Nov-Dec;36(6):610–6.
3. Hui Z, Jian-Shi H, Xiong H, Peng Lv, Da-Long Q. An analysis of the current status of hospital emergency preparedness for infectious disease outbreaks in Beijing, China. *AJIC.* 2007;35(1):62–7.
4. Maunder R, Hunter J, Vincent L, Bennett J, Peladeau N, Leszcz M, Dadavoy J, Lieve M, Verhaeghe RS, Mazzulli T. The immediate psychological and occupational impact of the 2003 SARS outbreak in a teaching hospital. *CMAJ.* 2003 May;168 (10):1245–51.
5. Asian Hospital and Healthcare Management. Infection control resurgence or reaction? Available from: http://www.asianhhm.com/facilities_operations/resurgence_reaction.htm (accessed June 27, 2012).
6. Health Canada. *Learning from SARS: Renewal of Public Health in Canada.* A report of the National Advisory Committee on SARS and Public Health. Publication Number: 1210, October 2003. Available from: http://www.phac-aspc.gc.ca/publicat/sars-sras/pdf/sars-e.pdf (accessed June 27, 2012).
7. The Joint Commission (TJC). Available from: http://www.jointcommission.org/ (accessed June 27, 2012).
8. Centers for Medicare & Medicaid Services. Available from: http://www.cms.gov/ (accessed June 27, 2012).
9. Centers for Disease Control and Prevention. National Healthcare Safety Network (NHSN). Available from: http://www.cdc.gov/nhsn/ (accessed June 27, 2012).

18 Reducing Zoonoses

Controlling Animal Importation

KAREN EHNERT AND
ROBERT KIM-FARLEY

THE NATURE OF THE PROBLEM

Sixty-one percent of human infectious diseases and 75% of emerging pathogens are zoonotic (e.g. SARS, avian influenza, West Nile virus, BSE), or capable of being transmitted between animals and humans (1). Liberalization of trade regulations, ease of transportation, and improved global communication have led to a threefold increase in global trade volume (2). With this growth of the marketplace, animal imports have dramatically increased, and with them the worldwide spread of zoonoses, emerging infections, and other animal diseases (3, 4). Over a billion live animals, about 588,000 per day, were imported into the United States between 2000 and 2004 (5). Many are imported for food, research, or exhibition; others enter the commercial pet trade. The lower costs of exotic pets and purebred dogs, especially in developing countries, along with relatively inexpensive shipping costs and high resale value, stimulate legal animal imports as well as smuggling (4). Due to the ever increasing volume of animal traffic, federal agencies are not able to inspect all imports, and so rely on risk-based procedures. Animals deemed to pose the greatest risk are inspected; others are admitted without examination.

The globalization of the animal trade has had substantial cost. Between 1995 and 2008, the impact of zoonotic epidemics exceeded $120 billion worldwide (6). Outbreaks restricted shipment of goods, travel, and employment, as health care costs increased for people and animals. The economic impact of outbreaks of SARS was over $50 billion, of foot and mouth disease in the United Kingdom reached $30 billion, and of avian influenza in Asia in 2003 cost $10 billion (6). Domestically, exotic Newcastle disease in birds was imported into California, probably from Mexico, and infected birds in four states (7). Nearly 4.5 million birds were destroyed and $138.9 million was spent to control this foreign animal disease. In another case, an imported Gambian rat was infected with monkey pox (8). The disease was transmitted to prairie dogs at a wholesale pet store, which resulted in infections in 47 persons who purchased or cared for these exotic pets. Imported dogs have been diagnosed with rabies (9), screw worm infestation (10), distemper, and parvovirus (11). In Los Angeles County, the last two rabid domestic pets were both imported, and entered the country while ill. As reports about diseases related to imported animals mounted, federal and local agencies began to recognize gaps in the live animal import regulatory framework that allow these kinds of problems to spread (7).

CONTEXT

In Los Angeles County, animal importation first became an issue during the exotic Newcastle disease outbreak and then again when there was a dramatic shift in local puppy importation. Earlier, most puppies were imported through airports for personal use, with only one or two per shipment. If an imported puppy did not meet the rabies vaccination requirements, a Centers for Disease Control and Prevention (CDC) confinement agreement was issued, in effect until 30 days after a valid rabies vaccination. Typically, owners complied with the CDC confinement agreement. In recent years, the number of imported puppies tripled, mostly in large shipments for the pet trade (2). Public health staff found that many of the puppies were sold prior to clearing the quarantine period and others could not be located due to false addresses on the confinement agreements. Some importers even falsified rabies certificates. As problems with legal imports increased, reports surfaced of puppies smuggled from Mexico dying within a few days of purchase. The new owners of these puppies, sold through classified ads or from the back of a car, could not contact the seller when the puppy became ill.

Due to the fact that these problems with puppy importation existed throughout Southern California, 14 animal control agencies and three health agencies formed the Border Puppy Task Force (BPTF) (2). The purpose of the BPTF is to share information and assess the increase in puppy importation in the region. The BPTF first conducted an assessment of animals imported through the two California-Mexico border crossings. The assessment identified more than 500 puppies imported within a two-week period, indicating that over 10,000 puppies may be imported through these crossings each year. However, currently no CDC staff are assigned at these border crossings, and so confinement agreements are rarely completed. The active investigation of potential puppy smugglers and enforcement of confinement agreements appeared to reduce the problem. In mid-2008, however, several dead puppies were found in shipments from Korea at the Los Angeles International Airport (LAX). An investigation ensued when one dead puppy was discovered to be only six weeks old, rather than the five months of age indicated on the health certificate. Examination of other shipments uncovered additional dogs with falsified ages on their health certificates in attempts to avoid the mandatory confinement period.

APPROACH TO THE PROBLEM

In 2008, Los Angeles County Veterinary Public Health and Rabies Control Program staff (VPH-RCP) met with CDC Quarantine Station (QT) officials at LAX to discuss animal importation problems. Although the VPH-RCP was interested in working with the CDC and other federal agencies to reduce the health impact of all imported animals, it was decided to focus on dogs and then expand to other species and agency collaborations in a phased manner. An investigation of dog importation identified that: the stated ages on some health certificates were different from age determined by physical assessment of the animal; also, some puppies were only five weeks old, which violated the Animal Welfare Act requiring them to be at least eight weeks of age to be shipped. Then, too, many had no food or water in their shipping cages, or were very ill on arrival. Some puppy shipments were quarantined at a nearby kennel until it could be determined that the puppies did not pose a public health threat. Because the importers refused to pay the kennel fees, the kennel owner declined to assist in any further dog importation quarantines.

These issues were identified because of the deaths of several puppies during shipment, which led to the cooperative investigation between CDC QT and VPH-RCP. At that time, CDC QT staff generally cleared animals through a review of paperwork only. Customs and Border Protection (CBP) officers monitored imported animals for overt signs of illness. Incorrect health certificates, such as of a dog's age, could lead to unvaccinated dogs not being confined after import, as required by law. Rabies vaccines may only be given to dogs three months of age or older, and in California, dogs may not be legally vaccinated until they are four months old. The initial age of vaccination is important, since a protective titer of rabies antibodies may not develop in younger animals due to interference with maternal antibodies.

Based on initial findings, VPH-RCP and CDC QT agreed that additional data were needed to determine if there was a major systemic problem with imported dogs and/or their paperwork, and whether their ongoing physical examination was warranted. But there were no additional funds or staff to work on this issue. Considering the limited number of staff in both programs, the numerous federal agencies involved in animal imports, and the need to have animal experts present during all inspections, it was determined that the survey could only be completed with the help of a broad coalition of partners. Thus the group created a unique federal-local collaborative to investigate and identify changes needed to protect the public (see Figure 18–1).

The new collaborative first focused on data to confirm or reject the hypothesis that imported animal health certificate fraud was a major problem. A three-week assessment was proposed for all animals imported through LAX. This focused on physical assessments of the puppies and reviewed the validity of accompanying documents. At LAX, several federal agencies oversee different aspects of animal importation. The CDC QT ensures compliance with CDC animal import regulations for dogs, cats, bats, primates, and certain African rodents. The United States Fish and Wildlife Services (FWS) regulates wild animals. The U. S. Department of Agriculture (USDA) monitors imported livestock and birds. CBP assists by monitoring the health of all imported animals, ensuring that animals are not released from the cargo areas until appropriately cleared. However, CBP officers have limited training in estimating animals' ages, identifying subtle signs of illness, or verifying species. Since each agency plays a key oversight role, a complete assessment requires their agreement and cooperation. Thus, the first meetings gained the cooperation of the federal partners. Once they agreed to collaborate, VPH-RCP staff contacted local animal care and control officials. The directors of the Los Angeles City Animal Services (LA Animal Services) and the BPTF both indicated their support.

The collaborative met to share their procedures, identify problems with health certificates, and develop an assessment. Each agency agreed to its role (see Table 18–1), and a complex project solution became possible with the buy-in from each and every agency.

■ IMPLEMENTATION OF SOLUTIONS

Animal importations are regulated by various federal agencies. Local agencies generally do not have an active role in the process. The concept of a federal-local

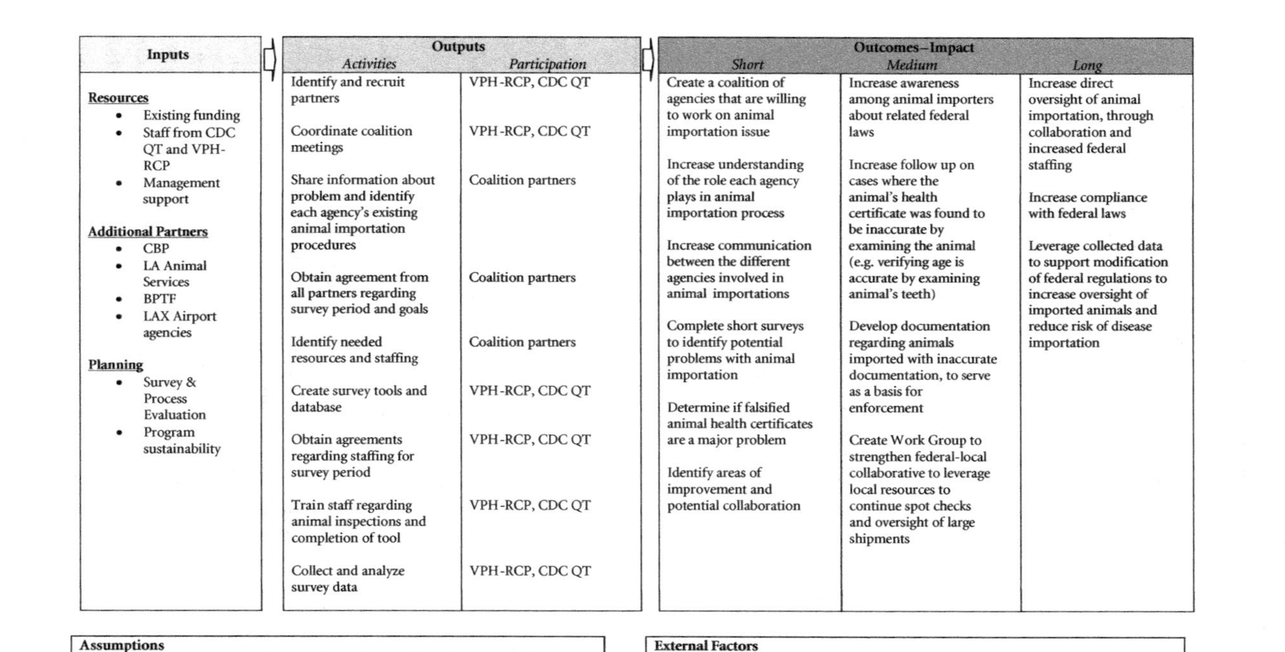

Figure 18–1 Animal Importation Collaborative at Los Angeles International Airport (LAX) Logic Model.
Logic Model Flowchart Template was obtained from the University of Wisconsin Extension at http://www.uwex.edu/ces/pdande/evaluation/evallogicmodelworksheets.html

TABLE 18-1 *Collaborative Partners' Roles During Animal Importation Assessment*

Agency	Role	Additional Support
CBP	Escort non-LAX survey staff into restricted cargo areas and provide access to imported animals	Provide animal importation manifest twice daily
CDC QT	Reviews health certificates and rabies vaccination documents for compliance with regulations Oversee release of imported dogs and cats after reviewing documents Determine action needed when sick or under-age dogs or cats are identified	Provide copies of the CDC Dog Importation Confinement agreements to survey staff
LAX Police	Provide general approval for non-LAX survey staff to access restricted cargo areas with CBP officers	
VPH-RCP	Provide the survey tool, train staff on form completion, collect completed forms, and enter and analyze the data Provide oversight of the survey and help coordinate response to any problems Provide staff to inspect animals and complete survey forms	Provide survey forms, clip boards, pens, and other office supplies to survey staff
LA Animal Services	Provide staff to inspect animals and complete survey forms	Provide command trailer Provide off-site animal quarantine
BPTF	Provide staff to inspect animals and complete survey forms	

partnership to address the issue is innovative. The BPTF had conducted two dog importation surveys at California-Mexico border crossings using local and federal staff. Thus, when VPH-RCP staff approached CDC QT staff about jointly investigating sick and under-aged puppies being imported through LAX, there was precedent for such a partnership.

The previous BPTF animal surveys served as a basis for developing the new initiative; however, working at LAX proved to be more complex than at the land border crossings. At the California-Mexico border crossings, the BPTF only needed agreement from the CBP, the overseeing agency. At LAX, however, numerous federal agencies oversee different aspects and species of animal importation. Communication among them is generally limited. Also, at border crossings the BPTF operated in a secondary screening area, after transport vehicles had been inspected by CBP. Cars were then sent to the screening area if the occupants reported or inspectors suspected that they were carrying animals. At LAX, animals were inspected in secure cargo areas, accessed by badged staff or special escort. Since only VPH-RCP staff obtained special LAX badges, federal agents needed to escort survey personnel during all inspections. During the BPTF surveys, individuals carrying sick animals could be denied entry into the United States. At LAX, the animals arrive from all over the world, some in transit for up to 24 hours. Such animals could not easily be returned to their origins, since they usually arrive unaccompanied. Return shipment could potentially be arranged, but lacking an easy mechanism to pay for such shipment, this generally did not happen.

Careful planning overcame many barriers to this federal-local collaborative (see Figure 18–1), including: clearly stating the mission; drafting specific procedures for the collaborative efforts, which outlined each agency's roles and responsibilities; creating staffing rosters; and obtaining special access to secure areas. To gain the confidence of all the federal agencies, it was clarified that the activities would provide support to them, not create negative reports about their work. Articulating how data could be beneficial was also important. Although some federal staff were needed, the impact on federal personnel was minimized by assistance from local animal control officers, health inspectors, and veterinarians. All personnel underwent background checks, either by their own agency or LAX, prior to accessing secure areas at LAX. Assessment staffing rosters went to all federal partners in advance of the survey to limit the risk in providing access to secure areas.

Even with careful planning, unforeseen issues arose. The LAX Parking Authority was not included in the preparatory meetings and was not aware of the project needs, so did not provide parking passes for the command trailer provided by LA Animal Services for office space and coordination. The matter was resolved, but demonstrates how complex conducting extensive surveys at airports may be and the difficulty in identifying all necessary partners.

One group deliberately excluded prior to the survey was the various airlines. The importers using one airline to ship dogs several times a month to LAX simply began using another carrier after VPH-RCP had conducted earlier spot inspections. When VPH-RCP approached the second airline, the importers switched carriers again. Due to the rapidity with which importers switched airlines to avoid animal inspections, it was decided that there would be no pre-notification of airlines about the surveys. It was initially proposed that no animals would be held, even with falsified paperwork. Confinement agreements would be issued for under-aged dogs. During previous investigations, medical and boarding fees quickly mounted after under-aged or ill puppies were held. Some importers refused to pay the fees and elected to abandon the puppies. To prevent similar problems during the assessment period, only very ill animals were impounded. But during one inspection, an animal control officer noted two dogs from South America that were covered with fleas and ticks, as well as having skin lesions. To safeguard the public, VPH-RCP issued an order that permitted the dogs to be taken to a local animal shelter for treatment before release to the owner. This was possible, since in Los Angeles County, special animal health ordinances give the health officer authority over infectious animal diseases. The health officer has authority to quarantine, examine, test, and destroy animals that may carry an infectious disease and pose a risk to the human or animal community. Related ordinances are an asset for the program, since they allow the local public health agency to support federal agencies when they encounter potentially infectious animals.

■ EVALUATION STRATEGY

Since the development of the collaborative, three separate animal importation assessments have been conducted; first to determine if there was a problem with health certificates that accompany imported animals, later to determine the impact of education and previous enforcement. During each assessment period and inspection, the officers examined both animals and related paperwork. Copies of manifests, shipping documents, and health certificates were kept for comparison with direct examination findings.

TABLE 18–2 *LAX Animal Importation Annual Assessment Results*

	First Survey	Second Survey	Third Survey
Length of Survey	3 weeks	2 weeks	2 weeks
# Animals Inspected	6048	118	337
# Dogs Inspected	183	118	126
# Multi-Dog Shipments (4 or more)	3	6	8
# (%) Dogs Younger than Listed Age	71 (39%)	12 (10%)	50 (40%)

Data were examined to determine if the percentage of animals and shipments with health certificate problems lessened after increased educational and enforcement efforts. The number of multi-dog shipments (4 or greater) increased during each subsequent survey, and those with incorrectly noted ages dropped between the first and second survey, only to rise again by the third survey (see Table 18–2). In 2008, the CDC QT identified 285 multi-dog shipments (4 or more dogs in a single shipment), totaling 2,878 dogs (12). By 2010, the number of large shipments decreased to 220, with 1,723 dogs. By 2011, only a few importers continued to bring in multi-dog shipments on a frequent basis.

During the surveys, almost half of the dog shipments came from countries considered "rabies free" (Australia, New Zealand, UK). These do not require proof of rabies vaccination prior to shipment; however, a current health certificate is required. No problems were noted with them. But problems arose for puppies imported from rabies endemic countries, with Yorkshire terriers from Korea and Brazil, and bulldogs from Hungary and Colombia being most problematic. The surveys revealed that falsified health certificates continue as a problem for multi-dog shipments, even after efforts to educate airline companies and importers. Due to the massive volume of imported wildlife, staff could examine only a small sample of those shipments. Reliance on health certificates only, without physical inspections of the animals from rabies endemic countries, poses a risk of rabies and other animal disease importations.

■ IMPACT

The LAX collaborative demonstrates the value of local and federal agency cooperation to oversee animal imports. The task force achieved more than its original goal to identify and document problems in the animal importation system. The initiative has been a conduit for increasing communication among separate oversight agencies, leveraging local resources, and creating more thorough follow-up on problematic shipments.

The first assessment uncovered major problems with falsified animal health certificates, specifically for large shipments of puppies. CDC QT staff continue to conduct spot checks of multi-dog shipments or those via frequent importers. The staff talked with airline peresonnel and importers to ensure awareness of legal requirements. They received additional information on how to estimate the age of dogs and symptoms of significant illnesses. Greater local follow-up verified importers' compliance with confinement agreements. However, subsequent surveys show that though the proportion of dogs with incorrect ages on their health certificates initially declined, they later increased again. CDC QT indicates no apparent increase in dog shipments through other airports, but an additional study will be undertaken to examine national data. It is possible that some puppy importers switched from overseas breeding to local kennels, which we surmise because following the first survey, VPH-RCP and CDC QT staff noted a large increase in shipments of older female dogs from countries where most of the imported puppies had originated. Although this could cause problems for local animal control agencies, such new facilities may be better regulated.

More shipments must be inspected to markedly reduce the problem of falsified health certificates, and expansion of the federal-local partnership should accomplish this. VPH-RCP staff obtained LAX badges so that they might assist with inspections in secure areas. The creation of an LAX Animal Importation Work Group will develop new protocols to increase cooperation among agencies and local assistance. VPH-RCP and CDC QT obtained a joint CDC public health associate for two years to bridge the two agencies. By participating in the third survey, investigating problem shipments, and overseeing local enforcement of CDC dog importation confinement notices, this associate has in-depth understanding of all steps in the process and provides recommendations on improving the system.

The U.S. Government Accountability Office (GAO) report on Live Animal Importation recommends greater federal interagency collaboration and has led to stronger support for expansion of this program (7). The LAX Animal Importation Collaborative serves as a model for federal-local partnership to address this issue and safeguard both animals and the public.

■ CONCLUSIONS

The experience of this collaboration on animal importation provides a number of important lessons and approaches, including:

Importance of a collaborative approach:

- Complex animal importation problems can only be addressed and mitigated through extensive collaboration among all local and federal agencies involved in the importation process.
- To maximize collaboration, it is important to emphasize positive solutions to problems rather than cite problems to criticize other agencies.
- Local agencies may provide valuable support to safeguard the country against imported animal disease threats by assisting in national efforts to enforce CDC dog confinement agreements, investigating reports of illness in imported animals, and alerting state and federal agencies when unusual diseases are identified.
- Local agencies in communities with international ports (especially air or land ports), should reach out to federal agencies to determine how best to support importation oversight or provide needed animal quarantine sites.

Quantification of the problem and highlighting the concerns regarding animal importation:

- Careful assessments can quantify a problem and be used to secure and maintain support.
- Recognition that animal importation sometimes serves as a conduit for the introduction of new diseases, foreign animal diseases, and zoonoses that endanger both humans and animals.

- Procedures for inspections, even those that are risk-based, may result in insufficient inspections of imported shipments.
- Official foreign certificates may not be accurate and, therefore, should not be used as the sole means to clear imported shipments.
- Strategically conducted surveys and follow-up monitoring help to quantify the magnitude of importation problems, and help to identify possible interventions.
- Local communities may be impacted if current animal importation screening methods fail to identify ill or unvaccinated animals.

Identification of obstacles and possible solutions:

- A mechanism for payment of quarantined animals needs to be identified to avoid animals being abandoned by shippers when local or federal agencies order animals to be quarantined. One solution could be to create or increase fees for importing animals; those fees then may be used to pay for the care of abandoned quarantined animals.
- The problems associated with animal importation also need to be addressed by federal policy and regulations since, by "hardening" surveillance and enforcement of animal importation regulations at one international airport, animal importers may simply shift their shipments to other, less monitored, airports. In some European countries, for example, governments have policies restricting the number of airports through which an animal from another county can be imported. In this way, it is possible to more efficiently monitor importations and to train staff who can estimate ages of animals and assess whether or not they appear ill.

ACKNOWLEDGMENTS

We thank Kimberly Crocker, Alberto Pina and Jackaleen Chapman, as well as the staff at CDC QT and VPH-RCP, for their assistance with creating this collaboration.

REFERENCES

1. Taylor LH, Latham SM and Woolhouse MEJ. Risk factors for human disease emergence. *Phil Trans R Soc Lond B.* 2001;356:983–9.
2. Ehnert K, Galland GG. Border Health: Who's guarding the gate? *Vet Clin Small Anim.* 2009;39:359–72.
3. Marano N, Arguin PM, Pappaioanou M. Impact of globalization and animal trade on infectious disease ecology. *Emerg Infect Dis.* 2007;13(12):1807–9.
4. Labonte R, Mohindra K and Schrecker T. The growing impact of globalization for health and public health practice. *Annu Rev Public Health.* 2011 Apr 21;32:263–83.
5. Jenkins PT, Genovese K, Ruffler H. *Broken Screens: The Regulation of Live Animal Importation in the United States.*Washington, DC: Defenders of Wildlife; 2007. Available from: http://www.defenders.org/resources/publications/programs_and_policy/international_conservation/broken_screens/broken_screens_report.pdf (accessed Feb. 16, 2008).
6. Marsh Report. *The Economic and Social Impact of Emerging Infectious Disease: Mitigation Through Detection, Research, and Response.* 2008. Available from: http://www.healthcare.philips.com/main/shared/assets/documents/bioshield/ecoandsocialimpactofemerginginfectiousdisease_111208.pdf (accessed May 16, 2011).

7. GAO. *Live Animal Imports: Agencies Need Better Collaboration to Reduce the Risk of Animal-related Diseases,* GAO-11-9. Washington, DC: November 2010.
8. Guarner J, Johnson BJ, Paddock CD et. al. Monkeypox transmission and pathogenesis in prairie dogs. *Emerg Infect Dis.* 2004;10(3):426–31.
9. McQuiston JH, Wilson T, Harris S, et al. Importation of dogs into the United States: Risks from rabies and other zoonotic diseases. *Zoonoses Public Health.* April 02, 2008. Published online. Available from: http://www.blackwell-synergy.com/doi/abs/10.1111/j.1863-2378.2008.01117.x (accessed April 6, 2008).
10. Wilson E, Eetherall K. Is it just another worble? *California Veterinarian.* Jan–Feb 2008;62(1):14–5.
11. Los Angeles County Department of Public Health, Veterinary Public Health and Rabies Control, unpublished data.
12. Centers for Disease Control and Prevention, Los Angeles International Airport Quarantine Station, unpublished data.

19 Safe Food Facilities

Reestablishing Public Confidence Through Letter Grades

HECTOR DELA CRUZ, TERRANCE POWELL, AND JONATHAN E. FIELDING

THE NATURE OF THE PROBLEM

In November 1998, a local CBS News exposé on unsanitary conditions at local restaurants captivated Los Angeles County (LAC) residents with images of vermin and alarming employee practices. The exposé used sensational video clips captured with an undercover camera to question the effectiveness and reliability of LAC Environmental Health (EH) restaurant inspections. Residents were led to believe that conditions reported were commonplace throughout LAC and that reports were not easily accessible.

Emotional public reaction to the exposé was shared by the County Board of Supervisors, who are vested with both administrative and legislative authority. While inspection results had always been available upon request, this constituted very limited transparency and offered little value to the restaurant-going public. Under this inspection system, the primary incentive for restaurant owners was to avoid code violations serious enough to lead to closure (1). The Board of Supervisors directed the LAC Department of Public Health (DPH) to rapidly restore public confidence through an improved inspection system with clarity and transparency of results to the general public.

CONTEXT

Although prior television news segments featured various aspects of restaurant inspections, none had piqued public interest like the CBS exposé. Not only did it raise the station's ratings, but CBS also capitalized on this popularity by running daily follow-up segments that continued to fuel public outrage.

Although LAC Supervisors historically considered the concerns of business owners before calling for policy changes in any of its enforcement divisions, the directive clearly reflected public sentiment, and the LAC Board of Supervisors did not solicit input from food industry stakeholders. Thus the department was operating in an unusual political environment where the revised program could be based solely on the best-known science and strong economic incentives, without concern for resistance from industry groups that recognized the need to restore public confidence in food service rather than negotiate or lobby for more lenient inspection standards.

APPROACH TO THE PROBLEM

A key aspect of the new program would address the misperception of secrecy and help to restore public confidence in the food inspection program. Essential were a system of public disclosure and ease of access to that information. The department leadership, working with EH, explored how to display the results of inspections in a manner easy for consumers to grasp. This led to the decision to implement an easy-to-recognize letter grading system, with the issuance of a letter grade to each food facility, based on its inspection score.

The model called for raising the visibility of the established practice of starting each food facility inspection with the score of 100 and deducting points for each problem based on its severity and link to risk of food-borne illness. Assuming that all residents could relate viscerally to grading letters widely used in the public school system, an ABC ranking was adopted, wherein inspection scores from 90–100 receive an "A," 80–89 a "B," and 70–79 a "C" (see Figure 19-1). Those with grades below 70, which were unlikely to remain open without fast and substantial improvements in food safety, received numerical grades.

Several other jurisdictions previously had adopted similar grading, but Los Angeles was the first to issue quantitative risk assessment grades to assure consistent results. Risk-based inspections place greater value on factors directly linked to the prevention of food-borne illnesses. Such risk factors include food from unsafe sources, inadequate cooking, improper holding temperatures, contaminated equipment, and poor personal hygiene (2). Therefore, higher numerical outcomes suggest that a food facility received fewer point deductions due to its superior food safety practices.

Since the existing inspection form was not designed for inspections to lead to final numerical scores and subsequent letter grades, EH redesigned it to create a risk-based scoring system that clearly prioritized food safety practices causally linked to food-borne illness (see Figure 19-2). The retooled inspection report form assigned point values to violation categories commensurate with their level of food-borne illness risk, as identified by the Centers for Disease Control and Prevention. For example, hand washing was divided into three violation categories, with each category assigned a risk-based point value. If a facility had no sinks available for hand washing, that was considered a high-risk violation and resulted in a six-point deduction. Facilities with only one hand washing sink inaccessible as a result of being blocked by hard-to-move items received a four-point deduction as a moderate risk violation. A low risk hand

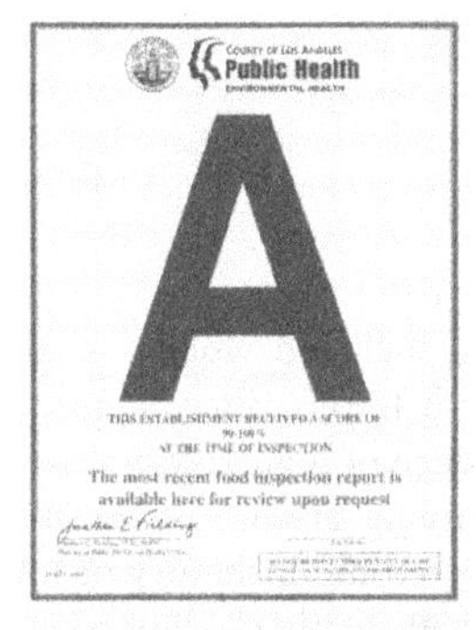

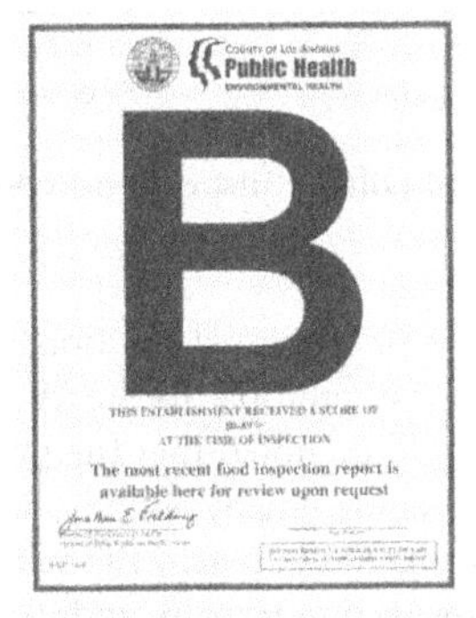

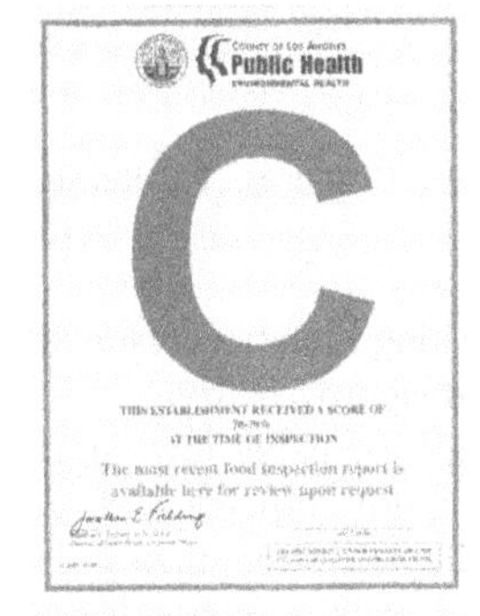

Figure 19-1 LAC Food Facility Letter Grades.

DATE VIOLATIONS CORRECTED | EHS INITIALS | OPERATOR INITIALS

SCORE | GRADE

TIME OUT: | TIME IN: | INSPECTION DATE: | COMPLIANCE DATE(S): | EHS: (PRINT) | EHS: (SIGNATURE) | BUS. E-MAIL ADDRESS: | TOTAL PAGES: | 004 | 002 | 001 | OTHER:

ZIP CODE: | POSITION: | SERVICE

CITY / STATE: | (SIGNATURE) | EMERGENCY PHONE #: | PROGRAM ELEMENT: | SITE #:

DBA / NAME: | ADDRESS: | PERMIT HOLDER: | RECEIVED BY: (PRINT) | BUSINESS PHONE #: | EXPIRATION YEAR:

ENVIRONMENTAL HEALTH OFFICE | PERMIT #: | SUBDISTRICT: | DISTRICT:

RETAIL FOOD OFFICIAL INSPECTION REPORT

COUNTY OF LOS ANGELES ❖ DEPARTMENT OF PUBLIC HEALTH
ENVIRONMENTAL HEALTH

☐ No Violations Observed At Time Of Inspection ☐ Complaint Allegations Not Observed

OUT=Out of Compliance **N/A**=Not Applicable **N/O**=Not Observed **COS**=Corrected On Site

SECTION I

(POINT VALUE – 6 POINTS FOR VIOLATIONS IN EACH CATEGORY IN SECTION I – MAXIMUM POINTS DEDUCTIBLE = 36) POINTS

OUT	N/A	N/O	COS	FOOD TEMPERATURES	OUT	N/A	N/O	COS	FOOD
1	2	3	4	1. Holding of PHF - Multiple Servings (Major)	37			40	10. Adulterated Food (Major)
5	6	7	8	2. Holding of Unpasteurized Pooled Eggs	41	42		44	11. Highly Susceptible Populations
9	10	11	12	3. Cooking	45	46		48	12. Unapproved Source - PHF (Major)
13	14	15	16	4. Reheating (Major)	OUT	N/A	N/O	COS	VERMIN
17	18	19	20	5. Cooling (Major)	49				13. Rodents (Major)
OUT	N/A	N/O	COS	EMPLOYEE HEALTH	53				14. Cockroaches (Major)
21			24	6. Disease Transmission – Carrier/ Wound (Major)	57				15. Flies (Major)
25			28	7. Hand Washing (Major)	OUT	N/A	N/O	COS	WATER / SANITIZATION
OUT	N/A	N/O	COS	SEWAGE	61	62	63	64	16. Cleaning / Sanitizing – Food Contact Surfaces (Major)
29				8. Sewage Disposal System (Major)	65			68	17. No Water / No Hot Water – Food Preparation Facility (Major)
33				9. Toilets (Major)					

SECTION II

(POINT VALUE – 4 POINTS FOR VIOLATIONS IN EACH CATEGORY IN SECTION II – MAXIMUM POINTS DEDUCTIBLE = 26) POINTS

OUT	N/A	N/O	COS	FOOD TEMPERATURES	OUT	N/A	N/O	COS	FOOD
69	70	71	72	18. Holding of PHF – Multiple Servings (Minor)	105			108	27. Risk For Contamination
73	74	75	76	19. Holding of PHF – A Single Serving (Minor)	109			112	28. Unapproved Source – Non-PHF (Minor)
77	78	79	80	20. Holding of Unpasteurized Raw Shell Eggs	113	114		116	29. Reused / Re-served
81	82	83	84	21. Cooling / Reheating – Improper Method (Minor)	OUT	N/A	N/O	COS	OPERATIONS
OUT	N/A	N/O	COS	FOOD STORAGE	117			120	30. Hazardous Materials / Chemicals (Major)
85			88	22. Improperly Covered / Labeled / Elevated	121		123	124	31. Employee Practices (Minor)
89	90		92	23. Raw/Ready to Eat Food – Exposed to Possible Cross-Contamination	OUT	N/A	N/O	COS	CONSUMER PROTECTION
93			96	24. Food Not Protected From Consumer	125	126	127	128	32. Gulf Coast Oyster Warning Signs
OUT	N/A	N/O	COS	PLUMBING / FIXTURES	129			132	33. Labels / Misrepresented – Consumer Foods
97			100	25. Backflow / Back Siphonage	133	134	135	136	34. Disclosure Notification
101			104	26. Critical Sink/Fixture (Hand Washing / Janitorial / Food Preparation)	OUT	N/A	N/O	COS	FOOD SAFETY CERTIFICATE
					137	138	139		35. Valid Food Safety Certification

SECTION III

(POINT VALUE – 1 POINT VIOLATION FOR EACH SUBCATEGORY IN SECTION III – MAXIMUM POINTS DEDUCTIBLE = 36) POINTS

OUT	FOOD / METHODS	OUT	VERMIN
141	36. Thawing	161	56. Rodents (Minor)
142	37. Adulterated Food (Minor)	162	57. Cockroaches (Minor)
143	38. Improper Inspection at Delivery / Transportation	163	58. Flies/Other Insects (Minor)
OUT	OPERATIONS	164	59. Open Door / Air Curtain / Not Fully Enclosed
144	39. Customer Self-Service Utensils	OUT	PLUMBING / FIXTURES / EQUIPMENT
145	40. Hand Washing (Minor)	165	60. Sinks / Fixtures / Supply Line
146	41. Hair Restraints / Outer Garments / Nails / Rings		
147	42. Shellfish Tags / Labels	166	61. Drain Lines / Floor Sinks / Floor Drains
148	43. Hazardous Materials / Chemicals (Minor)		
149	44. Spoils Area	167	62. No Hot or Warm Water (Minor)
150	45. Interior Premises / Linens / Living – Sleeping Quarters	OUT	VENTILATION / LIGHTING
151	46. Animal / Pets	168	63. Hood – Not Clean / Disrepair / Missing Filter(s)
OUT	UTENSILS / EQUIPMENT / SHELVING / CABINETS	169	64. Hood – Missing / Incorrect Type / Improper Installation
152	47. Disrepair	170	65. Ventilation – General
153	48. Cleaning – Non-Food Contact Surfaces	171	66. Lighting / Light Shields
154	49. Storage	OUT	TOILETS / DRESSING ROOMS
155	50. Unapproved Type / Improper Use / Improper Installation	172	67. Toilets / Toilet Rooms (Minor)
156	51. Wiping Cloths		
157	52. Cleaning / Sanitizing – Food Contact Surfaces (Minor)	173	68. Dressing Room / Personal Items
158	53. Thermometer	OUT	REFUSE / PREMISES / JANITORIAL
OUT	WALLS / CEILINGS / FLOORS	174	69. Janitorial – Storage & Conditions
159	54. Deterioration / Unapproved Materials	175	70. Refuse / Containers
160	55. Not Clean	176	71. Exterior Premises

See Reverse Side For The General Requirements That Correspond To Each Violation Listed Above | **PAGE 1**

ORIGINAL

Figure 19-2 LAC EH Retail Food Official Inspection Report.

washing violation resulted in a one point deduction and included violations such as unapproved drying devices (i.e. multiple use terry cloth towels versus approved single use paper towels). It should be noted that the presence of high-risk violations may also coincide with other enforcement actions, including closure of the food facility. To strengthen the risk-based approach, EH reassessed the inventory of LAC food facilities to establish an inspection priority and more efficiently use limited staff resources. The existing policy was that all food facilities receive the same number of annual inspections, regardless of their level of food handling and type of foods sold. This resulted in food facilities selling only pre-packaged foods (e.g., liquor stores) receiving the same number of annual routine inspections as restaurants offering a full menu of prepared dishes for breakfast, lunch, and dinner. Under the new policy, each facility is evaluated to assess its level of food handling and to determine an appropriate inspection frequency. Inspections now range from one to three per year. As added performance criteria, facilities ordered to close or with repeated inspection scores below a "C" within the past 12 months receive one more inspection in addition to their established inspection frequency until marked improvement is noted.

Providing the public with quick and easy access to inspection results is paramount for establishing program transparency. Signs advising concerned consumers to contact the local LAC EH office were developed to display with letter grades in all food facilities. In addition, inspection results were made available on the Department's web page, and LAC Code Title 8 was amended to require each facility to provide a copy of its most recent inspection report upon request for anyone to view. Thus facility operators were prevented from representing problems in their facilities as less serious than in reality because consumers could verify the facts on the inspection reports.

Food safety training for foodservice managers and employees can have positive impact on regulatory compliance (3, 4). A key element of the grading and enforcement program is to assure that each facility possess fundamental knowledge of food safety principals. LAC Code Title 11 was amended to require that each facility have at least one certified food handler (CFH) onsite during all hours of operation. The code required that CFHs successfully complete, every three years, an eight-hour course approved by the Department, inclusive of safe practices in food preparation and control of storm water pollution (1).

Although the political climate favored these sweeping changes exclusive of industry input, the Department solicited input from local and state food industry associations to lay a foundation for future partnerships addressing emergent food safety issues. Meetings were hosted to receive food industry concerns. Restaurateurs were particularly upset about a grading system that assigned letter grades based solely on their performance during the most recent routine inspection. Restaurateurs held that performance on any given day could be atypical for any number of unforeseen circumstances and that letter grades were unfairly based on a "snapshot."

Addressing this, the department agreed to include an optional "owner initiated inspection" (OII) feature in its proposal to the Board of Supervisors. This allowed each facility to request a new inspection if it received an undesirable grade during a previous routine inspection. These inspections require an additional fee, may only be requested once each 12 months, and lead to two unannounced supplemental inspections within 60 days. Both supplemental inspections result in newly posted grades, whether they are an improvement or a downgrade from the prior inspection.

Industry stakeholders also expressed concern about inconsistent code enforcement among food inspectors. Although LAC EH's three-month training program for newly hired inspectors helped establish core competencies, and supervisors were available to answer questions from line inspectors, examination of inspection results when inspectors switched territories suggested that this was a legitimate concern. Responding, the department established a quality assurance unit to better standardize enforcement, and an ombudsman to address complaints of serious inspector errors or unprofessional behavior.

IMPLEMENTATION

The State of California Health and Safety Code allowed for local jurisdictions to establish their own retail food facilities public disclosure grading programs. LAC Supervisors quickly passed Ordinance 97–0071 to amend LAC Code, Title 8, and authorize mandatory letter grading. The ordinance required letter grading at all facilities located in LAC's unincorporated areas, covering 2,600 square miles with over 1 million residents; however, executing the new requirement in the 85 incorporated cities within the department's jurisdiction required approval of each city council.

Initially, in cities where the ordinance had not been adopted, many restaurateurs took advantage of the fact that the grading program was voluntary and only displayed their letter grade if it was an "A", removing any "B," "C," or numerical grade. LAC EH addressed this by no longer requiring grade posting in cities where the ordinance for mandatory posting was not yet adopted. This decision increased demand by residents in those cities for their elected officials to adopt the ordinance, while food facility operators simultaneously urged the same city leaders to reject it. Letter grading proved popular with consumers, and residents prevailed. All cities adopted the ordinance with the exception of several having very few food facilities within their boundaries. These remaining cities have a combined total of only 0.4% of LAC's approximately 39,000 retail food facilities.

In the face of mandatory grading's influence on business, retail facilities were motivated to make sure the program treated all fairly and equally. Improving industry confidence in the inspection program was also a priority of the department. With the EH Division, DPH created the Bureau of Special Operations (BSO) and its component units, Quality Assurance and Compliance (QAC), Consultation and Techinical Services (CTS), and the Office of the Ombudsman. These new units centralized support services for stakeholders. Prior to establishing BSO, industry concerns regarding the inspection process and requests for consultative services were addressed by the same district offices responsible for routine and complaint retail facility inspections. BSO's creation allowed district offices to operate more efficiently, handling responsibility for investigating allegations of field inspector errors and for providing consulting services to the retail food industry.

QAC became the unit solely responsible for standardizing inspection protocols and grading. This centralized approach decreased the inconsistent application of laws and department policies, and also became an efficient alternative to disparate district efforts to improve standardization. In four years, QAC conducted over 447 field audits and reviewed office procedures of all 22 district offices to assure adherence to departmental policies. Within five years of inception, QAC, under direction of the Ombudsman, investigated and resolved 118 cases of citizen and industry complaints about the inspection process and/or personnel.

Inspection accuracy and comprehensiveness has always been a department concern. Preexisting unannounced field audits (conducted by supervision immediately following routine inspections by staff) provided only limited assurance that inspector demeanor and findings were consistent with policies regarding integrity and comprehensiveness. Additional measures were implemented to enhance this. Field reviews wherein supervisory staff conduct side-by-side inspections with food inspectors added one more element of consistency and training in the actual work environment. A policy mandating the routine rotation of inspection territories for inspection staff reduced subjectivity that can occur from over familiarity and/or personal relationships developed over time with facility operators. A 24-hour hotline allowed the public and facility operators to report complaints about facilities as well as inspection staff. As EH learns of issues from these complaints, it updates inspection policies and provides additional related staff training. The result is more consistent inspection protocols.

Centralizing standardizations into one unit provided EH with the ability to respond quickly and efficiently to a state standardization task force recommendation that called for local jurisdictions to standardize food inspections. QAC completed performance reviews of all supervisorial inspection staff to assure that their performance met state recommendations and to establish them as primary instructors handling performance reviews of subordinate inspection staff. Supervisors then conducted extensive trainings for their subordinate inspectors, including concurrent facility inspections, to assure full compliance with state recommendations and ensure food inspection program consistency.

Active management is essential to control food-borne illness risk factors. Regulators must assist operators in developing and implementing strategies to strengthen existing systems to prevent the occurrence of risk factors (2). Thus CTS helped industry representatives to establish controls and to understand the inspection process through multilingual outreach efforts. In its first four years, CTS:

- Developed and translated a 70 page inspection guidebook into Chinese, Japanese, Korean, and Spanish.
- Distributed the guidebook to owners and employees of over 38,000 food establishments.
- Conducted over 360 food safety and inspection workshops attended by over 10,000 industry stakeholders.
    - Over 70 workshops were conducted in a foreign language (Chinese, Korean, Japanese, Russian, Thai, and Spanish) and attended by over 1,700 stakeholders.
- Provided technical assistance and expertise by conducting over 1,500 consultations with stakeholders.
- Participated in 95 community fairs and professional expositions at which over 210,000 domestic food safety bulletins in several languages were distributed.
- Established partnerships with key organizations including: Asian Pacific Islander Small Business Association, Office of the Japanese Consulate, Japanese Restaurant Association, Black Restaurant Association, Korean American Business Association, Thai Restaurant Association, and California Restaurant Association.

■ EVALUATION STRATEGY

Two years after the new system was implemented, the LAC Board of Supervisors directed LAC EH to survey county residents about their opinions of the food facility grading system and whether it influenced their out-of-home dining habits. EH developed a questionnaire that included a telephone script and contracted with a private company to survey a random sample of 2,000 LAC residents in both English and Spanish. The company used random digit dialing to contact county residents and conducted the survey with adults who agreed to participate.

Survey results reflected a favorable response among residents, with 91% of respondents reporting that they liked the grading system. Public awareness of letter grades was also high, with 77% of respondents reporting that they noticed posted grades always or most of the time. Grading also restored public confidence, as 86% of respondents believed that grading had been very or somewhat effective in improving sanitary conditions in restaurants and food markets. Dining choices were also influenced by the grading system, with 88% reporting that they would eat or purchase food from an "A" rated facility always or most of the time, compared to 25% from a "B" rated facility and only 3% from a "C" rated facility.

A subsequent quantitative analysis explored the effect of increased consumer information on the behavior of food facilities. Jin and Leslie (2003) analyzed the effect of increased product information on facilities' product quality choices by studying the impact of LAC letter grading (5). Mandatory posting of grade cards for an "A" rated restaurant resulted in a 5.7% increase in revenue, compared to revenue before the introduction of grade cards. "B" rated restaurants increased revenue by 0.7% and "C" rated restaurants experienced a decrease of 1% in revenue (5). Jin and Leslie suggested that this underlying economic incentive influenced a restaurant's choice to increase hygiene quality.

Several restaurant chains responded to the grading system's popularity by instituting performance incentives tied to grade cards. Restaurants gave managers bonuses based on whether or not a food facility received an "A" grade. Many single site restaurants reported slower business if they received letter grades below an "A"; however, this effect was not consistent in all cities and neighborhoods. Many ethnic communities continued to patronize facilities posting "B" and "C" grades, especially Asian communities and neighborhoods with a limited choice of restaurants and food markets.

Comments from community stakeholders such as the American Chinese Restaurant Association attributed continued patronage at "B" and "C" restaurants to customer priorities for quantity and price versus food safety. Coalitions within the Chinese community, recognizing a prevalence of "B" and "C" restaurants and concerns over negative perceptions of Chinese restaurants, partnered with LAC EH to initiate food safety training courses and onsite consultations for Chinese restaurant operators.

■ IMPACT

Public outcry after the television exposé was the impetus for the program inception, and public approval drives its continued popularity. Following implementation of grading and its associated program enhancements, the State of California Health and Safety Code was amended to include key elements from LAC. California incorporated the mandatory food handler certification requirement (LAC Code Title 11 [1998]) into state law in 2000. Although it bolstered food safety efforts in many local jurisdictions, the state law was significantly less stringent than LAC's. LAC required each food facility to have a CFH onsite during all hours of operation, whereas state law called for each food facility to simply have a designated CFH and did not require one to always be present.

State law also adopted LAC's approach to food inspection reports, making it mandatory for all local jurisdictions to use risk-based reports. Many jurisdictions used LAC's report for reference in developing complaint inspection report forms.

Public disclosure aspects of grading also influenced disclosure regulations in state law, a further reflection of the public's healthy appetite for government transparency. internet disclosure of inspection results and onsite inspection report availability were added to the State Health and Safety Code, making LAC's practice and easily accessible consumer information a statewide mandate.

The impact of grading and increased transparency of inspection results is felt both locally and nationally. Locally, in 2010 DPH expanded the food facility grading system to include mobile food facilities. The grading system's popularity also led to a similar model for LAC EH's Recreational Waters program where letter grades are assigned to county beaches based on water quality. Nationally, the public disclosure trend in food inspections has grown, and jurisdictions such as New York City and Albuquerque, New Mexico, have adopted aspects of the LAC grading system.

The most important evaluation question is whether the new system could better protect consumers from food-borne illnesses. An analysis of hospital discharge data on food-borne disease hospitalizations found the grading program was associated with a 13.1% decrease in the number of food-borne disease hospitalizations in LAC the year following program implementation, compared to all surrounding counties (6). The decrease was sustained over the next two years, and the results strongly suggest that grading was an effective intervention for reducing food-borne disease. To the best of our knowledge, LAC's program is the first retail food facility environmental protection program to demonstrate health improvements. As the move toward public disclosure, transparency, and evidence-based interventions continues, the LAC model may serve as a very useful case study for jurisdictions considering similar systems.

■ CONCLUSIONS

This program yielded many important lessons:

- Never let a good crisis go to waste. A crisis may present an opportune political climate to implement sweeping changes to an outdated system.
- Communicate with stakeholders early to form productive and supportive collaborations. This also creates common ownership of new policies and programs.
- Develop clear messages and outreach to the public that clarify program processes and goals, including why specific efforts will benefit them.
- Solicit feedback from all stakeholders to make timely program adjustments.
- Public approval can be just as powerful as public outcry. Be creative in making visibility work to your advantage and maintain a high degree of program transparency of inspection outcomes and policies.
- Refine programs over time. A static program does not respond to changes in the regulatory landscape or maximize efficiency and effectiveness.
- Developing a program identity or brand popular with all consumers greatly increases the visibility of the public health function and helps dispel the assumption that we only serve the poor.

REFERENCES

1. Fielding JE, Aguirre A, Palaiologos E. Effectiveness of altered incentives in a food safety inspection program. *Prev Med.* 2001;32(3):239–44.
2. U.S. Department of Health and Human Services. *2009 Food Code.* Washington, DC: Public Health Service, Food and Drug Administration; 2009.
3. Henroid D, Sneed J. Readiness to implement hazard analysis and critical control point (HACCP) systems in Iowa Schools. *J Am Diet Assoc.* 2004;104(2):180–5.
4. Cotterchio M, Gunn J, Coffill T, Tormey P, Barry MA. Effect of a manager training program on sanitary conditions in restaurants. *Public Health Rep.* 1998;113(4):353–8.
5. Jin GZ, Leslie P. The effect of information on product quality: Evidence from restaurant hygiene grade cards. *Qtrly J Econ.* 2003;118(2):409–51.
6. Simon PA, Leslie P, Run G, Jin GZ, Reporter R, Aguirre A, Fielding JE. Impact of restaurant hygiene grade cards on foodborne-disease hospitalizations in Los Angeles County. *J Environ Health.* 2005;67(7):32–6.

20 Food Product Recalls

Effective Local Response

HECTOR DELA CRUZ AND
TERRANCE POWELL

THE NATURE OF THE PROBLEM

Producing food on the farm, field, or processing plant has always presented challenges in controlling biological, chemical, and physical contamination. When contamination does occur, timely identification and removal of implicated foods from commerce is necessary to ensure public health and safety. Food product recalls play a critical role in accomplishing this task.

The success of food product recalls depends upon how completely, rapidly, and effectively products are removed from commerce and residences. Federal and state agencies may expedite the process by communicating information to industry stakeholders, local government agencies, and the general public; however, their efforts do not guarantee product removal. A 2004 Government Accountability Office report revealed that the Food and Drug Administration (FDA) and U.S. Department of Agriculture (USDA) are unaware of how promptly and completely food recalls are executed (1). Verification checks of product removal can help ensure that recalled foods do not reach consumers and are necessary if recall information is not communicated in a timely manner, or if there is likely to be a failure to remove implicated foods from commerce when information is received. Verification checks and product removal are often the last safety net before recalled foods are consumed.

Although recalls that stem from illness outbreaks carry a high profile, a significant number of food recalls result from undeclared allergens (2) as the USDA recently issued instructions to its inspection program personnel in an effort to reduce allergen and other ingredient-related recalls (3). The number of food recalls addressed by Los Angeles County (LAC) Environmental Health Department (EHD) increased in recent years, with a dramatic recent rise that may be partially attributed to increases in the number of recalls for undeclared allergens. In 2009, EHD responded to 431 recalls, versus 87 recalls in 2008, and 78 recalls in 2007. Since the responsibility for removing recalled products rests primarily with the food industry that typically does not add staff solely to assure that recalled foods are removed from the distribution chain, the greater number of recall events increased the probability of recalled foods remaining in commerce, requiring EHD to conduct more recall verification checks.

CONTEXT

Recalls are classified by the FDA as class I, II, or III. *Class I recalls* involve a reasonable probability that the consumption of an implicated food product will cause serious adverse health consequences or death. *Class II recalls* occur when consumption of an implicated food product may cause temporary or medically reversible adverse health consequences or where such probability is remote. *Class III recalls* are situations in which consumption of an implicated product is not likely to cause adverse health consequences (4).

For all recall classifications, regulatory agencies and food industry share the task of providing timely recall information to affected food facilities and consumers. Federal, state, and local agencies accomplish this through press releases, public service announcements, and direct communication with industry stakeholders. Although emphasis is placed on communicating critical information, such news may not be communicated as expeditiously as needed to minimize consumption of the product, and it does not guarantee that corrective actions will be taken. Removing food from commerce falls squarely on the food industry, which bares sole responsibility for identifying, segregating, and verifying the exclusion of recalled foods. As the number of recalls increases, industry's responsibility becomes more labor-intensive and time-consuming, increasing the probability for errors. The net result is increased risk to consumers as recalled foods remain in markets and restaurants for longer periods of time.

Although federal and state laws do not require local jurisdictions to verify recalled food removal from commerce, EHD's experience with previous recall events uncovered numerous occasions when recalled foods were still offered for sale. These events led EHD to start recall verification checks for product removal, enhancing its existing services related to retail food inspections (managed by its Bureau of District Surveillance and Enforcement [DSE]) and wholesale food inspections (managed by its Food and Milk Program [FM]).

■ APPROACH TO THE PROBLEM

Historically, local enforcement agencies (LEAs) rely solely on producers, wholesalers, distributors, and retailers to effectively execute food recalls. In California, LEAs are not mandated to conduct verification checks or to report recall findings to the state Department of Public Health. As a result, the state receives a very limited amount of information from LEAs and does not generate verification check summaries for recall events. This has made it difficult to assess the efficacy of verification checks or to determine whether they add value to consumer protection efforts.

To address this gap in consumer protection, EHD developed a functional structure to assure timely and appropriate actions. A coordinated effort was established involving DSE's retail food inspection program and FM's wholesale food inspection program. Both programs were needed to assure that EHD's retail food inventory of over 39,000 facilities and wholesale food inventory of over 1,200 facilities would both be covered. This allowed for a single line of communication between facilities and the program responsible for their oversight.

EHD receives notification of recall events from state and federal agencies, in addition to industry partners. In the absence of passive notification, FM actively surveys internet websites to secure information related to current recall events. Upon notification of a recall event, the effort between DSE and FM requires that FM contact the state, manufacturer, and/or distributor to secure a list of where the implicated product was produced, stored, and sold in LAC. Once a list is secured, facilities on the list are contacted by FM via telephone surveys to facilitate communication of recall information, and to assess whether implicated product may still be in commerce. If facilities are not aware of the recall event, report having recalled food in commerce, or FM has reason to suspect that a facility is not forthright with its response, field verification checks of product removal are then conducted. In-person verification of product removal ensures that recalled foods are removed from commerce and eliminates uncertainty about recalled foods still being offered to consumers (see Figure 20–1).

Although DSE is intimately familiar with retail food facilities, its field inspection staff largely comprises new hires and less seasoned inspectors. By assigning to FM the initial task of following up recall notifications, EHD capitalized on the experience of seasoned staff already familiar with state, federal, and industry partners. FM's responsibility also simplified the flow of information within the department, helping to overcome the challenge of disjointed communication within a large agency of over 200 food inspection personnel.

To complement the structured recall response, a comprehensive recall database is being completed to give EHD the ability to electronically capture data related to telephone surveys and field verification check activities, in addition to providing information on recalled products and their manufacturers. EHD will use the data collected by analyzing how recall events are managed to identify ways to improve (i.e., analysis of staffing hours, cost effectiveness, and appropriate staffing levels). Additionally, EHD will be able to review a recall event's impact by geocoding. For example, if large amounts of recalled products are found on retail shelves of a community where Spanish is mainly spoken, it may reveal ways to improve recall communication.

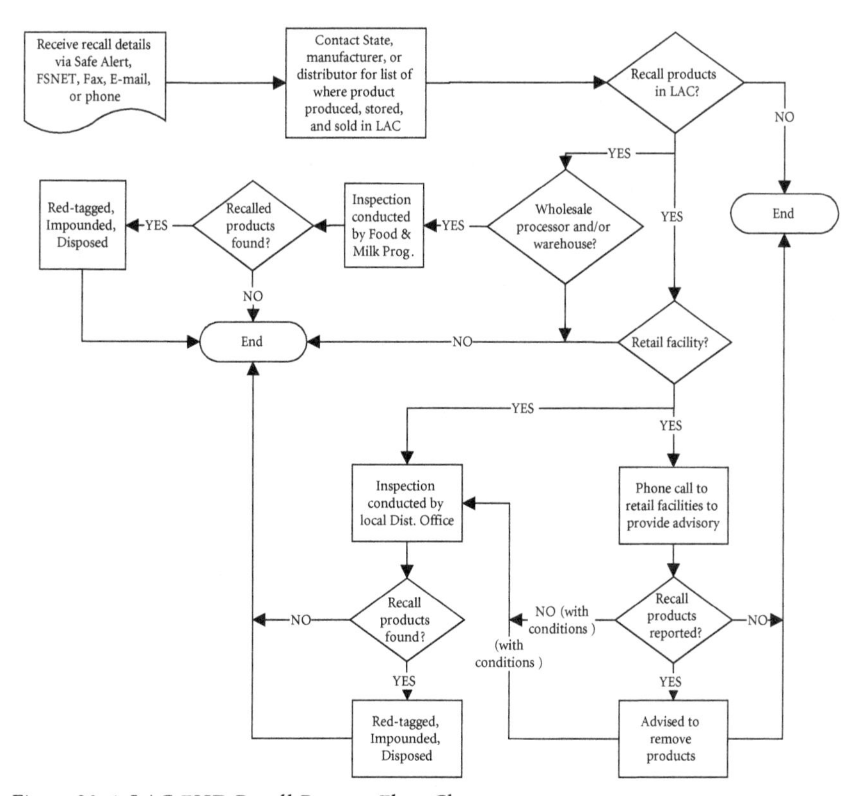

Figure 20–1 LAC EHD Recall Process Flow Chart.

IMPLEMENTATION OF SOLUTIONS

In 2009, EHD responded to 431 recalls, of which 410 were classified as Class I. The recalls involved foods possibly contaminated with such pathogens as *Salmonella*, *Listeria*, and *E. coli* O157:H7. FM conducted telephone surveys with 1,076 facilities, of which 200 (18.6%) reported having no knowledge of an ongoing recall event. Thus FM was the primary vehicle to report critical recall information in all 200 instances. Follow up verification revealed that product was still offered for sale in 8.8% of the facilities, leading food inspectors to order the removal of 1,661 pounds of recalled product from sale (see Table 20–1).

EHD's activities during a Class I spinach recall involving *E. coli* O157:H7 illustrated the significant role that LEAs can play in identifying and removing implicated foods during large-scale recall events (5). They also demonstrated how food facilities benefit from guidance and clarification from food inspectors during field verification checks.

Over 90% of 2,883 inspected food facilities removed both prepackaged and unpackaged spinach from sale. However, 2.1% of the facilities still offered prepackaged spinach, and 7.7% still offered unpackaged spinach. Food inspectors were successful in having 265 facilities remove 16,941 pounds of recalled spinach from sale in four days of verification checks (see Table 20–2).

In some cases, package labeling presented a problem. Although pre-printed packages sometimes listed spinach as an ingredient in mixed greens, spring mix, and herb salad mix, these same packages also read "ingredients may vary." Producers, wholesalers, and some retailers clarified the actual ingredients in the packages with a corrective sticker stating that the mix "contains no spinach." This resulted in conflicting ingredient statements on the same packages. Many retail operators were unsure if label modifications complied with state law and relied upon EHD food inspectors for clarification. The checks provided added value for affected facilities.

The benefits of EHD's functional structure are best illustrated by a Class I raw milk recall involving *Listeria monocytogenes*. Contrary to the passive recall notification for spinach, the raw milk recall tested FM's active surveillance for current recall information.

When EHD learned of the recall order, a list of affected food facilities was not yet available from the state. To expedite the notification process, FM used the manufacturer's website to locate LAC facilities where recalled products were sold.

TABLE 20–1 *LAC EHD Recall Response Activity for a Recent Year*

Recall Classification	# Recalls	# Facilities Contacted	# Facilities Aware of Recall	# Facilities with Product for Sale	Pounds Removed from Sale
Class I	410	934	767	77	764
Class II	15	69	61	0	0
Class III	1	0	0	0	0
No Classification*	5	73	48	18	897
TOTALS	**431**	**1,076**	**876**	**95**	**1,661**

* Recalls identified as "food safety" are not assigned a classification.

TABLE 20-2 *LAC EHD Spinach Recall Activity*

District (Field) Office	# Facilities Inspected	# Facilities with Prepackaged Spinach for Sale	Pounds Removed from Sale	# Facilities with Unpackaged Spinach for Sale	Pounds Removed from Sale
Alhambra	156	7	314	21	1043
Antelope Valley	71	4	81	4	87
East LA	268	2	7	13	285
East Valley	233	9	75	27	498
Hollywood-Wilshire	119	5	241	7	150
Inglewood	209	4	189	11	113
Mid-Valley	188	7	50	17	113
Mid-Wilshire	168	3	55	18	254
Northeast	310	10	2135	25	8346
Norwalk	152	1	27	25	1678
Santa Clarita	147	4	18	11	247
South Bay	225	2	23	17	258
Southeast	283	0	0	14	399
West	199	1	3	2	17
West Covina	155	2	73	11	162
TOTALS	2,883	61*	3,291	223*	13,650
		(2.1%)		(7.7%)	

* 19 facilities sold both prepackaged and unpackaged spinach.

This proved crucial in allowing EHD to mobilize staff 20 hours prior to receiving the state-promulgated list of affected food facilities. Additionally, certified farmers markets (CFMs) not included on the state list, but familiar to DSE as retail outlets for raw milk, were identified for telephone surveys and verification checks. CFMs are only set up and operated during specific days of the week and are not considered traditional brick and mortar fixed retail outlets; therefore, DSE's familiarity with their operation was valuable.

Unlike the high rate of removal of spinach before inspection, 11 of the 31 facilities (35%) inspected for verification of product removal still offered raw milk for sale. As a result, DSE food inspectors ordered the removal of 167 gallons of implicated raw milk products.

An incident involving product labeling also characterized the raw milk recall. DSE inspectors responded to a complaint alleging unlabeled containers of recalled raw milk for sale at a local CFM. Investigation of the CFM revealed that unlabeled containers of milk had been commingled with labeled containers of milk, resulting in uncertainty about the origin and safety of the unlabeled containers. Food inspectors ordered the unlabeled containers removed from sale due to misbranding.

■ IMPACT

Mixed industry response to verification checks ranged from cynical to grateful. Many distributors viewed local efforts to secure distribution lists as just a layer of regulatory involvement requiring response. In contrast, retailers typically appreciated receiving recall information, regardless of it calling for additional work. The difference may be attributed to retailers' commitment to customer service, and for larger chains, maintaining the image of quality associated with their brand.

Queries from the pending database should provide effective predictors of risk and aid in developing an algorithm to prioritize future response activities. These predictors may include identification of food products commonly purchased by specific demographic groupings (e.g., *queso fresco* soft cheese in Latino communities), enabling EHD to develop and provide critical information to susceptible populations during future events. Such information may also bring to light opportunities for partnerships that enhance best practices for food protection (e.g., coordinated effort with Latino Grocers Association to educate members about approved food sources and illegal *queso fresco* production). Proactive partnerships are expected to encourage industry stakeholders to increase product removal efficiencies and surveillance of recall information.

Consumers can eliminate or reduce risks from recalled foods, even after such foods enter their homes. EHD developed a web page that allows LAC users to identify current food recalls that could affect them. Visitors to this page can see the name of the recalled food, its recall date, the contaminant, and locations in LAC where the product was distributed. Additionally, site visitors may click on the associated contaminant to view details about it.

Centralizing information for recalls affecting LAC also creates opportunities to provide the same recall information via social networking outlets such as Facebook and Twitter. This has led EHD to explore expanding its consumer information efforts using social media.

■ EVALUATION STRATEGY

Verification checks performed by EHD remove significant amounts of recalled foods from commerce. But it is not clear if facilities unaware of a recall event would have received recall information prior to more sales without intervention from FM telephone surveys. Chain stores may be more aware of current recalls than independent ones, or prefer e-mail alerts to telephone warning (6). To analyze the efficacy of recall efforts, an evaluation is needed of methods to communicate recall information used by state and federal agencies. Such an evaluation will help define an LEA's role during recall events, and determine if additional actions are needed to assure recall information is understood by operators who do not speak English.

For EHD's current functional structure, completion of a comprehensive recall database will serve as the cornerstone for future quantitative evaluations. Although the presence of recalled foods found in commerce helps establish a value in recall verification checks, it remains to be seen whether EHD's current approach is fiscally sustainable in light of continued increases in the number and scope of recalls. Recent changes in federal laws must be considered in the possible reduction of recall events. EHD is completing its database and will commence a formal evaluation of its recall activities.

CONCLUSIONS

Important lessons learned from implementing this enhanced recall process:

- An agency may be able to add or enhance services and minimize the fiscal impact by coordinating the efforts of existing divisions.
- The expertise of existing personnel can be leveraged to simplify communication channels and streamline recall response activities.
- Providing recall services locally adds value to existing consumer protection activities. The current method of recall notification (i.e., federal and state web posting, industry notification to first-line distributors) does not guarantee product removal or public awareness.
- The honor system is not always reliable. Recall response should not solely rely on the food industry's efforts to remove products from wholesale distribution and retail sale.
- Recall events are expected to expand in scope. It is not uncommon for recalls to include previously unidentified foods using original recalled products as ingredients.
- Social networking outlets can provide additional means to effectively communicate consumer information now focused on agency websites.

REFERENCES

1. U.S. Government Accountability Office. USDA and FDA need to better ensure prompt and complete recalls of potentially unsafe food. GAO report October 05–51, 2004. July 29, 2011. Available from: http://www.gao.gov/new.items/d0551.pdf. (accessed June 18, 2012).
2. Vierk K, et al. Recalls of foods containing undeclared allergens reported to the US Food and Drug Administration, fiscal year 1999. *J Allergy Clin Immun.* 2002;109(6):1022–6.
3. U.S. Food and Drug Administration. USDA issues instructions to reduce allergen and other ingredient-related recalls. July 7, 2011. July 29, 2011. Available from: http://www.fsis.usda.gov/News_&_Events/NR_070711_01/index.asp (accessed June 18, 2012).
4. U.S. Food and Drug Administration. Background and definitions. June 24, 2009. April 28, 2011. Available from: http://www.fda.gov/Safety/Recalls/ucm165546.htm (accessed June 18, 2012).
5. U.S. Food and Drug Administration. FDA warning on serious foodborne E.coli O157:H7 outbreak one death and multiple hospitalizations in several states. Sept 14, 2006. May 12, 2011. Available from: http://www.fda.gov/NewsEvents/Newsroom/PressAnnouncements/2006/ucm108731.htm (accessed June 18, 2012).
6. Hanson H, et al. Evaluating the effectiveness of food recalls in retail establishments in New York City. *J Food Protect.* 2011;74.1: 111–4.

21 Sewage Discharge Response

Reforms in Reporting and Public Notification

BERNARD FRANKLIN AND
KENNETH MURRAY

THE NATURE OF THE PROBLEM: PUBLIC HEALTH IMPACTS FROM SEWAGE DISCHARGES

Several studies focus on the adverse health effects of bathers and swimmers' contact with sewage contamination in recreational waters. In 2004 the federal Environmental Protection Agency (EPA) estimated that each year 3,669 beachgoers become ill due to contact with sewage-contaminated waters (1). The most common associated illness is gastroenteritis, which can result in vomiting, diarrhea, fever, and headaches. Other less common illnesses involve infections of the ear, nose, eyes, and throat. These are most often caused by bacteria, viruses, and parasites. There is also some concern over illnesses caused by pharmaceuticals, synthetic hormones, and other pollutants in recreational waters, but those illnesses are not clearly defined. Most sickened people recover, but the elderly, children, and those with compromised immune systems are at higher risk for more serious consequences. A 2004 EPA study for Congress noted limited quantitative evidence linking adverse human health impacts with sewage discharges due to the difficulty of establishing a cause-and-effect relationship between waterborne disease outbreaks and sewage discharges. Although literature reviews do not reveal a direct link, the potential for illness from contact with sewage-contaminated recreational waters has been a concern for public health officials for decades. These concerns highlighted the need for health officials to set water quality standards that could be used to inform the public of health risks when sewage is discharged.

In 1999, an EPA-funded study of ocean waters adjacent to the Los Angeles County (LAC) coast looked at untreated runoff from storm drains and became the basis for necessary public health standards (1). The study reviewed the health risks of contact with recreational ocean water in the Santa Monica Bay and focused on identification of water quality indicators as predictors for illness; 17,253 people participated in the study. It focused on the use of total coliform bacteria, enterococcus bacteria, and fecal coliform *Escherichia coli* bacteria (*E. coli*) as predictive indicators of the risk of illness for participating bathers and swimmers. The following water quality limits and standards for use of recreational waters were established as minimum warning levels:

1,000 total coliform bacteria per 100 milliliters, if the ratio of fecal/total coliform bacteria exceeds 0.1; or
Total coliform bacteria: 10,000 organisms per 100 milliliter sample;
Fecal coliform bacteria: 400 organisms per 100 milliliter sample;
Enterococcus: 104 bacterial organisms per 100 milliliter sample.

The Los Angeles County (LAC) Department of Public Health (DPH) Environmental Health Division (EHD) is responsible for monitoring ocean water quality as required by the California Health and Safety Code, by Title 17 of the California Code of Regulations (2), and the California Health and Safety Code Sections 115880–115915 that were added in 1998 (3). These mandate testing of the ocean waters at public beaches for the established water quality standards. The ocean water monitoring program was developed in LAC after a series of sewage discharges either were not reported, or were reported late, and notifications not provided to the public in time to prevent its contact with the contaminated waters. A history follows of the events that led to development of the current LAC ocean water quality monitoring program.

■ CONTEXT: THE HISTORY OF SEWAGE DISCHARGE IN LOS ANGELES COUNTY

Following a 4,000,000-gallon sewage spill in 1987, the LAC Board of Supervisors (Board) passed a motion that directed the DPH to monitor surf zone ocean waters and to close beaches when waters became polluted. As a result of that discharge, the LAC Auditor-Controller started an investigation into the county's sewage spill reporting system. During the investigation, the Auditor-Controller noted numerous flaws in the communication protocols between local wastewater operators and EHD staff. The investigation revealed a lack of understanding at the local levels as to which agencies must be contacted immediately after a sewage discharge, and a lack of clear LAC policies about contacting first responders after normal business hours. The investigation revealed that over 11 million gallons from 208 discharges of untreated sewage had been spilled from wastewater treatment collection systems throughout the Santa Monica Bay watershed. Over 90% of these spills were not reported to the DPH. Although most spills are contained and are not a public health threat, rapid reporting is critical to mitigate those sewage spills that do have potential for adverse public health consequences.

On November 3, 2001, a 1,400,000-gallon sewage discharge occurred when a pumping plant failure went undetected for 15 hours. The Board was informed that the affected LAC departments and interested environmental groups had reviewed the incident and had developed procedures to improve the public notification of such discharges.

On August 8, 2006, a sewage discharge estimated at 20,000 to 30,000 gallons was not reported to EHD for 12 hours, causing a delay in public notification that put beachgoers at risk. The repeated lack of communication between agencies resulted in the Board passing a motion instructing the Auditor-Controller to perform a thorough review of the reporting system, and to provide recommendations for improvements. The Auditor-Controller's investigation found differences in sewage discharge reporting requirements between the various oversight agencies. Discharge permits issued by the Regional Water Quality Control Board (RWQCB) to the owner/operators of sanitary sewer collection systems and separate storm sewer systems require reporting to the local health officer "as soon as possible," but no later than 24 hours after knowledge of a discharge. Health and Safety Code Section 5411.5 requires "immediate" reporting of a sewage discharge to the local health officer (4), while the Water Code Section 13271 designates the California State Office of Emergency Services (Cal-EMA) as the entity to be notified in the event of a sewage discharge, not the local public health officer (5). The Auditor-Controller's report also noted the issue of sewer maintenance. The discharge permits of owners/operators of sanitary sewer collection systems and storm sewer systems require them to "properly" operate and maintain their systems. This vague requirement at times resulted in the improper operation/maintenance of sewer equipment. Several significant sewage spills were found to be caused by pumping station failures and not by their collection system stoppages.

The Auditor-Controller's report of the investigation detailed 15 recommendations to improve sewage spill reporting. Some of the key recommendations included: development of policies and procedures to centralize documentation and tracking of all reports of sewage spills; improvements in inter-jurisdictional communication between the DPH and other agencies; development of a regional call center; assignment of DPH staff to respond to sewage spill reports received after normal business hours; development of an educational program for wastewater personnel; amendments to state law to include a requirement that the local public health officer be immediately notified of a sewage spill; and the ability to impose civil fines on dischargers who fail to report.

■ APPROACH TO THE PROBLEM: ESTABLISHING A SEWAGE RESPONSE PROGRAM

In January 2007, the Board of Supervisors adopted a motion instructing the DPH to pursue all 15 recommendations from the Auditor-Controller to improve the sewage spill reporting process.

In response to the Board motion, EHD convened a stakeholder workgroup consisting of: interested environmental professionals; sewer system personnel; the LAC Departments of Public Works, Beaches and Harbors, and the Fire-Life Guard Division; the LAC Sanitation District; Los Angeles City Bureau of Sanitation; the Los Angeles Regional Water Quality Control Board; and community-based organizations such as Heal the Bay and the Surfrider Foundation. This workgroup met to develop reporting criteria, including a mandatory 15-minute time frame (subsequently amended to reporting within 15 minutes or when the collection agency verifies a discharge from its system) for reporting sewage spills to EHD, and a system to prompt rapid responses to reports of sewage discharges. Discharge reports came from several sources, including self-reporting by the sewage system operators to their permitting agencies and calls from the general public to emergency service centers such as "911." All of these types of calls are routed to the California Office of Emergency Services and the LAC Emergency Operator. EHD and the working group also raised awareness among potential dischargers through education efforts, and the Recreational Waters Program within EHD was established as the agency responsible for monitoring ocean water quality and for notifying the public when sewage spills occur.

All 88 incorporated cities in LAC were sent a "Sewage Spill Notification Chart" (see Figure 21–1) with procedures for reporting sewage discharges, including telephone numbers of state and county agencies that require sewage discharge reporting. Key components include immediate reporting of sewage discharges and timely public notification when an imminent public health threat exists from a sewage release. Once it has been determined that a discharge could potentially affect beach users, the beach is immediately closed, and ocean water sampling must also occur immediately.

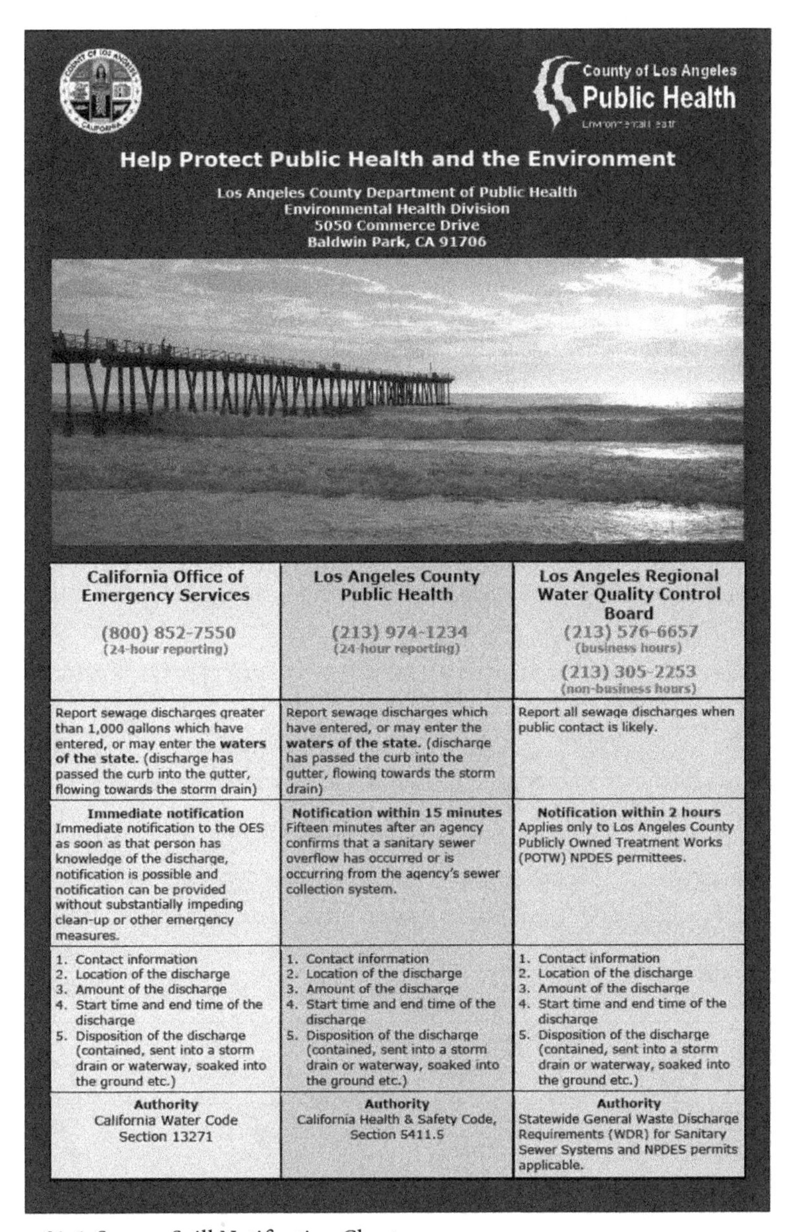

County of Los Angeles
Public Health

Help Protect Public Health and the Environment

Los Angeles County Department of Public Health
Environmental Health Division
5050 Commerce Drive
Baldwin Park, CA 91706

California Office of Emergency Services (800) 852-7550 (24-hour reporting)	Los Angeles County Public Health (213) 974-1234 (24-hour reporting)	Los Angeles Regional Water Quality Control Board (213) 576-6657 (business hours) (213) 305-2253 (non-business hours)
Report sewage discharges greater than 1,000 gallons which have entered, or may enter the **waters of the state.** (discharge has passed the curb into the gutter, flowing towards the storm drain)	Report sewage discharges which have entered, or may enter the **waters of the state.** (discharge has passed the curb into the gutter, flowing towards the storm drain)	Report all sewage discharges when public contact is likely.
Immediate notification Immediate notification to the OES as soon as that person has knowledge of the discharge, notification is possible and notification can be provided without substantially impeding clean-up or other emergency measures.	**Notification within 15 minutes** Fifteen minutes after an agency confirms that a sanitary sewer overflow has occurred or is occurring from the agency's sewer collection system.	**Notification within 2 hours** Applies only to Los Angeles County Publicly Owned Treatment Works (POTW) NPDES permittees.
1. Contact information 2. Location of the discharge 3. Amount of the discharge 4. Start time and end time of the discharge 5. Disposition of the discharge (contained, sent into a storm drain or waterway, soaked into the ground etc.)	1. Contact information 2. Location of the discharge 3. Amount of the discharge 4. Start time and end time of the discharge 5. Disposition of the discharge (contained, sent into a storm drain or waterway, soaked into the ground etc.)	1. Contact information 2. Location of the discharge 3. Amount of the discharge 4. Start time and end time of the discharge 5. Disposition of the discharge (contained, sent into a storm drain or waterway, soaked into the ground etc.)
Authority California Water Code Section 13271	**Authority** California Health & Safety Code, Section 5411.5	**Authority** Statewide General Waste Discharge Requirements (WDR) for Sanitary Sewer Systems and NPDES permits applicable.

Figure 21–1 Sewage Spill Notification Chart.

If a state standard for indicator bacteria is exceeded, then the beach remains closed until two consecutive ocean water re-samples are collected that meet state standards.

EHD assigned staff to respond to calls 24 hours a day, and developed two database applications to track reports of sewage discharges. The first is web-based and allows the public to view spill information, including: the reporting party, the location and cause of spill, the amount discharged/contained, and whether a spill has reached the ocean and warranted a beach closure. This system also allows EHD staff to update information via the internet on weekends and after workday hours. EHD and the Internal Services Department (ISD) developed an incident tracking system that is completely auditable (i.e., all calls/conversations related to a spill are time stamped and recorded). The current system allows the County Emergency Operator to electronically attach all calls/conversations related to a spill ticket (for a specific spill) with a click of a button. EHD tracks the calls as verification of the written information submitted by the reporting agency. Additionally, the ISD system interfaces with the EHD database, allowing data from the spill ticket to be "pushed" out to create the initial EHD system record. All the necessary information that is needed is recorded from the sewage collection agency using a "Sewage Incident Report" (see Figure 21–2). The second database system is maintained by the Recreational Waters Program and is used to produce reports for the DPH. These reports assess whether a sewage collection agency or city has been recalcitrant in reporting any sewage discharges from their collection system. EHD follows up with these agencies and cities to assess if changes or improvements need to be made to their sewage management infrastructure.

EHD addressed the lack of understanding of the reporting requirements by developing and distributing 17,000 educational brochures to public agencies that own

DATE OF DISCHARGE 1	TIME OF DISCHARGE 2	END DATE 3	END TIME 4	ISD INCIDENT # 5

LOCATION 6	CITY 7	ZIP 8

AGENCY REPORTING 9	PERSON REPORTING 10	PR PHONE 11

DATE AGENCY NOTIFIED 12	TIME AGENCY NOTIFIED 13	DATE AGENCY NOTIFIED EH 14	TIME AGENCY NOTIFIED EH 15
GALLONS DISCHARGED 16	GALLONS CONTAINED 17	GALLONS TO OCEAN / RIVER 18	DID SEWAGE ENTER OCEAN? 19

LOCATION SEWAGE ENTERED OCEAN 20
CAUSE OF DISCHARGE 21
EH ACTION 22
OTHER AGENCIES INVOLVED 23
COMMENTS 24

TODAY'S DATE 25	EHS SIGNATURE 26	PRINT NAME 27

OFFICE 28	PHONE 29

Figure 21–2 Sewage Incident Report.

ENVIRONMENTAL HEALTH
SEWAGE DISCHARGE INCIDENT REPORT
Category Glossary

1. DATE OF DISCHARGE: Date discharge occurred.
2. TIME OF DISCHARGE: Time discharge occurred in military time (or best approximation).
3. END DATE: Date discharge ended.
4. END TIME: Time discharge ended in military time (or best approximation).
5. ISD INCIDENT #: For internal Recreational Waters use only.
6. LOCATION: Location of discharge. Address or other most accurate coordinate.
7. CITY: Name of city where discharge occurred.
8. ZIP: Zip code of where discharge occurred.
9. AGENCY REPORTING: Agency reporting discharge to Environmental Health.
10. PERSON REPORTING: Full name of person reporting discharge.
11. PR PHONE: Telephone number of person reporting discharge.
12. DATE AGENCY NOTIFIED: Date the agency received notification or new about the discharge.
13. TIME AGENCY NOTIFIED: Time the agency received notification or new about the discharge.
14. DATE AGENCY NOTIFIED EH: Date the agency notified Environmental Health about the discharge.
15. TIME AGENCY NOTIFIED EH: Time the agency notified Environmental Health about the discharge.
16. GALLONS DISCHARGED: Total number of gallons discharged out of the wastewater system.
17. GALLONS CONTAINED: Total number of gallons contained or recovered (if any) from discharge and not in any other way dissipated into the local environment (e.g. soaked into soil).
18. GALLONS TO OCEAN/STORM DRAIN, RIVER: Total number of gallons not contained or recovered from discharge, and not in any other way dissipated into the local environment (e.g. soaked into soil).
19. DID SEWAGE ENTER OCEAN? Yes, No, or Not known.
20. LOCATION SEWAGE ENTERED OCEAN: Location where discharge entered ocean. Address or other most accurate coordinate.
21. CAUSE OF DISCHARGE: Reason why sewage discharged from the contained system.
22. EH ACTION: Action taken by Environmental Health (what is EH doing or has done to respond to the incident).
23. OTHER AGENCIES INVOLVED: All collaborating agencies involved in any aspect of the incident's mitigation effort (name and contact numbers, if available).
24. COMMENTS: Any additional notes, comments of information regarding the incident.
25. TODAY'S DATE: Date the report is being filled-out.
26. EHS SIGNATURE: Signature of EHS filling out report.
27. PRINT NAME: Printed name of EHS filling out report.
28. OFFICE: Office of EHS filling out report.
29. PHONE: Telephone of EHS filling out report (office and cell).

Figure 21–2 (Continued)

and operate wastewater collection systems in LAC. The brochures include notification criteria and contact numbers for reporting spills to the DPH, the State Office of Emergency Services, and the RWQCB. The DPH also distributed brochures to the owners of approximately 42,000 food facilities and 70,000 multiple family dwelling units. The brochures provided information on common causes of spills, spill prevention methods, the public health impacts of sewage spills, and related reporting requirements. A local service named "Dig Alert" also was established to provide information to callers about the location of underground utilities. A call to the "Dig Alert" system can identify the location of underground sewer lines and prevent the accidental rupture of these lines by construction crews and other diggers.

Since greater system maintenance is a key to reducing the occurrence of sewage spills, the CEO formed a Sewage Spill Prevention Program Committee to develop "best management practices" for maintaining sewer systems, and to provide related training to all cities in LAC. The committee consists of RWQCB staff, Auditor-Controller staff, and staff from the county's primary sewer agencies.

■ EVALUATION AND IMPACT

The number of sewage spills reported to EHD has increased dramatically since the new program started. In 2006, 26 sewage spills were reported; in 2007, 780 sewage spills were reported, a 3,000% increase. Clearly, EHD succeeded in educating sewage system agencies on the need to report spills and in improving the spill reporting process!

Primary reporting evaluation can be based on comparison of sewage discharges reported to the RWQCB and those reported to EHD. All RWQCB discharges reported by collection agencies are sent to the DPH and are compared with the DPH reports to determine if the discharge was unreported. Any unreported discharges are investigated by the Recreational Waters Program staff, and reporting procedures are reviewed to ensure that the collection agency understands the required reporting process.

Once the new system was implemented, the number of spills reported to the DPH increased more than 30-fold from 26 to 780. This increase reflected increased reporting of sewage spills, which resulted in timely notification of health risks to the public. The increase in reported spills to the DPH was the direct result of enhanced awareness among dischargers of the reporting requirements, as were improved inter-jurisdictional communication between the DPH and other agencies and increased availability of weekend/after-hours "on-call" response personnel within the DPH. Before the current reporting system was in place, EHD received irregular notification of sewage discharges and would not have been able to provide timely warnings of hazard to the public. Now the DPH can provide timely public notification of sewage discharges into recreational waters, and the public is alerted to potential hazards in time to protect themselves.

The sewage spill reporting procedures inform the public; increase awareness among dischargers of reporting requirements; improve inter-jurisdictional communication between the DPH and other agencies; and provide for the availability of weekend/after-hours "on-call" personnel within the DPH to respond to incidents.

These improvements were apparent from a sewage spill in South Pasadena early in 2011. A spill there of approximately 20,000 gallons entered a storm drain that eventually made its way to the City of Long Beach and led to the closure of that city's beaches. The spill occurred on a Saturday morning and was promptly reported by the South Pasadena Public Works Department to County DPH via the County Emergency Operator. Within 15 minutes of notification, EHD staff notified Long Beach Public Health on-call staff, which, in turn, made the determination to close the affected beaches. The effectiveness of this response on an early weekend morning was due to clear and rapid communications between the discharger, the county, and the City of Long Beach.

CONCLUSIONS

- Failure to report sewage discharges in a timely manner can potentially contaminate the receiving waters and have a negative impact on the public's health, as well as undermining public confidence in government agencies.
- The ability to quickly report and respond to sewage discharges is essential for the health of the communities of LAC, which share a 75-mile coastline.
- Developing a cooperative agreement regarding a response plan and method of notification among 88 cities and multiple agencies poses significant challenges. Nonetheless, at this time in LAC, any discharge of sewage, regardless of size or location, is quickly reported to the DPH. Any threat to public health can be quickly evaluated and reported to all appropriate agencies so that they can take timely corrective measures. With these discharge procedures in place, necessary actions can be implemented to ensure that our beaches are safe and public health is protected.
- The ability for local costal government agencies to monitor sewage discharges must be based on a mutual understanding between the health officer and sewage collection system agencies for the need to safeguard public health.

REFERENCES

1. Haile RW, Witte JS, Gold M, Cressey R, McGee C, Millikan RC, Glasser A, Harawa N, Ervin C, Harmon P, Harper J, Dermand J, Alamillo J, Barrett K, Nides M, Wang G. The health effects of swimming in ocean water contaminated by storm drain runoff. *Epidemiology.* 1999;10.4:355–63.
2. Title 17 California Code of Regulations Division 2. Water quality control plans. California Environmental Protection Agency: State Water Resources Control Board, March 2010. Available from: http://www.swrcb.ca.gov/water_issues/programs/ocean/docs/2009_cop_adoptedeffective_usepa.pdf (acessed June 18, 2012).
3. California AB 411. California State Legislation, October 1997. Available from: http://www.swrcb.ca.gov/water_issues/programs/beaches/beach_surveys/bills/ab_411_bill_19971008_chaptered.pdf (accessed June 18, 2012).
4. Sewage discharge reporting guidelines. Los Angeles County Department of Public Health: Environmental Health, Nov. 1, 2009. Available from: http://www.publichealth.lacounty.gov/eh/docs/ep_rw_SDRguidelines.pdf (accessed June 18, 2012).
5. Water Code Section 13260–13275. Official California legislative information. Available from: http://www.leginfo.ca.gov/cgi-bin/displaycode?section=wat&group=13001-14000-&file=13260-13275 (accessed June 18, 2012).

22 Contaminated Fish

Protecting Communities Through Community Education and Reducing Availability

MARITA SANTOS, JANICE LEWIS, AND JANET SCULLY

THE PROBLEM

For four decades, the Montrose chemical plant and other local industries dumped tons of chemicals into the sewage system in Los Angeles County (LAC). The contaminated wastewater made its way through the sewers into the ocean, where it settled onto the Palos Verdes Shelf. Discharged chemicals included the pesticide DDT (dichlorodiphenyltrichlorothane) and PCBs (polychlorinated biphenyls), which were used in electrochemical insulation. Subsequently, both DDT and PCBs have been deemed hazards to human health and wildlife (1) and have been banned from use.

The Palos Verdes (PV) Shelf is located off the PV Peninsula on the southern coast of LAC (see Figure 22–1) between Point Fermin and Point Vicente. The 43-square-kilometer area contains contaminated sediment on both the continental shelf and the continental slope. It is among the largest DDT- and PCB-contaminated sediment sites in California. High levels of DDT and PCBs were found in the active biological zone of the PV Shelf sediment, and fish in the area tested positive for DDT and PCBs (1). Based on the health risks, a fish consumption advisory was issued by the California State Office of Environmental Health Hazard Assessment (OEHHA) (2, 3) and in 1990 the California Department of Fish and Game banned commercial fishing of white croaker, the most significantly tainted fish, in the PV Shelf waters. The ban extended from Point Vicente to Point Fermin, and from the shoreline to three miles off the coast (1).

In August 1997, the PV Shelf was designated as a Superfund site, providing the U.S. Environmental Protection Agency (EPA) with authority and management responsibility over the location (2). That year, EPA formally included the PV Shelf as part of the Montrose National Priority List (NPL) (1). Also in 1997, Heal the Bay (a nonprofit environmental advocacy organization) performed a study which found that white croaker purchased in retail markets contained levels of DDT and PCBs similar to those found in fish caught from the PV Shelf. This raised concern that white croaker caught by sport fishermen were being sold at commercial fish markets. To address the issue, in March 1998 the California Department of Fish and Game revised the white croaker bag limit for sport fisherman from "unlimited" to "10 fish per day."

Historically, the waters of the PV Shelf have been used extensively for recreational and commercial fishing, as well as for subsistence of local people and families (1). Fish contain important nutrients, such as protein and omega-3 fatty acids, and

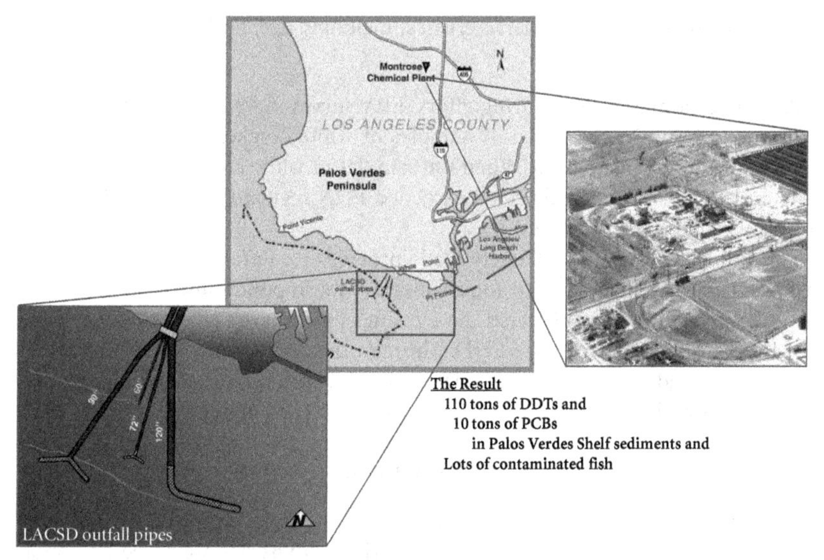

Figure 22–1 Palos Verdes Superfund Site.

are part of a well-balanced diet (4), but industrial contamination of local waters has compromised this food source. Thus, the LAC Department of Public Health (DPH) implemented projects to manage the risk associated with eating locally caught fish (1).

Through a cooperative agreement with the EPA, the LAC DPH's Environmental Health Division (EHD), implemented a Removal Action Plan. Through this plan, the EHD inspected specified markets and collected fish samples to determine whether contaminated fish from PV Shelf waters were reaching consumers through local markets. The EHD's Toxics Epidemiology Program conducted public health outreach and educational components of the cooperative agreement, and the EHD continues as an active partner in developing and implementing programs to reduce the risk of exposure to contaminated fish.

■ CONTEXT

The white croaker (also called "kingfish" or "tomcod") found in the PV Shelf region has high levels of DDT and PCB because it feeds directly off the contaminated sediment concentrated on the ocean floor and has a high percentage of body fat; DDT and PCBs tend to build up in fatty tissues. Consumption of DDT and PCBs has been associated with increased cancer risk and with liver and central nervous system damage (1), particularly in vulnerable populations such as children and pregnant women (3).

The risk to health of eating white croaker depends on the:

- Types and quantities of chemicals found in the fish;
- Amount consumed;
- Frequency of consumption;
- Preparation and cooking methods;

- Individual consumer characteristics, including age, body size, and health status (3).

As part of a market monitoring effort, EPA surveyed 68 markets in Los Angeles and Orange Counties, in which 30 samples of white croaker were collected at 6 of the markets on repeated visits. When the samples of white croaker were analyzed for DDT and PCBs, the levels detected exceeded FDA regulatory levels and the results led to subsequent interventions.

The California Health and Safety Code provides for enforcement officers in local health agencies to inspect retail food facilities and impound any food suspected of being contaminated or adulterated. As a result of the survey, the EPA entered into a cooperative agreement with the EHD. Through the cooperative agreement, the EPA and EHD created a direct working relationship focused on outreach to market owners/operators and the inspection and monitoring of LAC markets.

■ APPROACH TO THE PROBLEM

OEHHA issues local fish advisories that recommend limits on the amount of specific locally caught fish that a person should eat. These advisories are based on contamination studies performed in the PV Shelf. EPA implemented a PV Shelf Institutional Controls Program (ICs) to feature public education and outreach, increase enforcement of existing commercial and recreational fishing restrictions, and to monitor markets and ocean fish quality. The EHD actively supports the public education and outreach portion, which relies on collaboration among EPA and several federal, state, and local agencies, environmental groups, and community-based organizations. To facilitate this coordination, the EPA created the Fish Contamination Education Collaborative (FCEC), of which the EHD is an active partner.

FCEC was established to educate the public about the health risks posed by contaminated fish and to encourage the public to become wiser consumers. The cornerstone of the FCEC is its partnerships with local health departments, community-based organizations, and other agencies. The program goal is to educate the most vulnerable populations, including women of childbearing age, pregnant women, and children, so that they are aware of local fish contamination and can make informed decisions about fish they eat. As part of the FCEC, the EHD's role is to provide public education and outreach to LAC, especially to vulnerable populations, and to provide monitoring and enforcement for LAC markets.

EHD inspectors monitor and inspect markets to enforce applicable fish advisories. The Toxics Epidemiology Program participates in outreach and education efforts through health fairs and community events and offers training about fish consumption advisories to public health nurses and other health care providers, such as obstetrics and gynecology and pediatric practitioners.

■ IMPLEMENTATION OF SOLUTIONS

Some 400 public health nurses and EHD inspectors have been trained about fish consumption advisories and local fish contamination issues. The Toxics Epidemiology Program collaborated with several other programs within the DPH, including the Maternal, Child and Adolescent Health Program, Comprehensive Perinatal Services Program, the Child Health and Disability Prevention Program, and the Nutrition Program, to develop effective ways to address fish contamination issues. These groups are connected to over 360 obstetricians and more than 1,200 pediatricians throughout LAC, many of whom provide care to the most vulnerable populations. Educational materials regarding fish consumption advisories and contamination issues have been distributed to over 1,000 other medical providers, and free in-services with continuing education units were offered to practitioners.

As part of the outreach and education program, packets of educational materials, written in several languages, were distributed to market owners and operators. Pamphlets supplied by the EPA and FCEC informed readers about local fish contamination.

An Enforcement Program was created, and 12 health inspectors attended a four-hour EPA workshop on monitoring the sale of white croaker in markets. A train-the-trainer course on fish also addressed contamination issues. EHD inspectors incorporated white croaker inspection into their routine inspection of a group of selected markets. White croakers were impounded and sent for analysis to an independent laboratory under contract with the EPA if the vendor did not have invoices documenting that the fish came from an uncontaminated source. Results of these laboratory tests were then publicized. If a market owner did not present a purchase invoice during the inspections, the white croakers were confiscated and the owner/operator was required to attend an office hearing.

■ EVALUATION STRATEGY

Since the initial interventions, environmental health inspectors now re-survey the markets every six months and distribute fish education brochures with their contact information. The number of markets inspected has changed over time because some of the original markets went out of business and additional markets were added. The following are the preliminary results of five rounds of inspections:

- Round I: 5 of 35 inspected markets (14%) sold white croaker; 2 of these 5 markets (40%) presented proper product invoices at the time of the inspection.
- Round II: 0 of 32 inspected markets (0%) sold white croaker.
- Round III: 0 of 22 inspected markets (0%) sold white croaker.
- Round IV: 5 of 37 inspected markets (14%) sold white croaker; 4 of these 5 markets (80%) were different from the markets that sold white croaker during the Round I inspections. All 5 markets (100%) presented proper product invoices at the time of the inspection.
- Round V: 1 of 37 inspected markets (3%) sold white croaker. This market was new to the list of inspected markets. It is unknown whether it presented proper product invoices during inspection.

■ CHALLENGES OF THE FISH IDENTIFICATION PROJECT

- Accurate identification of white croaker was a new skill for health inspectors. EHD collaborated with California Department of Fish and Game to conduct joint market inspections with the EHD in Round II and later rounds to provide training and quality assurance.

- Inspectors who joined the project after its inception did not receive the initial fish identification training. To address this issue, additional training in fish identification was provided for these inspectors.
- It was difficult to determine the legitimacy of purchase invoices provided by market owners and operators. Valid product purchase invoices verify that suppliers obtained the fish within approved areas outside the catch ban area. On several occasions, market owners presented questionable invoices that were handwritten or written in different languages. These invoices were referred to CDFG for verification of legitimacy.
- Many fish suppliers named on the invoices were located outside LAC. Inspectors relied upon other health departments and CDFG for help in verifying fish species and the validity of product invoices.

IMPACT

The proportion of inspected markets selling white croaker decreased from Round I (14%) to Rounds II and III (0%). The five markets that sold white croaker in Round I were re-inspected six months later in Round II and then re-inspected six more months later in Round III. No white croaker was sold in the five markets or any other markets that were inspected in Round III.

Five of 37 markets (14%) sold white croaker in Round IV; however, four of them were new to the inspection program. When they were re-inspected in Round V, none was selling white croaker. The only market selling white croaker in Round V was new to the inspection program. The percentage of owners/operators presenting invoices at the time of market inspections increased from 40% in Round I to 100% in Round IV. Market owner/operator awareness of local fish contamination issues also increased; 40% of market owners/operators responded "Yes" to the question "Are you aware of the local fish contamination issue and the white croaker advisory?" in Round I, compared to 70% in Round V.

CONCLUSION

The DPH, the California Department of Fish and Game, and the U.S. EPA, along with various community-based agencies representing the diverse LAC cultures, have formed partnerships to protect Los Angeles consumers from local fish contamination. The Fish Contamination Education Collaborative exemplifies how federal, state, and local governments can work together, along with community-based organizations, to address a local health problem.

REFERENCES

1. Site Overview of Palos Verdes Shelf, USEPA Region 9 Superfund. Available from: http://yosemite.epa.gov/r9/sfund/r9sfdocw.nsf/7508188dd3c99a2a8825742600743735/e61d5255780dd68288257007005e9422!OpenDocument (accessed Dec. 14, 2010).
2. Cleaning up the Palos Verdes Shelf. Available from: http://www.epa.gov/region9/superfund/pvshelf/ (accessed Dec. 14, 2010).
3. Office of Environmental Health Hazard Assessment (2009, June). Available from: http://oehha.ca.gov/fish/so_cal/pdf_zip/SoCalAdvisoryl61809.pdf (accessed Aug. 30, 2011).
4. American Heart Association. Available from: http://www.heart.org/HEARTORG/GettingHealthy/NutritionCenter/HealthyDietGoals/Fish-and-Omega-3-Fatty-Acids_UCM_303248_Article.jsp (accessed Dec. 14, 2010).

PART FOUR
Emergency Response

23 Emergency Management

Building an Effective Structure for Local Public Health

MICHAEL CONTRERAS, BENJAMIN BRISTOW, ALONZO PLOUGH, AND KIM HARRISON EOWAN

THE PROBLEM

Landmark Southern California wildfires in 1970 resulted in the loss of 16 human lives, 700 structures, and over 500,000 acres, at a cost of over $200 million. These devastating losses and expenditures illustrate the challenges of inter- and intra-agency coordination. Post-incident investigations revealed disorganized responses characterized by unclear lines of authority, a dearth of reliable information, incompatible communication systems, and unspecified incident objectives.

In response, Congress provided funding for establishing a unified command structure for consistent use in emergency response. An early system, FIRESCOPE, designed by the U.S. Forest Service with state and local partners, became the prototype for what is now known as the Incident Command System (ICS) (1, 2).

More recently, the ICS expanded beyond its initial focus on wildfire management. ICS is now a standardized incident management system, uniformly used by local, tribal, state, and federal agencies. It divides emergency response into five manageable functions essential for emergency responses: command, operations, planning, logistics, and finance and administration (see Figure 23–1 and Box 23–1). ICS allows for integrating diverse resources and personnel within a common organizational structure, enables a coordinated response among agencies and jurisdictions, and establishes common processes for planning and managing resources (see Box 23–2).

Initial structures prompted "traditional" emergency responders such as fire and law enforcement. Common ICS terminology now enables diverse groups of partners to join in a variety of functions emphasizing an "all-hazards" perspective. ICS is flexible and scalable to fit incidents of varying scope and nature—from biological, chemical, and radiological events to earthquakes, wildfires, and natural disasters.

Emergencies can have significant impacts on individual and population health. Thus public health departments are essential participants and, at times, leaders in ICS activation.

In theory, ICS implementation within local public health departments seems straightforward: design an organizational chart using ICS methodology, insert personnel into logical ICS roles on the chart, train personnel on their respective roles, and practice during exercises or real-world events. However, for many agencies, adapting emergency response structures to the ICS system has been challenging to implement. The default ICS structure presents numerous problems for the public health practitioner. System characteristics exemplified by a rigid centralized

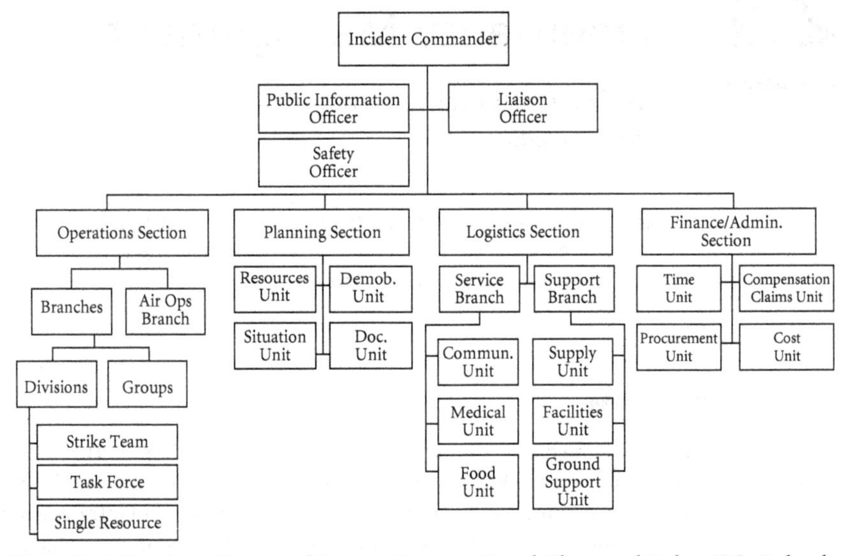

Figure 23–1 Incident Command System Organizational Chart and Roles, U.S. Federal Emergency Management Agency (FEMA) (2).

BOX 23–1 ■ Incident Command System Roles, U.S. Federal Emergency Management Agency (FEMA) (2)

- Incident Commander: Responsible for all aspects of the response, including developing incident objectives and managing all incident operations
- Command Staff
  - Public Information Officer: Develops and releases information about the incident to the news media, incident personnel, and other appropriate agencies and organizations
  - Liaison Officer: Serves as point of contact for assisting and coordinating activities between the IC/UC and various agencies and groups
  - Safety Officer: Develops and recommends measures to the IC/UC for assuring personnel health and safety, and to assess and/or anticipate hazardous and unsafe situations
- General Staff
  - Operations: Responsible for all operations directly applicable to the primary mission of the response
  - Planning: Collects, evaluates, and disseminates tactical information related to the incident; prepares Incident Action Plans
  - Logistics: Provides facilities, services, and materials for the incident response
  - Finance and Administration: Responsible for all financial, administrative, and cost analysis aspects of the incident

BOX 23–2 ■ Incident Command System (ICS) Management Characteristics, U.S. Federal Emergency Management Agency (FEMA) (6)

- Common Terminology
- Modular Organization
- Management by Objectives
- Incident Action Planning
- Manageable Span of Control
- Incident Facilities and Locations
- Comprehensive Resource Management
- Integrated Communications
- Establishment and Transfer of Command
- Chain of Command and Unity of Command
- Unified Command
- Accountability
- Dispatch/Deployment
- Information and Intelligence Management

decision-making hierarchy, action orientation, and reliance on staff cross-training are not characteristic of usual public health practice. Early efforts using decision protocols borrowed from fire and law organizations; these imposed vernacular and cultural norms onto public health emergency response that confused participants about appropriate roles and actions. This, in fact, led to misinterpretation of ICS goals. For ICS to function in public health and emergency response contexts, these issues had to be addressed.

CONTEXT

In 1999 the Centers for Disease Control and Prevention (CDC) awarded the first public health preparedness grants to states. These grants signaled national recognition of the role of public health agencies in emergency management. The level of funding and impetus to respond increased after the 2001 anthrax attacks on media outlets and the US Senate (3, 4). At the time, the CDC refined their funding strategy to provide grants directly to four major metropolitan areas, including Los Angeles County. A significant gap then became clear in national health security, as few public health agencies were equipped to respond to targeted biologic attacks.

The federal preparedness grants mandated many new capabilities to improve bioresponse, including a directive to incorporate ICS for public health emergency response. In California, a long established emergency management system also required that public health departments integrate the range of bioterror response operations into local processes.

APPROACH TO THE PROBLEM

Initially, ICS tried to superimpose fire and law enforcement response models on public health practice without noting the differences in mission and focus of a health protection agency. For example, the standard ICS chart includes a position for an "Air Operations Unit" (see Figure 23–1). Air assets are valuable, although critical questions of their value in public health operations were not addressed. (How would such assets be used? What would be the mission tasking? Who would control them? Where are they relevant to public health?)

The ICS system was assumed by federal planners to be perfect. Forgotten was that fire and law ICS models were developed from analysis of past responses of enforcement agencies.

The Los Angeles County (LAC) Department of Public Health (DPH) Emergency Preparedness and Response Program (EPRP) was tasked with adapting existing ICS models to meet the needs of a local public health department. General objectives were to align ICS structure with public health work culture and expertise, to develop supporting response plans, and to implement and exercise the system within the DPH (5).

Development of the Public Health Emergency Management Framework

Early efforts to implement a public health ICS structure revealed no unifying DPH framework to codify and guide the organization's operational response.

Efforts to develop a framework began with interviews with DPH executives and senior program managers assigned to emergency response roles. It was important to incorporate their advice regarding the roles of public health subject matter experts (SMEs) in emergency responses. Among the questions asked: What did they see as their specific tasks? How would they use personnel? How did they view their leadership roles? What support did they need to perform their roles during an emergency? What thresholds did they consider before declaring a public health emergency? These discussions with DPH managers gave insight into fundamental problems hindering the ICS implementation process. The results indicated that early efforts might best be focused on tactical issues, such as which program's resources best aligned with necessary responses to specific hazards. This saved for later the larger challenge of defining how the department would write specific procedures for emergency management.

Managers very clearly understood their roles in day-to-day operations, but were less clear regarding their ICS assignments. Some saw the ICS structure as simply a CDC pro forma requirement with no added value. Others ignored the ICS structure and operated as if conducting day-to-day functions. Many were unclear which events required ICS responses.

Formerly, the department dealt with many incidents, such as infectious disease outbreaks, with no dedicated management structure. Existing program roles and structures sufficed, and for some, ICS simply added unneeded layers to a smoothly working process. These interviews raised the issues and preconceptions that needed to be addressed in order to develop a shared understanding of a workable emergency response framework.

■ THE EVOLUTION OF A RESPONSE FRAMEWORK

The LAC DPH Emergency Management Framework developed from five concepts:

1. ICS supports effective public health practices.

2. Public health professionals are assigned to public health emergency response tasks.
3. Scientific and clinical assessment of risk and vulnerability drive response strategies.
4. The major public health emergencies fall into definable clusters that allow for pre-planning.
5. The threshold for the declaration of an emergency requiring activation of ICS is based on the scale of resources required to respond.

These core concepts form the basis of all department emergency management structures. The concepts cleared up misconceptions, aligned the missions of the Department, provided a standard process for public health from which to operate, removed the stigma of reaction, and defined a public health emergency.

ICS Supports Effective Public Health Practices

Differing missions and cultural mores between public health processes and ICS provided the first challenge: how to reconcile ICS with DPH core values and culture. ICS implementation conveyed ICS as a superior management approach compared with usual public health practices. Enthusiastic to implement a system that worked in other response settings, emergency managers failed to appreciate the different practice context of public health. A major lesson was that ICS must be grounded in and adapted to the needs of the organization in which it is being implemented.

The revised ICS strategy recognized that what informed public health practice—the best science backed by research—can be integrated with an emergency management system such as ICS. The department then moved forward with a base from which to develop a public health hybrid ICS.

Public Health Professionals Are Assigned to Public Health Emergency Response Tasks

In many ICS structures, personnel fill numerous assignments. The fire captain may be assigned as the logistics chief or the police sergeant may be assigned to planning, and each works well in these roles. For public health—a field populated by both generalists and specialists—this concept does not always work. Public health professionals are critically thinking, analytical scientists trained to prioritize, compare, and contrast potential solutions to a health incident. Their decision processes often take time, which can be impractical in the context of a rapidly evolving health incident. Occasionally public health professionals use different skill sets from those of personnel in action-oriented response organizations. However, public health decision process are often streamlined and accelerated, as in the response to a food-borne outbreak or the severe acute respiratory syndrome (SARS) epidemic.

At the DPH, ICS roles that do not require the scientific, clinical, and analytical skill sets of a public health practitioner are assigned to administrative staff. Non-professional staff fill the positions responsible for ordering DPH supplies managing logistics, and other support functions. If a need arises for more general administrative personnel than the DPH can support, it turns to other LAC departments for additional personnel to handle tasks in finance or logistics. This ensures that department SMEs focus on its operations, plans, and risk communications.

An area of improvement that should be noted is that in order to improve public health ICS efficiency, SMEs must exercise and drill to develop "rapid cycle assessments" of complex incidents and to make timely decisions that could be refined as situations develop and better information becomes available.

Scientific and Clinical Assessment of Risk and Vulnerability Drive Response Strategies

A challenge with ICS in public health is the need to make immediate decisions during emerging events. The response community is action oriented and usually a checklist suffices to detail progress. However, public health demands data analysis to determine potential courses of action. Decisions come after practitioners are relatively confident that all available and relevant data are included in an assessment. Processes and scientific methods that comprise the "norm" for public health have been used and validated for decades; however, in the emergency response context, these practices may appear onerous or as lacking urgency. Tensions often arise between making a timely versus a fully informed choice; consequences of misplaced decisions include engaging complex systems that are often hard to reverse. Although these decision processes may not operate like the algorithms used to fight a wildfire, they are central to effective assessment and taking of protective actions. Thus, established emergency management processes, science, investigation, and discussion must be a part of ICS and response protocols within a public health department.

Major Public Health Emergencies Fall into Definable Clusters That Permit Pre-Planning

Some clusters of possible public health threats call for similarly organized responses. Flexible plans can be developed for situation-based adaptations. For example, no agency planned for the particular strain during the 2009–2010 H1N1 pandemic; but preexisting plans existed for an influenza pandemic, and those plans helped guide the response. Most public health emergencies can be clustered into categories for which developed plans are flexible and scalable. All, however, change and adapt to the specific context of actual responses.

The DPH is developing a manageable number of plans, each to cover several anticipated needs. One example is LAC's "Bio Response Plan," which describes intervention strategies based on the known elements of disease spread. It provides strategies for a variety of biological agents and details protocols for possible distribution of medical countermeasures, isolation/quarantine, and other scenarios. These macro-level plans do not include detailed task assignments. Instead, they provide frameworks from which a response structure can be developed and implemented for a specific incident.

The Threshold for Declaring an Emergency Requiring ICS Activation Is Based on the Scale of Resources Required to Respond

Executives and managers first struggled to define conditions under which the DPH would declare an emergency. With no definition, it is difficult to know when to activate the ICS structure. Defining an emergency for the DPH became a central feature of the Public Health Emergency Management Framework.

There are many ways of defining an emergency, such as scope, scale, and severity, but the process requires an agreed-upon principle to trigger the need to establish an ICS system. If one considers the use of severity in a disease outbreak, the problem presented by the definition becomes clear: What is severe in the context of public health? How extensive must an outbreak be or have the potential to be to constitute an emergency? Does the outbreak need to be life-threatening, or is it enough that it will make people severely ill? This line of questioning can grow *ad infinitum* as different scenarios play out in the realities of public health practice. Other criteria for further lines of questioning include anticipated complexity of the response effort, access to appropriate personnel, and political considerations. Obviously, seeking a definition of a public health emergency should not leave users with more questions than answers.

In traditional emergency management practice, the dictum is that the need for resources determines the need for additional response elements and size of the structure. The scale of an event and new information drive these decisions. Therefore, the need for resources beyond the usual capacity of an individual DPH program determines the need to create an emergency management structure.

A disease outbreak may be initially managed at the program level with minimal staffing. If the outbreak becomes larger in scale or if an increased severity is defined, the need for additional resources may overwhelm the program's management capability and may evolve into a broader emergency.

Adopting this definition, the DPH no longer had to determine in advance the particular "trigger point" for an emergency. Instead, the definition of an emergency requiring a specialized management structure became grounded in real-time need for resources.

■ EVALUATION STRATEGY

Since the framework is a base from which strategies and tactics are developed, evaluation is conducted when core concepts are validated during emergency response operations. A review of how the framework was applied allows us to test the concepts' validity.

The H1N1 pandemic prompted the DPH's first major activation of the Public Health Emergency Management Framework. When first cases presented in Mexico, the communicable disease epidemiologist warned the DPH of potential dramatic expansion. Discussion focused on the need for coordination and a singular departmental response. As policy makers and managers traded potential scenarios, it became clear that DPH resources would likely be stretched. Given the framework's resource-need-based definition of an emergency, the DPH quickly activated the ICS structure. The framework's definition of an emergency removed confusion over the need to implement the system and clarified the task ahead for DPH personnel. This allowed the DPH to work as a collective response unit focused on critical objectives.

Throughout the H1N1 response, every one of the framework concepts was evaluated and validated. These have proven invaluable as the base from which public health emergency operations function.

Framework in Action

The Public Health Emergency Management Framework is the basis for the organizational response structure. Illustrations of how the framework has adapted to good public health practices can be found in the DPH ICS model's Operations and Planning Sections.

Operations Section: Health Education Branch

Growth of the Health Education Branch exemplifies the two framework conditions of "ICS supports effective public health practices" and "Public health professionals are assigned to public health emergency response tasks."

The Health Education Administration (HEA) program promotes health education communications, an engaged health education workforce, and successful partnerships. For the ICS purist, this role belongs to the public information officer (PIO) and is not part of Operations (see Figure 23–1 and Box 23–1). However, in practice, health education is clearly a function of Operations. These educators are highly skilled in their craft and regularly work with field operation units to target public health messages to population groups such as schools and first responders. Assigning this unit to the Operations section simply extends the normal course of business into an emergency operation effort.

While HEA could be assigned to the PIO unit, this would disrupt the flow of standard practice, since the PIO does not develop health education materials in its daily work. In an emergency, the PIO maintains approval authority over developed messages to ensure a consistent message, but HEA's work is done with a substantive understanding of the underlying science to inform the messages, adhering to established health education standards. Having the messages developed by this branch frees the PIO to concentrate on media and joint information disbursal during an emergency.

Planning Section: Strategic Planning Branch

The Planning Section exemplifies two framework concepts: "scientific and clinical assessment of risk and vulnerability drive response strategies" and "the major public health emergencies fall into definable clusters that allow for pre-planning." The need to ensure the scientific process is included in emergency management structure led to developing a Strategic Planning Branch within the Planning Section. In traditional ICS, the Planning Section does not have branches.

The DPH codified this concept in a Public Health Strategic Planning P (see Figure 23–2). The Public Health Strategic Planning P expands upon the traditional ICS tactical Planning P by adding an outer strategic loop where science, investigation, and discussion reside (2). By making strategic planning a critical part of the event response, the DPH placed the analytic strength of public health practice at the core of emergency response operations.

Using Strategic Planning P to frame emergencies allows a readily accepted process for pre-planning. Planners and operators thus can identify incidents and set a macro-level plan after the normal processes of public health. The DPH can identify key situational awareness issues and use the Strategic Planning P to develop a macro operational plan. Therefore, as emergencies develop, but no detailed plans are yet available, the incident manager can easily identify key units, assign mission tasks, and ensure that his/her intent is being carried out.

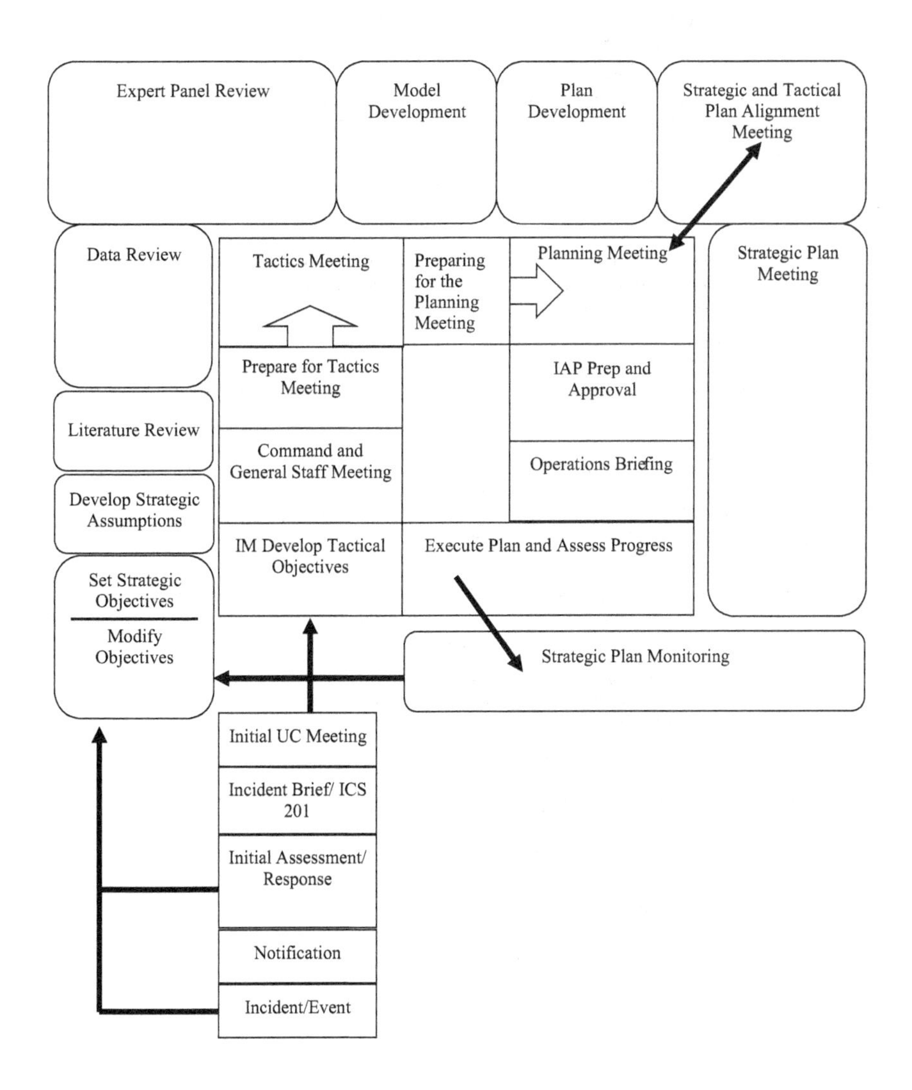

Figure 23–2 Public Health Strategic Planing P.
Adapted from the “Planning P,” U.S. Federal Emergency Management Agency (2).

Purpose: The Public Health Strategic Planning system provides for public health practice to be applied to the effective management of a public health emergency.

The Strategic Planning Cycle (outer cycle) is a 7–14 day cycle, which uses data sets and analysis from ongoing tactical response operations to refine strategic objectives and adjust projections. The Strategic Planning Cycle is linked with the traditional tactical Planning P (inner cycle).

A strategic incident plan may be developed in anticipation of an event, such as pandemic influenza, or as need arises. In most cases, public health planners could develop the strategic plan ahead of an event. This helps determine best operational objectives to apply to an event or incident type.

1. Develop Strategic Objectives
Set broad strategic objectives for an incident to be used as the starting point for understanding the problem; to establish macro level goals for response, and to refine them as they move through the strategic planning cycle. Referencing back to existing operational plans (i.e. Pandemic Influenza Plan) for scenario assumptions is a critical step in this process.

2. Develop Strategic Assumptions
Identify macro level parameters (such as availability and efficacy of resources) specific to hazard, threat, and/or response capabilities associated with the current incident.

3. Literature Review
Review journals and texts to establish a baseline of best practices and to develop an understanding of the incident type.

4. Data Review
Review existing public health data sets to develop a clear picture of at risk populations. During an event new data sets may need to be developed to better evaluate event changes, but base line data sets establishes the discussion framework.

5. Expert Panel Review
Planners meet with subject matter experts and review data and literature to determine best actionable evidence. By utilizing experts from outside the agency planning can also develop a snapshot of community needs.

6. Model Development
Modeling, when utilized to plan an incident, provides a test bed for assumptions and objectives. Existing model parameters—intervention strategies, pathogen transmission and severity and response variables—are adjusted, which gives planners a 'best practice' analysis. This identifies interventions strategies forming the Strategic Plan's foundation.

7. Strategic Plan Development
Plan is written and prepared for approval. It identifies necessary tasks to achieve strategic and mission objectives to control the incident and assigns tasks as Missions to elements of the Department. Data collection methods and reporting processes are identified.

8. Strategic and Tactical Plan Alignment Meeting
Tactical and strategic planners meet and ensure that the tactical operations plan meets the mission requirements established by the Strategic Plan. Once accomplished, the Planning Chief signs the document.

9. Strategic Planning Meeting
Planning Section Chief introduces the plan to the IM to ensure the command intent and strategic objectives are met.

10. Strategic Planning Monitoring & Evaluation
Planners use identified data sets and processes captured from the tactical operations to verify that these are achieving stated Strategic and Operational Objectives.

Cycle returns to modifying the objectives and begins anew

Figure 23–2 (Continued)

■ IMPACT

The development and implementation of an effective Emergency Response Framework has improved integration throughout all response efforts and has allowed public health personnel to understand their roles and responsibilities in ICS. Overall, the framework ensures that the DPH is an effective LAC emergency response agency.

The framework resolves misconceptions and integrates public health practice and ICS. Using the framework as a guide, the DPH develops strategies and tactics for a range of incidents and events. This is evident through responses to LAC wildfires and water contamination incidents. The Public Health Emergency Management framework ensures that the DPH is engaged and prepared to respond to events that threaten the public's health.

New confidence in the DPH's response capabilities is evidenced by the emergency response community's acknowledgement of the department's leadership role during drills, exercises, and real events such as the H1N1 pandemic. The DPH also has succeeded in garnering public resources from local property taxes to increase preparedness capability.

■ CONCLUSIONS

Lessons Learned

The DPH's experience of integrating ICS into the culture and mission of public health indicates that public health agencies implementing ICS should consider the need to:

- Build on and flex to fit existing organizational cultures rather than replacing them;
- Engage and educate managers and staff unfamiliar with emergency response;
- Routinize and exercise implementation of ICS (see Chapter 24); and
- Continually assess levels of organizational acceptance.

Looking Forward

A Public Health Emergency Management Framework has proved invaluable to the DPH. As planning efforts move forward, the framework continues to:

- Prioritize public health practice as the key element to response;
- Clarify public health roles and responsibilities;
- Clarify what constitutes a public health emergency;
- Adapt the ICS emergency management structure to benefit public health practice;
- Foster a deep involvement in emergency planning and response throughout the DPH; and
- Develop a greater commitment to emergency response from public health practitioners.

REFERENCES

1. Incident Command System (ICS) Overview, U.S. Federal Emergency Management Agency. Available from: http://www.fema.gov/emergency/nims/IncidentCommand System. shtm#item1 (accessed May 2, 2011).
2. ICS Review Document, ICS Resource Center, Emergency Management Institute, U.S. Federal Emergency Management Agency. Available from: http://www.training.fema.gov/EMIWeb/IS/ICSResource/assets/reviewMaterials.pdf (accessed May 2, 2011).
3. Centers for Disease Control and Prevention. Recognition of illness associated with the intentional release of a biologic agent. *MMWR*. 2001;50:893–7.
4. Jernigan DB, Raghunathan PL, Bell BP, et al. Investigation of bioterrorism-related anthrax. *Emerg Infect Dis*. 2002;8:1019–28.
5. Fielding JE, Plough AL. Public health preparedness in a large county department of public health. In: Levy B, Sidel V, editors. *Terrorism and Public Health*, 2nd edition. New York: Oxford University Press; 2012.
6. ICS Management Characteristics, Emergency Management Institute, U.S. Federal Emergency Management Agency. Available from: http://www.fema.gov/emergency/nims/ICSpopup.htm#item14 (accessed July 22, 2011).

24 Employees as First Responders

A Framework for Emergency Readiness

MICHELLE BOSSHARD, BENJAMIN BRISTOW, NOËL BAZINI-BARAKAT, AND ERNESTO HINOJOS

THE NATURE OF THE PROBLEM

Local and state public health departments (PHDs) are the lead agencies responsible for preparing for and responding to the health threats of emergencies, such as pandemics, natural disasters, and acts of terrorism. In Los Angeles County (LAC), both natural and man-made disasters, can cause many deaths and leave millions of survivors homeless, economically devastated, or injured with long-term effects. Globalization brings populations closer together and increases the risk of widespread transmission of novel infectious diseases, while the risk of diseases used as weapons of war creates new challenges (1).

Growing Emergency Readiness Demands

The twenty-first century has already seen the SARS epidemic of 2002–2004 and the H1N1 influenza pandemic of 2009–2010. The events of 9/11/2001 and the anthrax attacks of 2001 remind us of the imminent threats of terrorism, including the use of biological, chemical, and radiological agents as weapons of mass destruction (2, 3). After 9/11, ongoing threats of bioterrorism brought increased focus on the nation's public health system. Public health needs to be an integral part of the first responder team. Release of unknown biological or chemical agents would put local public health departments at the forefront of responders (4, 5).

Mobilizing Public Health as a First Responder Team

Centers for Disease Control and Prevention (CDC) Public Health Emergency Preparedness (PHEP) funding supports the rebuilding of both local and state public health infrastructures. PHDs need new strategies to improve public health workers' understanding of their roles so they could respond to emergencies effectively. The LAC Department of Public Health (DPH) approached workforce development for emergency preparedness and response by creating and implementing a Public Health Employee Emergency Readiness Framework (PHEERF).

■ CONTEXT

Los Angeles County Readiness Barriers

The DPH and other local health departments assessed emergency readiness within their regions. As a large urban region, LAC is a high-risk terrorism target and also is at high-risk for earthquakes, wildfires, mudslides, floods, and hazardous material spills. The region's large and mobile populations from Latin America, Southeast Asia and elsewhere also increase the risk of communicable disease epidemics.

Further challenges are due to LAC's geography, which spans over 4,000 square miles, with 21,000 miles of roadway and over 10 million residents. The DPH faces its own infrastructural challenges as well, having about 40 public health programs staffed by some 4,000 public health workers. In emergencies, each needs to be assigned incident management and response roles outside their normal day-to-day departmental duties (see Chapter 23). To attain operational readiness for a timely response amidst such complexity, the DPH set top priority on developing a systematic approach to prepare employees for emergency response.

Emerging Solutions Across the Nation

A core objective was to develop a public health workforce capable of rapidly moving from day-to-day operations to an emergency management structure akin to the first responder community. Following 9/11, the need to quickly distribute information and materials for workforce readiness left no time to create a standardized national-level plan. A patchwork of mandated trainings emerged, and local health departments were responsible for the planning, implementation, and evaluation of emergency preparedness workforce development.

Preparing the workforce for first responder activities called for new first responder skills as well as skills specific to public health emergency response. For example, mass dispensing of medications as countermeasures against pandemics or acts of terrorism at points of dispensing (POD) sites demands the coordinated response of a most of the public health workforce (see Chapter 27) (6). Public health professionals needed training, practice, and competence in these specialized skills. Further, key personnel needed to be able to quickly mobilize and operate remote Emergency Command Centers (ECCs) and a central Department Operations Center (DOC)/Emergency Operations Center (EOC).

Fostering the Paradigm Shift in Los Angeles County

In early 2003, PHDs across the nation struggled to grasp what competencies were needed to prepare all levels of staff to respond effectively to a bioterrorism event or other public health emergency. The DPH conducted a needs assessment to determine the challenges to staff involvement as first responders. This included questions on members' willingness to report to work in an emergency and being designated as disaster service workers (DSWs) under the California Emergency Services Act. The assessment revealed fear and anxiety over such responsibilities among the workforce, suggesting significant barriers to workforce willingness to report for emergency-related activities.

The results of the needs assessment provided the Office of Organizational Development and Training (ODT) within the DPH the chance to develop emergency preparedness trainings for all employees to increase understanding of worker roles in emergencies plus increase willingness to report to work in the event of an emergency. These trainings paved the way for further training development on emerging concepts in public health emergency preparedness.

Need for a Readiness Framework

Although the initial training curricula represented progress, a systematic approach had yet to be developed to link the other emergency response components, including emergency readiness competencies, Incident Command System (ICS) structure (see Chapter 23), preparedness exercises, and resources. ICS is a management tool for organizing emergency personnel, facilities, equipment, and communications—a national system that the DPH uses to guide the hierarchical staffing in emergencies. Such resources include emergency supply kits for home and car, building evacuation or safety procedures, up-to-date notification phone trees, and operations plans at worksites.

■ APPROACH TO THE PROBLEM

Breaking the Silos: The Genesis of a Readiness Framework

There is a growing need to prepare the public health workforce for its role in emergency preparedness at both local and national levels, but there are limited opportunities to effectively communicate and enhance synergy among colleagues.

Recognizing the expanded role of first responders and the need to organize and systematize the mandated competencies, trainings, and exercises, the department charged ODT with developing and implementing the PHEERF. ODT promotes workforce excellence through training and organizational solutions. In collaboration with the Department's Emergency Preparedness and Response Program (EPRP), a multidisciplinary, intradepartmental committee—The Emergency Preparedness Training and Exercise Committee (EPTEC)—was established to guide training exercises. The purpose is to unify staff training so that each reinforces the other for all public health staff.

To support information sharing at a national level, the Director of ODT established and currently chairs the Public Health Emergency Preparedness Training Collaborative (PHEPTC), a best practice-sharing network with over 200 members (10). Its goal is to enhance information sharing and standards of practice among public health emergency preparedness trainers.

Defining the Public Health Employee Emergency Readiness Framework

The PHEERF structures and links competencies, trainings, exercises, and resources to assure competent staffing based on the Federal Emergency Management Agency's (FEMA) Incident Command System (ICS) (7). A literature review showed that other local health departments addressed each construct independently rather than as parts of a cohesive system.

Five Core Constructs of the Emergency Readiness Framework

Initial planning noted five core components of an emergency readiness framework. These include 1) tiered staffing levels, 2) comprehensive competency objectives, 3) the need for more than federal and state mandated training, 4) exercises, and 5) resources to meet the identified readiness competencies.

Tiered Staffing Levels

A tiered staffing framework with four levels recognized the need to provide subsets of DPH staff with additional skill sets to enable specialized ICS roles in an emergency (see Chapter 23). The staffing framework was modeled after the chain of command hierarchy used in ICS. Competencies for each of four staffing levels was adapted from CDC recommendations (see Table 24–1) (8). Individuals in the higher levels are expected to achieve competencies within their own level in addition to the levels below. The number of staff assigned to each level assures adequate coverage for the diversity of emergency response scenarios.

TABLE 24–1 *Tiered Employee Emergency Readiness Competencies (adapted from [8])*

Staffing Level 1
1. Describe the public health role in emergency response in a range of emergencies that might arise.
2. Maintain knowledge in areas relevant to emergency response.
3. Describe the organization's role, chain of command, and management system in emergency response.
4. Identify and locate the department's emergency response plans.
5. Describe his or her basic functional role(s), which is to show up in an emergency response, and demonstrate his or her role(s) by participating in regular drills.
6. Demonstrate proficiency in the use of communication equipment used for emergency communication (phone, fax, radio, etc).
7. Describe one's communication roles in emergency response: within the agency, media, general public, personal (family, neighbor).
8. Apply problem-solving to unusual challenges within own functional responsibilities.
9. Solve problems under emergency conditions.
10. Maintain situational awareness.
11. Manage behaviors associated with emotional responses in self and others.
12. Demonstrate respect for all persons and cultures.
13. Act within the scope of one's legal authority.
14. Maintain personal/family emergency preparedness plans.
15. Employ protective behaviors according to changing conditions, personal limitations, and threats.
16. Collect data according to protocol.

(*continued*)

TABLE 24-1 *(Continued)*

Staffing Level 2

Level 1 Measures Plus:

17. Describe the chain of command and management system for emergency response in the jurisdiction.
18. Assure that knowledge/skill gaps identified through emergency response planning, drills and evaluation are filled
19. Manage the recording and/or transcription of data according to protocol.
20. Refer matters outside one's scope of legal authority through the chain of command.
21. Report unresolved threats to physical and mental health through the chain of command.

Additional Skills for Public Health Professionals within Specific Disciplines:

22. Demonstrate readiness to apply professional skills to a range of emergency situations during regular drills.

Additional Skills for Technical Staff and Specialized Teams:

23. Demonstrate the use of equipment (including personalized protective equipment) and skills associated with his or her functional role in emergency response during regular drills.
24. Describe at least one resource for backup/support in key areas of responsibility.

Staffing Level 3

Levels 1 and 2 Measures Plus:

25. Describe your management role in the chain of command and management system for emergency response in the jurisdiction.
26. Demonstrate effective leadership in a crisis, keeping focused on key information and decision points.
27. Communicate public health information accurately to POD staff and to the ECC and DOC during planning, drills, and actual emergencies.
28. Demonstrate basic knowledge in response to various hazards, and identify key system resources for effective response.
29. Facilitate collaboration with internal and external emergency response partners.
30. Report information potentially relevant to the identification and control of an emergency through the chain of command.
31. Contribute expertise to a community hazard vulnerability analysis (HVA).
32. Contribute expertise to the development of emergency plans.
33. Participate in improving the organization's capacities (including, but not limited to programs, plans, policies, laws, and workforce training).

Staffing Level 4

Levels 1–3 Measures Plus:

34. Assure that the program and the department practice all parts of emergency response.
35. Evaluate emergency response/drill to identify internal and external improvements.
36. Assure that plans for emergency drills, exercises and departmental response address knowledge and skill gaps previously identified.
37. Communicate public health information, roles, capacities, and legal authority to emergency partners.

(continued)

TABLE 24-1 *(Continued)*

38. Apply communication strategies, including principled negotiation, conflict resolution, and active listening in interactions with individuals and groups.
39. Build relationships with and between internal and external stakeholders to address community issues, including emergency preparedness and response.
40. Understand one's general tendencies for responding to different people and situations.
41. Understand how one's personal perspective affects one's thinking and approach to public health issues.
42. Manage one's emotions to respond positively and flexibly in different situations.
43. Manage information related to an emergency.
44. Use principles of crisis and risk communication.

IMPLEMENTATION OF SOLUTIONS

Training Integration into the Public Health Employee Emergency Readiness Framework

ODT developed locally relevant required training for staff in each tier of the emergency readiness framework to complement state and federal requirements, for example FEMA courses (see Table 24-2). Training requirements for each employee are determined by their staffing placement. Hence, the amount of training required is inversely proportionate to the staffing level in which members are placed (see Figure 24-1).

"Just in Time Trainings" (JITT) are pre-developed and can be rapidly tailored with high yield content for a specific, unfolding, public health emergency, for example a POD, how a POD is organized and operates, understanding ICS and how it is used in a POD, and the POD layout (see Chapter 27).

Since first responders need to be effective leaders in emergencies, leadership offerings were added. New courses focused on leadership competencies, strategic and systems thinking, team building, crisis management, effective communication, and clarifying objectives.

Exercise Integration into the Public Health Employee Emergency Readiness Framework

A core concept in implementing PHEERF is that employees need more than just mandatory training sessions during non-emergency time to become competent first responders. Exercises and drills assure mastery of material learned. Annual drills include phone notifications, reporting through the ICS chain of command, and staging employee evacuations. Trainings include annual communications and protective equipment drills for specialized level two staff; biannual POD/ECC exercises for level three staff; and biannual DOC/EOC exercises for level four staff.

The department embraces a "family first" view, recognizing that employees are more likely to report for emergency duties if they know that their family and loved ones are safe and prepared for disasters. All employees receive extensive training in personal/family preparedness at their new-hire orientation.

TABLE 24-2 *Public Health Employee Emergency Readiness Framework Required and Optional Trainings*

Staffing Level	Required and Optional Trainings
Level 1: **All DPH Staff** **~4000 staff**	**Required Trainings:** • Disaster Service Worker (DSW) Training Part 1 *(replacing PREP 101: Intro to Emergency Preparedness)* • DSW Skills Inventory • Standardized Emergency Management System (SEMS): A Basic Introduction • FEMA IS 100.a: Introduction to Incident Command • FEMA IS 700.a: National Incident Management System, An Introduction • Prep U 102 Online Annual Refresher Course (in development) • Just-In-Time Training (JITT) *(in response to an event/exercise)* - POD 101 **Optional Trainings:** • Seven Habits of Highly Effective People • Emotional Intelligence
Level 2: **POD/ECC Unit Leaders, Group Supervisors and Specialized Teams** **~1600 staff** (staff in specific payroll items from within DPH divisions listed in Level 3)	**Level 1 Trainings Plus:** **Required Trainings:** • FEMA IS 200.a: ICS for Single Resources and Initial Action Incidents • Targeted training for specific disciplines *(discipline unit as lead)* • Targeted training for specialized teams *(team coordinator as lead)* JITT *(in response to an event/exercise)* **Optional Training:** • Public Speaking Level I and II **Supervisor Training:** • Supervisor Development Program • Project Management
Level 3: **POD/ECC Section Chiefs & Command Staff** **~520** (Pre-identified staff from the following DPH divisions: Environmental Health, Community Health Services, Acute Communicable Disease Control, Emergency Preparedness & Response Program, Health Facilities, Toxics Epidemiology Program, Veterinary Health Program, Quality Improvement Division)	**Level 1 and 2 Trainings Plus:** **Required Trainings:** • Prep 301: Chemical Disasters • Prep 302: Radiation Emergencies • Prep 303: Bioterrorism • Prep 304: Natural Disasters (to be developed) • JITT *(in response to an event/exercise)*
Level 4: **DOC/EOC Staff** **~67** (Pre-identified staff listed in the DPH Emergency Desk Operations Manual)	**Levels 1–3 Trainings Plus:** **Required Trainings:** • ICS 300: Intermediate Incident Command System • ICS 400: Advanced Incident Command System • FEMA IS 800.B: National Response Plan (NRP), An Introduction • Department Operations Center—ICS Role Specific Training • Prep 400 courses *(to be developed)* • Crucial Conversations **Highly Recommended Trainings:** • Crucial Confrontations • Seven Habits of Highly Effective People • Emotional Intelligence

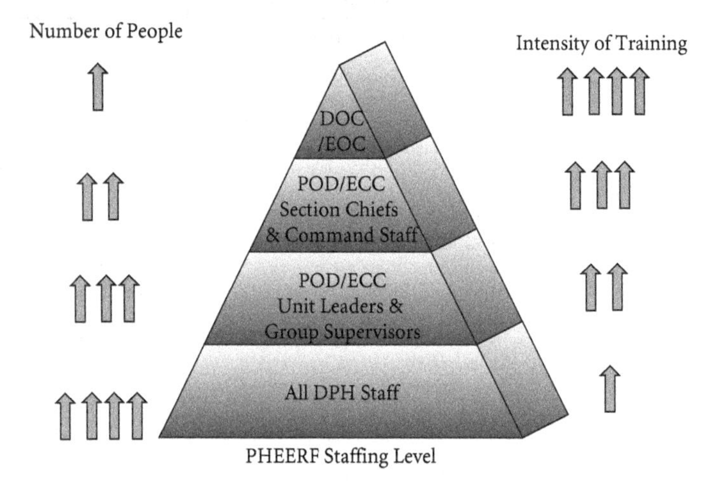

Figure 24–1 Relationship Between Staffing Level and Amount of Training Required. Note: Staffing level is inversely proportional to the amount of training required.

Methodology of Employee Emergency Readiness Framework *Implementation*

Once the department's executive staff approved the framework, EPRP and ODT notified all staff in writing of their ICS role and PHEERF staffing level. A training memo followed to each employee tailored to his or her staff level. Software for administering, documenting, tracking, and reporting of training programs and e-learning content—the department's Learning Management System (LMS)—is used to register learners, schedule resources, control and guide study units, and analyze and report performance.

■ EVALUATION STRATEGY

ODT regularly evaluates the PHEERF at individual, program, and Department levels. ODT evaluates its offerings using Donald Kirkpatrick's Learning and Training Evaluation Model (9). The model includes evaluation at four progressive levels that are distinct from the four tiered staffing levels:

Level 1. Measures the reaction of the student (What did the student think about the course?).
Level 2. Measures learning (What increase in knowledge occurred?).
Level 3. Measures changes or improvements (Was behavior or attitude improved or skill applied in the workplace?).
Level 4. Measures results (What effect did the improved behavior, attitude, or skill of the student have on business or environment?).

A Kirkpatrick Model evaluation analysis was conducted after the DPH 2009 H1N1 pandemic response. Results provide a practical readiness example and demonstrate the impact of the PHEERF implementation (see Box 24–1).

BOX 24–1 ■ The Public Health Employee Emergency Response Framework in Action: The 2009 H1N1 Response

The 2009 H1N1 influenza pandemic represented the first major departmental activation of ICS for emergency response following implementation of the PHEERF. The Department directly provided H1N1 influenza vaccine to over 200,000 individuals at 109 PODs over six weeks (see Chapter 27). Staff were assigned to roles based on their designation at one of the four staffing levels. In addition to the baseline training required at each level, the POD workforce was given extensive "Just in Time Trainings" (JITT) to ensure POD operational success. These trainings included an online POD overview training, a six-series vaccine administration training for clinical staff, volunteer management training, and refresher trainings regarding family preparedness.

Analysis of evaluations submitted by the POD workforce demonstrated the value of the systematic approach to workforce development represented in the PHEERF. Over two-thirds of POD workers reported feeling more adequately prepared as a result of their training to serve in a POD. Two-thirds of POD workers felt an increased willingness to participate in the next response following their POD training and experience and three quarters felt that the training and response helped them better prepare their families for an emergency. The systematic framework provided by the PHEERF, in conjunction with the department's "family first" perspective, were credited for the high levels of willingness, preparedness, and competence among the POD workforce.

Incorporation of the Employee Emergency Readiness Framework into Performance Measures

Its commitment to quality improvement embraces ODT's four performance measures, three of which are specific to the PHEERF.

1. Percent of DPH staff who state they are willing to report to work in an emergency;
2. Percent of DPH staff with at least six months of employment who have completed all mandatory level one courses in the Public Health Employee Emergency Readiness Framework;
3. Percent of designated DPH staff employed for at least 12 months who have completed all of the mandatory level four courses in the PHEERF;
4. Percent of DPH staff who were competent after completing Emergency Prepardness trainings at their highest certification level.

An annual public health "report card" with these performance measures provides transparency and ODT accountability for achieving quality in emergency preparedness.

ODT's Strategic Plan Incorporates the Employee Emergency Readiness Framework Evaluation Measures

Each performance measure is embedded in ODT's annual strategic plan. This plan incorporates fiscal year goals and objectives and performance measures. It is used as a guide in managing the status of each goal and in quantifying progress toward the PHEERF aim for DPH employees to have increased willingness and readiness to respond to public health emergencies. (See examples of specific PHEERF goals and objectives in the strategic plan in Box 24–2.)

Installing PHEERF staffing groups within the LMS allows ODT to evaluate individual and staff learners' progress. This enables ODT to measure and evaluate training compliance and progress.

■ IMPACT

The implementation of the PHEERF has resulted in a more systematic, cohesive and strategic way to build competencies of public health first responders. The DPH is on the path to preparedness and is more effectively able to respond to public health threats in Los Angeles. Numerous accomplishments have been acknowledged in creating a monumental paradigm shift toward achieving operational emergency readiness department-wide (see Box 24–3).

Box 24–2 ■ Examples of Employee Emergency Readiness Framework Goals Incorporated into ODT's Strategic Plan

- Increase awareness and understanding of the PHEERF among DPH employees; facilitate ongoing communication and collaboration with emergency preparedness training colleagues through the Public Health Emergency Preparedness Training Collaborative (PHEPTC) group
- Enhance internal communication, collaboration and planning through the ongoing meetings of the DPH Emergency Preparedness Training and Exercise Committee (EPTEC)
- Write a journal article for publication on the development, implementation, and best practices of the DPH Employee Emergency Readiness Framework
- Establish ongoing communication and collaboration with DPH divisions and programs to identify new and existing targeted trainings for specific disciplines and specialized teams within the DPH
- Increase willingness to report to work during an emergency among DPH staff
- Increase in the number of staff whose duty statement reflects their duties in emergency response
- Increase in the number of designated DPH staff with at least 12 months of employment who have ever completed all of the mandatory level four courses in the PHEERF;
- Increase in the number of DPH staff with at least six months of employment who have ever completed all of the mandatory level one courses in the PHEERF
- Increase in the number of staff who participated in an emergency preparedness drill or exercise
- Increase in the number of internal phone tree tests to contact employees in the event of an emergency
- Increase in the number of DPH staff who were competent after completing emergency preparedness trainings at their highest certification level

Box 24–3 ■ Accomplishments Demonstrating the Paradigm Shift Toward Department-Wide Operational Emergency Readiness

- Moved away from silos to departmental cohesion
- Provided a user-friendly and natural classification system influenced by the ICS hierarchy to enable easier familiarity of the PHEERF levels
- Established the first collaborative decision-making body, EPTEC, solely focused on systematizing ICS staffing, trainings, and exercises
- Received DPH Health Officer buy-in and executive staff team approval
- Achieved organization and systematization of staff members, trainings, exercises, and resources into a hierarchical order paralleling the ICS hierarchy and linked to CDC competencies
- Achieved branding and buy-in of PHEERF across the department through staffing notifications and intranet posting
- Developed a system to measure PHEERF staffing level group compliance through development of a certification process using the Learning Net Encouraged greater accountability toward staff compliance through training notifications and incorporation of PHEERF into the Learning Net system
- Shared PHEERF across the globe at various national conferences such as the American Public Health Association (APHA), National Association of County and City Health Officers (NACCHO), Strategic National Stockpile (SNS) Conference
- Adaptation of our framework from other local agencies around the nation
- Achieved increased staff willingness to report to work
- Achieved enhanced operational readiness and response to emergencies

CONCLUSIONS

An emergency readiness framework to develop all employees as first responders has proved invaluable to the DPH. Lessons learned from its implementation include:

- A systematic approach to workforce emergency readiness permits integration of emergency response training, disaster exercises, emergency management education, leadership development and public health practice.
- The PHEERF's standardized structure around each component of readiness has better prepared its leading first responder team in public health emergencies.
- Educating and empowering the public health workforce for family preparedness increases willingness to report to work during emergencies.
- The nature of a department-wide, systemized approach to workforce readiness encourages intra-departmental response entities to work cohesively.
- Appointment of staff to ICS positions and PHEERF levels, in addition to further grooming staff via training, encourages a sense of pride and buy-in to the roles appointed and the overall readiness goal.
- The development of a tracking/certification system for each PHEERF level, such as a Learning Management System, enables efficient, qualitative analysis and evaluation of performance measures.

■ REFERENCES

1. Fielding JE, Shultz E, Bazini-Barakat N, Davenport D, Freedman J, et al. Integrating local, state, and federal responses to infectious threats and other challenges facing local public health departments. In: Katona P, Sullivan JP, Intrillgator MD, editors. *Global Biosecurity: Threats and Responses*. London; New York: Routledge; 2010; 230–49.
2. Centers for Disease Control and Prevention. Recognition of illness associated with the intentional release of a biologic agent. *MMWR*. 2001;50:893–7.
3. Jernigan DB, Raghunathan PL, Bell BP, et al. Investigation of bioterrorism-related anthrax. *Emerg Infect Dis*. 2002;8:1019–28.
4. Gerberding JL, Hughes JM, Koplan JP. Bioterrorism preparedness and response: Clinicians and public health agencies as essential partners. *JAMA*. 2002;287(7):898–900.
5. Butler JC, Cohen ML, Friedman CR, et al. Collaboration between public health and law enforcement: New paradigms and partnerships for bioterrorism planning and response. *Emerg Infect Dis*. 2002;8:1152–6.
6. Hupert N, Cuomo J, Callahan MA, Mushlin AI, Morse SS. Community-based mass prophylaxis: A planning guide for public health preparedness. AHRQ Publication No. 04-0044, August 2004. Agency for Healthcare Research and Quality, Rockville, MD. Available from: http://www.ahrq.gov/research/cbmprophyl/ (accessed June 21, 2011).
7. Incident Command System (ICS) overview, U.S. Federal Emergency Management Agency. Available from: http://www.fema.gov/emergency/nims/IncidentCommandSystem.shtm#item1 (accessed May 2, 2011).
8. Columbia University School of Nursing, Center for Health Policy. Bioterrorism and emergency readiness: Competencies for all public health workers. November 2002. Available from: http://www.nursing.columbia.edu/chp/competencies.html (accessed April 2, 2011).
9. Kirkpatrick D. Techniques for evaluating training programs. In: *Evaluating Training Programs*. Alexandria, VA: American Society for Training and Development; 1975.
10. Public Health Emergency Preparedness Training Collaborative (PHEPTC). Available from: http://publichealth.lacounty.gov/odt/PHEPTC.htm (accessed April 3, 2011).

25 Responding to Potential Emergencies

The Threat Assessment Unit

BENJAMIN BRISTOW, DICKSON DIAMOND, MOON KIM, AND ALONZO PLOUGH

NATURE OF THE PROBLEM

The anthrax attacks in the United States in 2001 created a public health emergency caused by the intentional release of infectious products (1). These attacks, occurring shortly after the terrorist attacks of September 11, 2001, heightened awareness of the real threat of biological, chemical and radiologic agents as potential weapons of mass destruction (WMDs) and highlighted the need for a greatly expanded response role within public health (2–4).

Many potential agents of bioterrorism are infectious diseases that also can be acquired naturally by humans. Distinguishing acquisition from natural sources versus intentional terrorist actions became a public health priority for epidemiologic and environmental investigations (5). Unlike overt acts of terrorism using explosives, the covert nature of bioterrorism requires robust laboratory and surveillance system support to identify such acts at the earliest opportunity. Further, stockpiling and planning for the mass dispensing of countermeasures (such as antibiotics, vaccines, and antivirals) became necessary for agents likely to be used in bioterrorism (Centers for Disease Control and Prevention [CDC] Category A Agents). CDC Public Health Emergency Preparedness (PHEP) grant funding provided the resources for local public health departments to develop such capabilities.

Following the 2001 anthrax attacks, public health managers quickly recognized the special need for planning and partnership development across multiple agencies to represent law enforcement, intelligence gathering, traditional first responder, and public health. All would be necessary to prevent, respond to, and mitigate the risk from acts of terrorism (6, 7). These agencies, with different roles, objectives, resources and cultures needed to enhance their abilities to effectively communicate and partner before, during, and after an act of terrorism.

CONTEXT

Public health, law enforcement, and the intelligence communities found significant areas of overlap in their day-to-day activities regarding suspicious substance ("white powder") investigations and distinguishing naturally acquired disease from acts of terrorism. New systems were needed to facilitate sharing potentially important information among the response agencies. This was particularly so, given the collective professional expertise required to identify public threats. Mechanisms needed to be developed to facilitate joint epidemiologic and criminal investigations of suspected acts of terrorism.

Early attempts to formalize partnerships among federal, state, and local law enforcement, fire, and public health professionals to deal with early threat detection led to creation of the Los Angeles Terrorism Early Warning Group (TEW). This partnership provided the Department of Public Health (DPH) with the opportunity to effectively communicate public health's role as first responders in terrorism prevention. It also supported clearer communication with law enforcement agencies previously unfamiliar with the abilities of public health. The TEW facilitated partnership development between the DPH and the local Federal Bureau of Investigation (FBI) field office to support the development of joint protocols for detecting and responding to potential WMD threats.

Subsequently, the TEW merged with additional local and federal agencies to form a "Fusion Center" called the Joint Regional Intelligence Center (JRIC) to facilitate information sharing and joint analysis across multiple agencies of the intelligence, law enforcement and first responder communities (7, 8). The DPH's membership in the TEW created the means for partnerships in the JRIC and the vehicle for sharing information obtained by the DPH for use by the center for analysis to inform decision making for taking appropriate coordinated actions. JRIC expanded typical public health outbreak investigations by cross-checking information with known threats to a location, business, or population to confirm or rule out terrorism. Further, reports of an unusual disease presentation could be actively investigated if linked with intelligence suggesting a threat.

■ APPROACH TO THE PROBLEM

Recognizing the expanded role of public health in acts of terrorism, the DPH created a Threat Assessment Unit focusing on WMDs to serve as the interface of the DPH with law enforcement and intelligence agencies. This unit's goal is to build and enhance strong partnerships among the public health, law enforcement, and federal security agencies and to coordinate intelligence resources for the early identification of threats.

Creating such a unit required departmental leaders who understood the complex interface of public health with law enforcement and intelligence communities and the importance of their active collaboration to facilitate the development of a practical organizational structure.

The intelligence community and law enforcement enterprises function differently from traditional public health personnel; operating under strict chains of command, information is often protected by *Secret* and *Top Secret* clearance requirements. Essential DPH personnel had to obtain *Secret* and/or *Top Secret* clearance before significant partnership and information exchanges could occur. The Threat Assessment Unit's director, a former physician with an appropriate clearance level from both the FBI and the Central Intelligence Agency (CIA), was selected to bridge the cultural divide.

For the Threat Assessment Unit to function effectively, it needed an operational unit to facilitate connections among the local FBI field office, the JRIC (a multi-agency collaboration including such agencies as the FBI, Department of Homeland Security, and Local Law Enforcement), DPH Threat Assessment personnel, and DPH leaders (9). The operational unit formed to ease this process was the Public Health WMD Technical Advisory Group (TAG). The Los Angeles County TAG is the only known example of a formal operational unit between a local public health department and an FBI field office. The TAG comprises a core group of DPH personnel who possess locally relevant subject-matter expertise. TAG members are expert in the medical and epidemiological recognition of biological, chemical, and radiological threats, impact prediction, and mitigation strategies (see Figure 25–1). The TAG can offer public health expertise specific to the Los Angeles County (LAC) area, such as diseases endemic to the region, normal patterns of disease outbreaks, the presence of naturally existing toxins (e.g., ricin) and vulnerable targets (e.g., facilities processing hazardous substances or using multipurpose materials such as radiological sources).

Three key positions within the TAG provide the main interface for DPH with the JRIC and the local FBI field office. DPH personnel hold the TAG coordinator and public health WMD medical intelligence analyst positions. The third position, FBI WMD coordinator, represents a critical non-public health TAG member. The TAG coordinator serves as the public health bridge with the local FBI field office, triaging information in both directions. The FBI WMD coordinator, functions in a similar capacity between the FBI field office and the DPH. The Public Health WMD medical intelligence analyst represents the DPH personnel detailed to the JRIC and provides the TAG, through TAG's coordinator, with relevant law enforcement and situational awareness information.

Other DPH TAG members carry out role-related duties in addition to their regular DPH work responsibilities. TAG members fill functional positions based on their professional expertise (e.g., infectious disease, chemical/toxins, radiation, environmental threats) and work in multiple programs across the DPH, each possessing at least a *Secret*-level security clearance. In the event of TAG activation, members are pulled from normal day-to-day management chains to be part of the higher priority

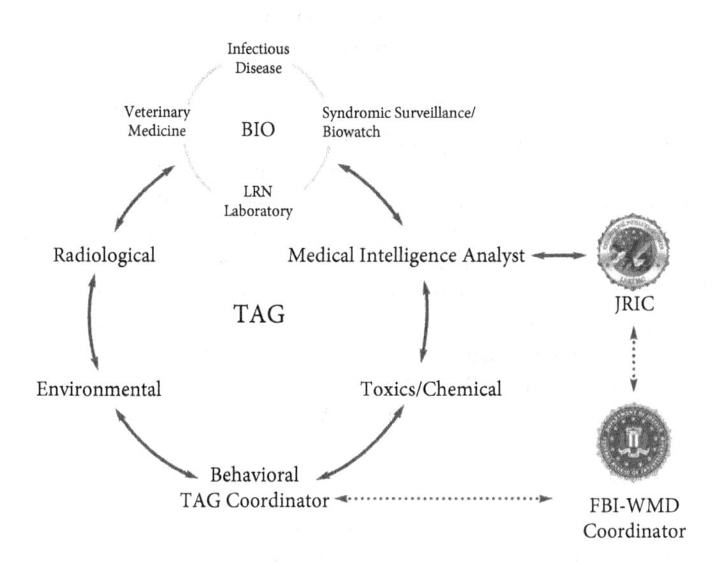

Figure 25–1 Public Health Technical Advisory Group.

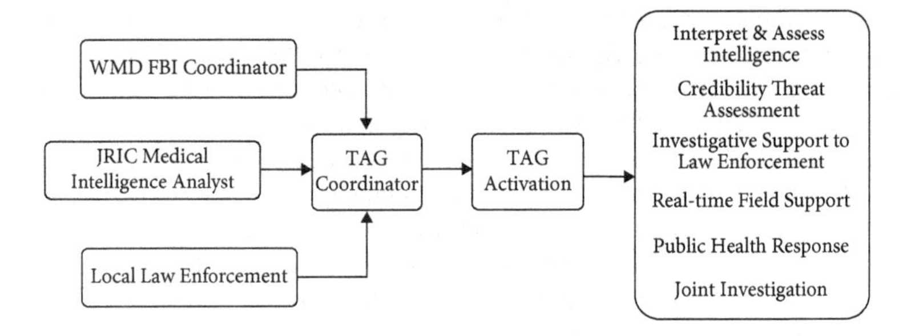

Figure 25–2 External Law Enforcement TAG Activation.

Threat Assessment Unit's management structure. The primary mission of TAG is to recognize, interpret, and assess threat information in the form of medical, epidemiologic, and WMD intelligence; the point is to determine its significance as an indicator of a potential or an emerging terrorism threat. TAG assists law enforcement in determining the credibility of a WMD threat and can serve to "rule-out" terrorism versus naturally acquired disease. TAG may recognize public health implications of a threat that are not apparent to the traditional first responders at the scene of an incident. TAG bridges law enforcement and public health needs on a 24/7 basis, is available to provide real-time subject matter expertise to an on-scene field operation, and can recommend further actions that may clarify or mitigate the health or medical aspects of a possible terrorism threat.

In order to ensure a public health presence at all threat incidents, the DPH created a WMD Incident Response Team (IRT) composed of mid-level public health practitioners with a 24/7 response capability. The primary purpose of the IRT is to be immediately available, on-scene, at a WMD threat incident and to provide a direct link to TAG. Having the on-scene presence of public health personnel at all threat incidents in LAC by way of the IRT compliments the Threat Assessment Unit's ability to build and reinforce working relationships with other first responder organizations.

When TAG is activated, a conference call is convened between TAG members, the FBI WMD coordinator, local law enforcement, and the DPH representative at the JRIC fusion center, permitting real-time sharing of relevant unclassified intelligence, situational awareness, and group analysis of possible health and medical threats. The DPH, the FBI, local law enforcement, or the JRIC fusion center may initiate a TAG call (see Figures 25–2 and 25–3). Multiple avenues of TAG activation allow a "low threshold" for initiating interagency communication. Through this system, the public health TAG coordinator and FBI WMD coordinator rely on their respective agencies to flag any information that may warrant a TAG call.

■ IMPLEMENTATION OF SOLUTIONS

The DPH's Threat Assessment Unit is based within the Emergency Preparedness and Response Program. It is responsible for administering the DPH's coordination with other agencies for the early detection, assessment, and investigation of

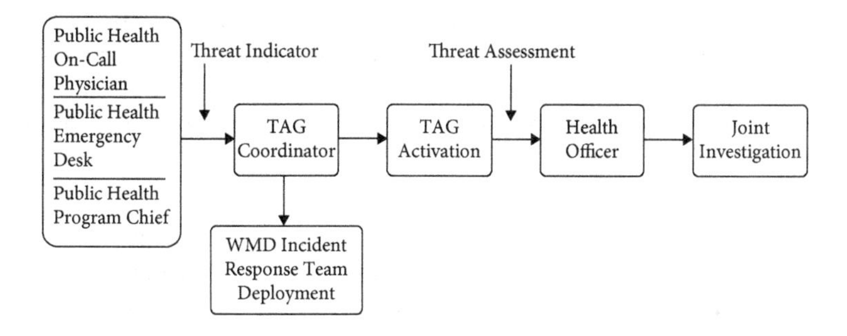

Figure 25–3 Internal Public Health TAG Activation.

terrorism acts that may pose a public health threat. To accomplish this, the Threat Assessment Unit has six core responsibilities:

1. Establishes and maintains working relationships with federal, state, and local law enforcement and intelligence agencies;
2. Coordinates the DPH WMD TAG;
3. Oversees DPH participation in the JRIC;
4. Provides situational threat awareness and intelligence to DPH decision makers and maintains DPH capabilities for handling classified intelligence;
5. Takes action to facilitate information sharing, joint analysis, investigation, and response between the DPH and other agencies to threats of WMD;
6. Collaborates with law enforcement and intelligence agencies in the development of joint WMD response protocols.

The Director of the Threat Assessment Unit leads the DPH TAG, and functions as TAG's coordinator. The public health WMD medical intelligence analyst position is filled by a public health nurse stationed full-time in the Situational Awareness Watch Unit of the Intelligence and Analysis Section within the JRIC.

As the medical and public health subject matter expert for the JRIC, the public health WMD medical intelligence analyst assesses unclassified and classified WMD threat intelligence, reviews law enforcement tips and leads, and analyzes epidemiological information from the DPH, including outbreak investigations and syndromic surveillance data. The analyst looks for commonalities among this interagency threat information, attempting to recognize possible links that might provide an early warning of an emerging terrorism event. This position also serves as a conduit for the exchange of threat information between the JRIC and TAG, drawing on TAG for its subject matter expertise, while updating TAG with relevant threat information.

TAG is composed of a number of specialists, including a medical toxicologist, radiation expert, environmental systems specialist, bioterrorism laboratory response network (LRN) expert, veterinarian, infectious disease physician, medical epidemiologist, WMD psychiatrist, and pharmacist. The Director of the DPH's Emergency Preparedness and Response Program also sits on TAG. Having members of DPH leadership as members of TAG provides an immediate pathway for communication to key DPH decision makers. All TAG members have a minimum *Secret* security clearance and have received training on protocols for communicating, handling, and safeguarding both sensitive and classified information.

TAG activations have varied widely, but in all cases have demonstrated the DPH's value in joint investigations with law enforcement and FBI to rule out bioterrorism. Example TAG activations include:

- The simultaneous notification of TAG coordinator by the JRIC, and the FBI WMD coordinator by local law enforcement, of a possible breach to an LAC reservoir. It was necessary to rapidly determine known intelligence regarding threats to water systems, threat agents which could pose a health hazard if introduced to the water system, and methods for detecting such threat agents. TAG provided real-time subject matter expertise to on-scene first responders including how to test and sample for specific biologic, chemical, and radiological agents. Additionally, TAG reviewed syndromic surveillance data from the geographic area that the reservoir services. Through TAG efforts, it was determined that no public health risk actually threatened the water system.
- TAG was notified by U.S. Postal Inspectors of a letter to a local hospital containing threatening language at the same time that several hospital employees developed symptoms and localized rashes after exposure to the letter. A joint investigation followed by TAG and law enforcement with some TAG members on-scene and others, such as the LRN expert, preparing a laboratory to test the letter. On-scene TAG members medically evaluated the symptomatic employees and assisted law enforcement by assessing whether the letter could have caused the rashes. When the medical assessment by TAG subject matter experts was combined with law enforcement information specific to the letter's threat language, TAG determined that the exposed individuals' symptoms were unrelated to the letter and that the letter contained no substances posing a health threat.
- The DPH's notification and subsequent activation of TAG followed the first human case of plague reported in a LAC resident since 1984. Plague, caused by the organism *Yersinia pestis*, is a CDC Category A bioterrorism agent for which any case requires immediate investigation, intervention, and notification of appropriate authorities. The TAG and the department's medical epidemiologist assigned to the case assessed details in conjunction with the FBI WMD coordinator. This joint investigation caused TAG to conclude that the individual had acquired the disease naturally and that this case was not the result of an intentional bioterrorism act.
- The FBI WMD coordinator's notification and subsequent activation of TAG followed the LAC hospital admission of a Russian woman and her adult daughter. They were recent international travelers who claimed that they had been intentionally poisoned with the heavy metal thallium. TAG's medical toxicologist and FBI personnel jointly interviewed the two women and determined that although they did have thallium poisoning, the incident did not pose a public health threat.

■ EVALUATION STRATEGY

The department signed a memorandum of understanding (MOU) with the Los Angeles field office of the FBI and the LAC Sheriff's Department addressing joint bioterrorism investigations. The MOU formalized the department's and FBI's relationship and created protocols for initiating and conducting bioterrorism investigations. This agreement provided a legal and theoretical framework to enhance interagency cooperation in the event of a bioterrorism threat.

The framework was tested in a full-scale functional exercise between the DPH and the FBI to check both DPH and FBI capabilities to jointly investigate bioterrorism attacks. The scenario involved patients presenting with pneumonic plague without clear risk factors or history to indicate a naturally acquired source. Through TAG, the FBI learned of the plague outbreak and a joint investigation began. The DPH then conducted active surveillance, drafting a health alert to hospitals including a case definition that resulted in the identification of new cases to be interviewed for epidemiologic data to locate the exposure source or potential site of biologic agent release. Case information was shared with the FBI via pre-established protocols to protect medically sensitive information. The FBI considered these new cases as suspected subjects for investigation, and conducted background checks for relevant intelligence to also determine a possible dissemination device.

As cases were identified by the DPH, FBI special agents and DPH epidemiologists teamed up to conduct joint interviews at the bedsides of simulated patients at three LAC hospitals. Existing protocols between the DPH and the FBI Los Angeles Field Office were used for team questioning these patients, including criteria for sharing personal medical information and sensitive law enforcement intelligence.

Information gathered by FBI agents from patient interviews was used by the FBI to develop priority intelligence reports and generate additional leads to investigate further. Information captured by DPH epidemiologists characterized the outbreak, provided descriptive epidemiology, and aided data analysis of risk factors to locate a common exposure source.

The primary mission of the DPH was to prevent the spread of disease caused by release of a bioterrorism agent. That of the FBI was to apprehend those responsible. Protocols developed jointly by the DPH and the FBI field office eased information flow between agencies, allowing the DPH to identify the point source of the release through outbreak investigation and epidemiologic methods, and for the FBI to identify likely suspects with a nexus to terrorism.

This exercise is now a model used by both the FBI and the CDC to train local public health and FBI personnel in sharing information and conducting joint investigations.

Formalized partnerships and subsequent field exercises are solidified by sustained interagency collaboration. The DPH teamed with the FBI field office to host a regional conference convening eight additional Southern California health jurisdictions to establish regional protocols for sharing, assessing, and responding to WMD threats. Later, the DPH was invited by the FBI to participate in a national-level exercise to test interagency collaboration in response to the threat of an improvised nuclear device in LAC. TAG members were detailed to the FBI Joint Operations Center, supported FBI field operations, and linked to the department's Operations Center to support the public health response.

Challenges for successful TAG implementation have centered around: getting TAG members and general public health personnel to embrace the concept of a "low-threshold" for TAG activation; understanding, using, and adhering to TAG and intelligence community chains of command; and accepting varying levels of reliability of information obtained by the intelligence community. For TAG to embrace the "low threshold" for activation concept, members receive extensive training in the "terrorist mind-set" and in the epidemiologic investigation techniques needed to rule out terrorism for infections by Category A Agents. In public health investigations, information often comes from reliable, trusted sources. This contrasts to information from the intelligence community, which often comes from unreliable sources including potential enemies of the United States who may have ulterior motivations for providing true or false information. DPH TAG personnel receive extensive training in interpreting intelligence reports and are well acquainted with the notion of "credible intelligence."

IMPACT

The Threat Assessment Unit, through TAG, developed strong pre-event relationships with the law enforcement and intelligence communities that are crucial for the success of any early detection, response, and mitigation effort against WMDs. Each TAG activation presents new opportunities to enhance partnerships and further align activities around common goals. Day-to-day relationship building through collaboration, exercises, and TAG activation strengthens overall capacity to prepare and respond to public health emergencies created by terrorism events.

Public health personnel physically detailed to the JRIC further allow law enforcement and intelligence partners to appreciate the role of public health in early detection, investigation, and mitigation of the health consequences of terrorism. Enhancing external partnerships, TAG facilitates coordinated deployment of department resources because TAG members are based throughout DPH programs.

CONCLUSIONS

A dedicated Threat Assessment Unit within the DPH has created critical infrastructure for early detection and response to new threats of WMD terrorism. Key lessons learned:

- Public health needs new expertise and needs to prioritize WMD threats as a key aspect for protecting public health and safety.
- The capacity to detect and mitigate the health consequences of terrorism requires an organized and ongoing system for sharing information with law enforcement and other intelligence agencies.
- Promoting the role of public health as a first responder, along with educating law enforcement and the intelligence community about what public health does and why, assists with partnership development.
- A coordinated department system for assessing and responding to threats and acts of terrorism is enabled and facilitated by subject matter experts who linked with their law enforcement and intelligence partners.
- Training and education among partner agencies enhances and improves terrorism detection and mitigation strategies.

REFERENCES

1. Centers for Disease Control and Prevention. Recognition of illness associated with the intentional release of a biologic agent. *MMWR*. 2001;50:893–7.
2. Jernigan DB, Raghunathan PL, Bell BP, et al. Investigation of bioterrorism-related anthrax. *Emerg Infect Dis*. 2002;8:1019–28.

3. Perkins BA, Popovic T, Yeskey K. Public health in the time of bioterrorism. *Emerg Infect Dis*. 2002;8:1015–18.
4. Gerberding JL, Hughes JM, Koplan JP. Bioterrorism preparedness and response: Clinicians and public health agencies as essential partners. *JAMA*. 2002;287(7): 898–900.
5. Dembek ZF, Kortepeter MG, Plavin JA. Discernment between deliberate and natural infectious disease outbreaks. *Epidemiol Infect*. 2007; 135: 353–371.
6. Butler JC, Cohen ML, Friedman CR, et al. Collaboration between public health and law enforcement: New paradigms and partnerships for bioterrorism planning and response. *Emerg Infect Dis*. 2002;8:1152–6.
7. U.S. Department of Justice. *Fusion Center Guidelines: Developing and Sharing Information and Intelligence in a New Age*. August 2006. Available from: http://www.it.ojp.gov/default.aspx?area=nationalInitiatives&page=1181 (accessed Mar. 16, 2011).
8. Surdin A. FBI, state, local officers join under one roof. *Los Angeles Times*; July 28, 2006.
9. Dickson D, Kim M. A public health model for WMD threat assessment: Connecting the bioterrorism dots on the local level. In: Katona P, Sullivan JP, Intrillgator MD, editors. *Global Biosecurity: Threats and Responses*. London; New York: Routledge; 2010:217–29.

26 Radiation Risk

Development of a Multi-Agency Radiation Response Plan

KATHLEEN KAUFMAN

NATURE OF THE PROBLEM

Prior to 9/11, the radiation protection community had thought it was unlikely that a terrorist would use radiation in an attack. Most people harbor a high fear level about anything involving radiation, and it was thought that this would be true for terrorists as well. After 9/11, it became apparent that terrorists could use any disruptive means available and that fear of radiation not only would not deter terrorists from using radiological materials, particularly in a "dirty bomb" radiation dispersal device (RDD), but would actually enhance the effect they sought—a fearful population. Exploding an RDD could cause enormous economic consequences, both in disruption of commerce and clean-up costs. Fear of the possibility of terrorists using an improvised nuclear device (IND, or nuclear bomb) also increased, and the unthinkable became a scenario for which citizens and governments should develop response plans (1).

In response to such risks of a terrorist attack, in 2004, Los Angeles County (LAC) had conducted or participated in several large-scale RDD exercises. During those exercises, responders were confused as to which organization was supporting related activities, such as surveying both injured and non-injured victims, as well as responders, for contamination. It quickly became clear that a more organized and effective response required clarification of the roles and responsibilities of agencies likely to respond to a significant radiological incident, that is, an incident that overwhelms the first agencies on-scene and therefore requires additional resources to mitigate the situation.

Historically, LAC Radiation Management (RM) had responded to incidents where the initial reports were inaccurate. For example, radiation levels were almost always either significantly higher or lower than the initial responders from the police or fire department had reported. This was certainly understandable because these responders received little training and had minimal experience using radiation detection instruments. So when a true event arose, they generally were not comfortable or prepared to use instruments that they may not have used in years.

LAC RM recognized the problem, had a "vision" for how all agencies' actions could be better integrated into one response plan, and received a grant from the Centers for Disease Control and Prevention (CDC) for its development. The plan, which is called the Multi-Agency Radiation Response Plan (MARRP) (2), addresses what to do in case of a major release of radiological materials, a radiological exposure device (RED), and/or RDD. While many parts of the plan could be used to respond to an IND detonation, such an extreme incident would require a more robust response that the MARRP plan was not written to cover.

CONTEXT

In LAC, responders can access widely varying levels of radiological expertise. The LAC Department of Public Health is fortunate to have a radiation control program and local radiation staff who can quickly respond to a radiation incident. But other programs, such as fire department hazardous materials teams, can perform many of these activities, particularly under the guidance of radiation control directives. During RDD exercise planning meetings with several agencies, activities that would require radiation monitoring were discussed. Examples of such activities include monitoring both injured and uninjured victims for contamination and performing decontamination if necessary, monitoring and decontaminating first responders, and determining which locations, if any, would need to be evacuated after a radiological event (1, 3). The initial expectation was that each agency understood the activities for which it had responsibility. However, as the exercises unfolded, it became clear that we had gaps where, for example, victims needed to be surveyed for contamination but no one with radiologic expertise was doing that job, and there were overlaps where too many people were performing a single function. The incident commander (IC) is the person responsible (1) for the overall management of an incident, directing appropriate assets to the right locations. Sometimes this person received contradictory advice regarding what areas would need to be evacuated and what areas would not. This can be frustrating to all, and unless sorted and prioritized for action, the health and safety of the public and the responders could be jeopardized in a real event.

As a consequence of the experience gaps uncovered, an integrated plan was developed to outline the activities that would have to be performed after a significant radiological event (2). This plan specified which agencies could best perform each function. In our decision-making process, we also considered which agency could most likely be on the scene quickest to carry out those activities. Radiation control program has the best expertise to perform certain actions, but in some cases they likely will not be on the scene quickly enough to be the most effective primary responsible agency.

Compounding the response difficulties in LAC is the fact that it contains 88 incorporated cities, many of which have their own fire and/or police departments. Having thousands of responders with so many chains of command makes the integration of any effective response particularly difficult, and particularly important.

APPROACH TO THE PROBLEM

In a radiation emergency, the primary response goals (1) are to:

1. Protect the health and safety of responders, victims, and the public from short-term and long-term radiation exposure;
2. Provide medical treatment to victims with injuries;
3. Contain the radioactive materials to the extent practicable;
4. Protect the environment and property, including critical infrastructure, to the extent practicable.

During exercises, LAC RM recognized the gaps and overlaps that reduced our effectiveness in ensuring that primary response goals were achieved. The vision was to determine the various activities that would need to occur after a significant radiological incident (primarily an RDD), decide which organizations could best support those activities, partner with them, and provide them detailed guidance on how to perform the specified activities. This plan was meant as an umbrella plan that would not replace existing response plans but would supplement them with more instructions. Based on the problems identified in our initial exercises, to assure "buy-in" it was clear that partners needed to participate in the development of the plan, and over 30 organizations did so. In addition to the LAC RM program, some other participants included: the State Radiologic Health Branch, the California Highway Patrol, the California Office of Emergency Management, the California National Guard, the LAC Sheriff HazMat, LAC Fire, Los Angeles City's police and fire departments, the Long Beach police and fire departments, the County coroner's office, County Department of Health Services, the County Department of Public Social Services, the Los Angeles and Long Beach port police, and the Red Cross. Our federal partners included the Department of Energy, the Federal Emergency Management Administration, the Department of Homeland Security, the Federal Bureau of Investigation, the Environmental Protection Agency, and the Coast Guard. In order for the plan to be useful to all these organizations, and particularly to the responders within these organizations, it was essential that it be written in plain language and avoid technical radiological jargon. The goal was to provide simplified guidance procedures that could be easily understood and used by responders and other decision makers.

Although general plans were already available (3), they were not coordinated, and none provided the level of description necessary to tell responders the activities that would likely be needed, how to complete those activities, and what levels of radiation contamination are "acceptable," meaning that they present an acceptable risk. While the plan can certainly be used for training purposes, it is meant to be a grassroots-level operational plan consistent with the National Incident Management System (NIMS). The first of the MARRP's two parts, Volume I, the *Responder Field Manual*, contains the essential radiological information for implementing safety procedures during an incident. It is designed as a stand-alone document, created in black and white and shaded tables so it can be copied easily and legibly. It was purposely featured at the front of the MARRP to facilitate quick access during an emergency. It contains 13 Activity Playbooks that describe scenarios likely needed to be conducted after an incident, and includes information cards and position job aids. Volume II, the *Extended Plan*, provides more detailed information, including color versions of the tables. Three major parts of Volume II include: 1) a Basic Plan, 2) Response Planning Guides, and 3) Attachments. The Basic Plan provides the necessary framework to support the remainder of the MARRP. The Response Planning Guides provide additional details to supplement the Activity Playbooks found in Volume I. Since radiological issues are complex, additional useful information is included and can be used for training and planning purposes. The attachments include handouts for the public, forms, and further information referenced in the plan all compiled in one easy-to-find location. With nearly 100 representatives providing input to the MARRP, an attempt to reach consensus was a priority and a challenge. The process started with a meeting of the major agencies. Large charts on the walls featured the chronology of an RDD and each agency was asked what they would be doing five minutes after detonation, 15 minutes after detonation, and so on. During this process, the activities were refined into requisite response actions that would need to take place, the agencies best prepared to perform those actions, and estimates of how quickly they might reasonably be available. Additional meetings, including sub-group meetings, were conducted over the following nine months. Drafts were distributed and comments solicited from the participating agencies. The contractor tracked the comments and changes and continually modified the plan. The 13 Activity Playbooks were the product of this collaborative effort, with each agency contributing its particular expertise to the overall project.

Responders need specific guidance regarding many complex radiological issues that challenge even the most experienced radiation experts. It was essential to include all the information a person responding to either the event, or subsequent activities such as population monitoring, would need in order to independently carry out their role. Thus technical guidance was provided and was simplified so that responders could easily understand it and use it during an incident.

■ IMPLEMENTATION OF SOLUTIONS

The development of a new County plan was easier in this case because so many of the participants knew one another personally, having worked together before on past radiation responses, training, and exercises. Therefore, we did not have to confront what could have been the hurdle of building trust and assuring that new "teammates" knew and respected their compatriots' levels of expertise. In forming the new plan, it was still important to maintain that trust and to push forward into new areas that would have to be confronted in various real radiological responses. It was important for everyone to have an opportunity to voice their concerns and opinions. Agencies each needed to "own" the plan. Experience shows that they would be unlikely to use the new plan if they felt it was thrust upon them. Each agency's input was incredibly valuable since each approached an activity from a unique perspective and with varying expertise. For example, an action plan may have made perfect sense to radiation control staff, but firefighters could tell if an action differed from the method approved for firefighters, and the problem needed to be approached differently. It certainly would have driven partners out of the room had radiation experts started discussions about arcane efficiency factors of outdated radiation detection instruments! Therefore, radiation experts did not discuss the arcane radiation measurement issues, but instead focused on pragmatic concepts needed for an adequate response.

While the purpose of the planning meetings was to involve all stakeholders, they also provided valuable participant training. It was extremely helpful for everyone to hear what each agency would be doing at specified times after an RDD detonation. Such sharing not only supported the plan's development, it also brought our groups closer together and helped us understand the challenges that each would face and what actions we could take to support each other. One lasting effect of writing the plan together is that the resulting cohesion of responders will be invaluable should we have a real incident.

Volume I of the MARRP begins with three Information Cards designed to be immediately useful after a large radiological event (2). The first two Information Cards, *First 30 Minutes of Radiological Response* and *Radiological Response Rules of Thumb*, are designed to give responders a quick primer on the most critical considerations related to a radiological incident, particularly those relating to health and safety concerns. A third Information Card, *Radiological Instrument Summary,* provides a brief summary of common radiological instruments to remind responders about the various tools they may use during an incident.

The MARRP provides seven position job aids: incident commander, operations section chief, planning section chief, public information officer, safety officer, liaison officer, and, decontamination team leader. Each job aid provides primary and secondary priority actions, and may be used as a check-off sheet to ensure that important activities are appropriately prioritized and are being addressed.

Each of the 13 Activity Playbooks describes an activity, the resources needed to complete the activity, and the names of the organizations having primary, secondary, or tertiary responsibility. Playbooks explain what to do, how to do it, action levels, and other considerations. In addition to continuous page numbering throughout the whole document, each activity also has its own page numbering (i.e., page 3 of 5) so that responders can know whether they have a complete Playbook. Because each Playbook is meant to be a set of stand-alone instructions, many tables are duplicated in Volume I if they are applicable to more than one activity. The 13 Playbooks are:

1. Exclusion Zone Operations
2. Initial Incident Control Zones
3. Monitoring Responders and Equipment for Contamination
4. Monitoring Injured Victims for Contamination
5. Monitoring Uninjured Victims for Contamination
6. Advanced Radiation Measurements
7. Alpha Radiation Detection and Considerations
8. Crime Scene Investigations
9. Monitoring People for Contamination at Public Reception Centers
10. Monitoring Public Property for Contamination
11. Public Protective Action Guide-Evacuation and Shelter-in-Place
12. Traffic Control Considerations
13. Hospital-Based Operations and Medical Considerations.

The entire MARRP is available on the web at http://publichealth.lacounty.gov/eprp/docs/LACMARRP/LACo%20MARRP%20VOL%20I%20Feb%202009.pdf and http://publichealth.lacounty.gov/eprp/docs/LACMARRP/LACo%20MARRP%20VOL%20II%20Feb%202009.pdf

■ EVALUATION STRATEGY

Fortunately, there has not yet been a significant radiologic event in the county that would test the effectiveness of the MARRP. However, the plan was evaluated by conducting a tabletop exercise with support from the U.S. Environmental Protection Agency. During the exercise, several tables represented assigned actions such as the setup of exclusion zones or hospital-based operations and medical considerations (where a particularly lively discussion took place). The incident command was represented by a table in the middle of the room. The outcome of the tabletop exercise did not result in substantive changes to the MARRP. Although it would be useful to conduct additional tabletop test exercises, or even full-scale exercises, each exercise requires extensive planning and skilled execution. Since 2009, additional Playbooks for MARRP have been suggested. For example, almost all of the agencies who participated in the plan's development are part of a county-wide telemetry system, whereby radiation measurements are sent over cellular data frequencies to a common platform and the measurements acquired are displayed in real-time on a county map. The number of instruments capable of inclusion in this system varies by agency, but LAC RM has about 50 instruments, including 21 portal monitors that can participate. Portal monitors look similar to the magnetometers used to detect metals at airports, but are used to detect radiation contamination instead. The result of this system is that LAC can better "footprint" a plume to give managers more accurate data than is available from software modeling. Issues of data sharing are being worked on; another Playbook is needed to describe how this is going to occur, what data will be shared, and with whom. An additional Playbook is needed to describe how to handle pets, including large animals such as horses, after a radiological incident. The MARRP includes a discussion of reception centers and includes a flow diagram developed by the CDC for an area for pets, but the topic is important enough to warrant its own Playbook.

IMPACT

Collaboration among so many different agencies that do not regularly communicate with one another in the normal course of business can result in a more effective response. In this case, it has created many unforeseen opportunities to work together that likely would not have happened without the collaborative development of the MARRP. For example, for certain inspections performed by LAC RM where security of radioactive sources is of particular importance, the staff now perform the inspections with either the Los Angeles City Police Department's HazMat officers or the LAC Sheriff's HazMat deputies. The Long Beach Fire Department now keeps three LAC RM portal monitors on their vehicles. A significant radiological event will require an "all hands on deck" response, and just knowing each other's faces and names is an important start to a trusting and mutually supportive relationship. The MARRP is reportedly being used as a template in other states, so they can develop their own integrated response plans. The concept of an integrated response can obviously be used for any response that is best handled by multiple agencies.

CONCLUSIONS

A plan that integrates so many different agencies' responses to a significant radiological event and that provides such a level of detailed guidance had not been written before. This is a first. Some key lessons learned include:

- When developing the MARRP it was important to focus on radiation issues only. It does not cover everyone's job duties but informs them about what would be different in a radiological event.
- It was phenomenal to have all these agencies working together to solve a common LAC problem. Constructive engagement around an important threat built real esprit.
- Multi-agency/multi-jurisdictional participation from all levels was crucial to ensure that the plan would work.

- Although there was initial concern that partner agencies would argue over who would perform what jobs, to our amazement there was very little disagreement. This may be attributable to the fact that most of the team had previously worked together on actual responses and therefore had a good understanding of each agency's capabilities.
- Participants must be knowledgeable about how their respective agencies will respond to radiation exposure events and have the authority to make decisions at the "boots on the ground" level of the plan. The planning group, which sometimes had as many as 100 participants, was engaged, thoughtful, energized, and focused. We attribute that to the fact that we all recognized the importance of having a response plan, and to having the participation of decision makers and those with actual response experience representing each organization. They inserted doses of "reality" to each step and, as a result, the plan is very operationally oriented rather than just being a conceptual document.
- Faster progress was made when the issues were kept simple, and, generally speaking, less is better. Too much information put the participants in overload mode.
- Having someone, such as a hired consultant, to keep the development of the plan orderly and the comments organized, is essential. The MARRP would not have been completed within a reasonable time frame had this not been the case.

Developing the plan together gave the participants a greater appreciation of what each agency will do in any emergency. That knowledge is likely to assist all parties when responding to any incident.

REFERENCES

1. National Council on Radiation Protection. Report #165. *Responding to a Radiological or Nuclear Terrorism Incident: A Guide for Decision Makers.* Bethesda, MD: National Council on Radiation Protection and Measurements; 2010. Available from: http://www.ncrppublications.org/Reports/165 (accessed June 26, 2012).
2. MultiAgency Radiation Response Plan, Los Angeles County, 2009. Available from: http://publichealth.lacounty.gov/eprp/docs/LACMARRP/LACo%20MARRP%20VOL%20I%20Feb%202009.pdf (accessed June 26, 2012).
3. National Council on Radiation Protection. Report #138. *Management of Terrorist Events Involving Radioactive Material.* Bethesda, MD: National Council on Radiation Protection and Measurements; 2001. Available from: http://www.ncrppublications.org/Reports/138 (accessed June 26, 2012).

27 Dispensing Emergency Medications and Supplies

Points of Dispensing

CATHERINE KNOX AND
DEBORAH DAVENPORT

THE PROBLEM

The 9/11 terrorist attacks in 2001 and the subsequent anthrax attacks in the nation's capital thrust public health departments across the country into immediate first responder roles. Shortly after, the federal government designated public health as the primary agency to rapidly provide mass prophylaxis to large populations—seen as an essential part of the nation's ability to address future security threats. The Los Angeles County (LAC) Department of Public Health (DPH) thus was charged with developing extensive emergency response plans to accommodate its 10.8 million residents. LAC's complexity and diversity among 88 cities, over 140 unincorporated areas, 83 school districts, and populations using some 100 foreign languages required collaborative DPH plans and responses. Addressing them all, it drew heavily on its established Incident Command System (ICS), the emergency response and communication arrangement used since 2001 by local, state, and federal law and fire departments but not by public health (see Chapter 23). Another resource was LAC Community Health Services (CHS), which provides public health field and clinical services for the DPH's communicable and chronic disease control programs. During the 2009 H1N1 pandemic, CHS's experience and links with LAC communities enabled the DPH to deliver influenza vaccine through many points of dispensing (POD) operations. To assure that the DPH could respond quickly to changing plans, CHS had already practiced using walk-through and drive-through POD models for emergency response and drew on a long history of experience with seasonal flu outreach (1). It also had established close ties with the LAC first responder community. The 2009 H1N1 pandemic provided the first opportunity for the DPH to respond department-wide to a real public health emergency.

CONTEXT

In April 2009, the World Health Organization declared the H1N1 pandemic. The DPH activated its Department Operations Center (DOC) and CHS investigated over 400 respiratory outbreaks throughout the spring and summer. By early fall a vaccine was developed and the DOC was operating "virtually." Teams planned to vaccinate an estimated 1.3 million residents, primarily those without access to clinical care services. Questions arose about which districts were in greatest need, how many PODs would be needed, how many staff would be necessary to operate this many PODs, quantity of vaccine doses required to ensure effective protection, and who would qualify for vaccination if supply ran short. Should LAC activate

PODs to distribute the vaccine or could other distribution methods be used, such as through primary care providers, schools, pharmacies, or urgent care centers? Previously, the City of Los Angeles had conducted three major seasonal flu POD exercises that stretched the department's emergency response POD capability. But most cities and unincorporated areas had not partnered with the DPH to activate local POD sites. It was clear that the DPH alone could not effectively implement this new campaign, so it became a priority for the four CHS Area Health Offices to engage their local cities in the mass vaccination effort. For success, local partners were critically needed, and multiple community resources became essential leverage. Planning a massive campaign in the face of constantly changing conditions created enormous challenges for everyone. DPH leadership discussed when to activate Continuity of Operation Plans (COOP) so that staff could focus resources on what lay ahead, simultaneously continuing to provide essential public health services.

■ APPROACH TO THE PROBLEM

The initial Incident Action Plan (IAP) for the mass vaccination strategy employed several tactics at once. The amount of vaccine allocated to LAC from the Centers for Disease Control and Prevention (CDC) let DPH distribute 70% to private and public partners, including community clinics, private physicians, and large health care organizations and hospitals. Since pregnant women were at high risk, particular efforts also were made to reach obstetricians (whose response was disappointing.) The tactic of using mainly community providers was called the Push Model. The remaining 30% of vaccine, an anticipated 1.3 million doses, was to be distributed through the mass vaccination PODs in partnership with local LAC cities and unincorporated areas; this was called the Pull Model (2) and was targeted to the uninsured and underinsured.

However, the department quickly learned that it also would become a point of access for the insured whose clinical providers did not have vaccine. As CHS was busily recruiting POD partners and POD sites, the CDC still had not released its recommendations for the number of vaccine doses necessary to realize protective immunity. It was assumed that children under nine years of age would require two doses, since this was a novel virus and seasonal flu guidelines would apply. It was unclear whether the same principle might apply to adults, too, since those under 65 were also "naïve" to the H1N1 virus. These unknowns caused POD sites to be planned to provide two vaccine opportunities, that is, two vaccinations per person at the same location three to four weeks apart, each site capable of vaccinating approximately 500 people per hour for eight hours. After incorporating assumptions about the number of patients to be immunized, adherence to dose recommendations and calculation of patient flow rates by the number of sites and hours of operation, CHS estimated that 250 POD events would be needed between mid-October and December. Due to uncertainty about the number of doses needed, and the types and timing of vaccines available, internal discussions focused on a POD implementation plan that could be expanded or contracted, depending on supply, need, and demand.

In addition to POD site selection, the DPH developed plans to recruit and train staff, and to establish public information messaging, health education, and continuity of operations. Curricula were developed to enable CHS nurse and health educator trainers to reach external partners who would work in the PODs (see Chapter 24). Just-in-Time Training (JITT) curricula were updated to address the H1N1 scenario.

All DPH staff, and particularly licensed staff not working routinely in clinical roles learned POD procedures from experienced CHS field and clinic staff. Area Health Offices (AHOs) activated their COOP Plans to provide essential community services, including the ongoing field follow-up for H1N1 case and contact control, while allotting enough staff to also organize and run the PODs. To assure that operations were scalable, a POD Assignment Staff System (PASS) was set up to recruit and assign people from other DPH programs to fill the many POD positions. External partners included the American Red Cross, the local Medical Reserve Corp, nursing school students, and other allied health professionals, and all were trained on POD procedure and vaccine administration. As quickly as CHS identified POD sites and event dates, the AHOs submitted partially completed organization charts along with additional staffing requirements to be met through external resources or PASS. The original POD Plan Organization Chart later was modified with additional clinical staff to ease greater throughput (see Figures 27–1 and 27–2). The Planning section was removed as the DOC managed this function, and the Dispensing and Evaluation Units were expanded to adjust for client volume.

Planning assumes an efficient generic pattern and flow for PODs, but in practice each POD's convenience and setup often fell short of ideal due to logistical issues such as patient flow, clinical supply access, and staff safety unique to each location. Creativity was required to adapt the POD generic footprint to the physical spaces available.

Public messaging about where to get vaccinated was problematic due to the uncertainty of vaccine availability and the large number of stakeholders. Never before had the DPH engaged so many cities simultaneously in a unified effort, or provided a department-wide response to a public health emergency.

The complexity grew as more cities and external partners were recruited, placing additional pressures on CHS field staff who had to leverage relationship building and maintenance in support of departmental priorities, and prudent use of available funding. The DPH induced some reluctant municipalities that were concerned about costs to participate. The DPH did engage most of the LAC cities in this endeavor, mainly because the cities understood growing public concern about the virus and wanted to demonstrate support for public health safety.

■ IMPLEMENTATION OF SOLUTIONS

The original POD schedule was based on initial CDC advisories about undelivered vaccines. Due to delay, PODs could not open until October 23, which meant, despite increasing public concern, canceling PODs scheduled before that date. This delay, along with new vaccine clinical trial findings that eliminated the need to provide a routine second dose, reduced to 109 the originally planned 250 POD events. Instead of delight, confusion about the reason for this change drew concern and disappointment from cities whose PODs were canceled, so efforts were made to adjust the overall schedule to include at later dates PODs in as many of those cities as possible.

CHS was concerned that POD cancellation could have negative ramifications long after the H1N1 campaign wound down because building relationships with local stakeholders takes time, expertise, and trust. Thus the CHS AHOs quickly moved to open communication with the impacted cities and adjusted scheduled sites and dates.

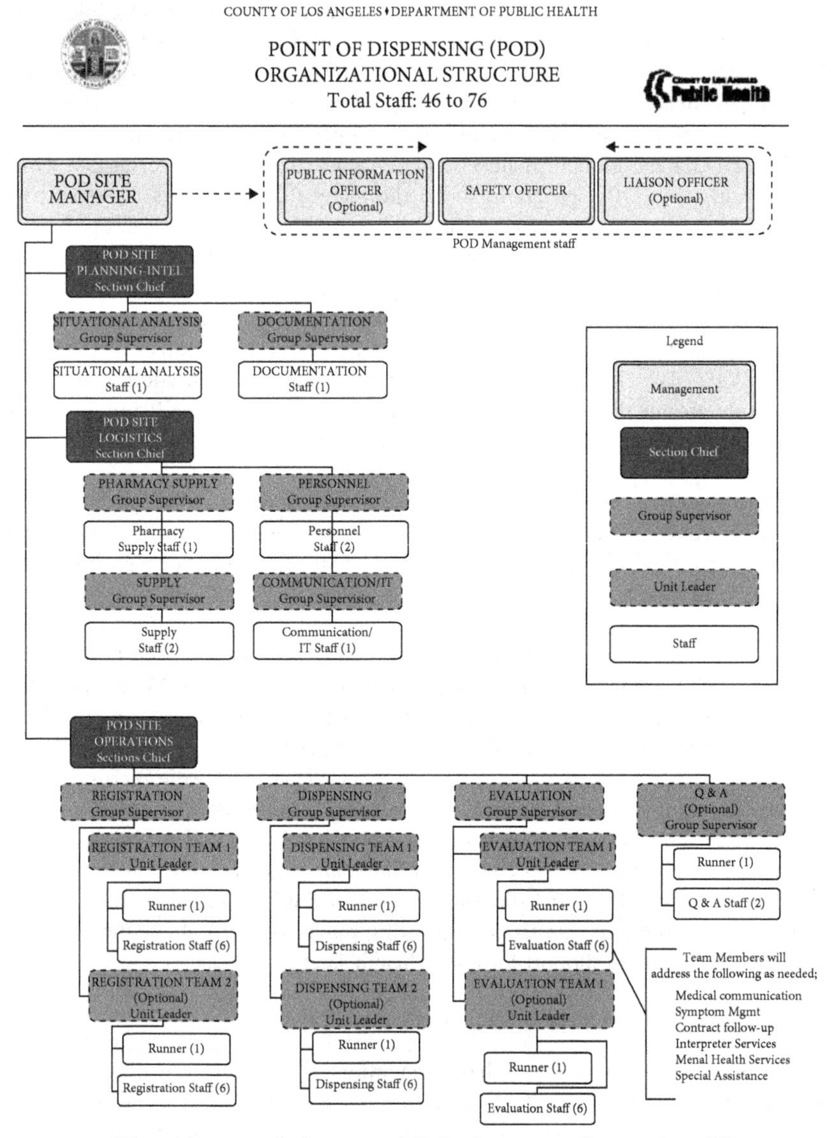

Figure 27–1 Point of Dispensing Organizational Structure.

Because of uncertainty about demand and vaccine delivery, the POD schedule was posted only in two-week increments on the department website to control messaging and manage expectations. As a consequence, some planners and community partners felt that some sites were not advertised in a timely manner. Both media influence and perceived shortages of vaccine amplified public fears. When the DPH opened the first two PODs on October 23, the lines were long, and the people were anxious. Many came to the PODs because they were afraid they could not get the vaccine through

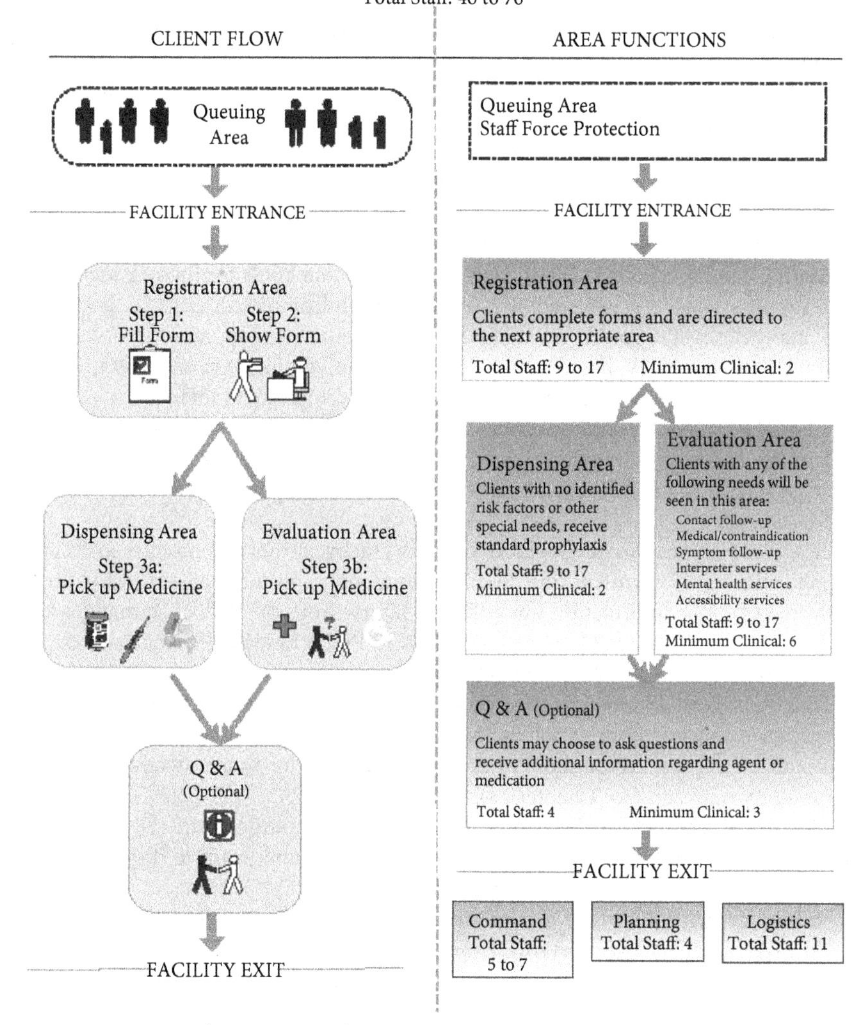

Figure 27–2 Point of Dispensing Flow Diagram.

their regular providers, and pregnant women came because their obstetricians did not have the vaccine. A combination of perceived threat of influenza, limited quantities of vaccine, and new eligibility criteria (seniors were not prioritized to receive H1N1) created waves of public fear, anger, and occasionally panic.

After initial outreaches, it was clear that rapid screening of those seeking vaccine at the PODs was critical to prevent crowd control issues. Several methodologies determined need for different vaccines (child, adult, LAIV, preservative free) as did eligibility based on CDC criteria. Many of those presenting did not meet the criteria and those crowds, in several instances, required intervention by local police or sheriffs. The best methods used color coding for types of vaccine needed, and eligibility screening by licensed staff who clearly understood valid candidates and exceptions based on patient histories. POD Command Staff exercised flexibility and capacity to modify operational tactics as new DOC directives arrived. Because the vaccine supply was limited, monitoring and aligning vaccine supply with demand became critical. Each POD received a specific vaccine allotment one hour before the POD opened its doors. Most caches included a mix of multidose trivalent influenza vaccine (TIV), live-attenuated influenza vaccine (LAIV, Flumist), preservative-free TIV (adult and pediatric pre-filled vials). A standard shipment of 2,300 doses of the various formulations went to each POD, so respective staff had to determine where to cut the line of waiting clients to prevent them from waiting for hours only to discover that available supplies had been depleted. This created an enormous challenge to determine how many doses staff could provide for pregnant women (preservative free), children (Flumist and some TIV, based on the child's age and vaccine recommendation), and seniors who adamantly claimed they were primary caregivers to infants.

The DOC issued several directives to pre-identify eligible clients waiting in line before the POD officially opened—some more successful than others, and over the next six weeks, as public demand slowed and vaccine supply increased, the situation self-corrected.

The Planning Section developed an inventory/delivery tool that monitored vaccine supply, number of clients in line, hourly throughput, and number of vaccine doses delivered (3). This information was collected hourly from the POD Commander and reported to the DOC. On October 24th, 2009, 13 PODs ran simultaneously throughout the county (see Table 27–1). Not clearly anticipated was low vaccine uptake in the African American community that fell significantly below demand by other populations. Since vaccine, such as for flu, was known in this population to have a poor acceptance rate, this factor should have been the basis for more effectively tailored community outreach (see Chapter 14).

POD Logistics were challenged, as this was the first time that the DPH had had to manage and move such a large inventory of supplies and forms to disparate communities and ensure adequate resources for every POD.

Inventory control became a huge issue, especially when tensions ran high from stress over rapidly changing events. Contributing factors to the logistical complexity included a large variety of printed materials in 15 languages, extremely tight truck delivery schedules when multiple PODs went active simultaneously across LAC's notoriously unpredictable traffic, and with POD staff moving to set up dispensing stations before the POD Logistics staff had fully accounted for supply stocks.

These challenges were resolved through corrective actions to improve inventory management and to review setup procedures with site managers. As public perception waned about the severity of the pandemic, demand for vaccine diminished and PODs were discontinued.

■ EVALUATION STRATEGY

During the six-week campaign, the DOC was activated daily when PODs occurred. The DOC conducted daily briefings within the ICS structure. The Intervention

TABLE 27–1 *Pod Throughput Tally Tool*

DOSES GIVEN a/o 16:00/10–24–09														
	Adv. Park	Balboa Sports Center	Beach Cities Health Dist.	Herald Cmmty Center	Harvard Rec Center	Concourse Med Ctr	Chevy Chase Rec Ctr	Entrprse Park	Granada Hills Rec Ctr	Lincoln Park Center	Oakwood Rec Ctr	Wilmn. Rec Ctr	Wood HillsRec Ctr	TOTAL
Vaccine Doses Administered														
H1N1														
MDV	1,529	1,850	2,574	2,880	759	2,984	895	257	1,012	1,028	1127	1542	1609	20046
LAIV	163	150	0	470	261	0	159	37	248	175	189	326	304	2482
P-Free Peds	60	0	0	0	0	0	0	12	0	0	0	0	0	72
P-Free Preg	0	120	0	69	14	0	0	13	0	0	60	49	60	385
Seasonal	0	0	0	100	0	0	0	0	0	0	0	0	0	100
Total Seasonal	0	0	0	100	0	0	0	0	0	0	0	0	0	100
Total H1N1	1,752	2,120	2,574	3,419	1,034	2,984	1,054	319	1,260	1,203	1376	1917	1973	22985
Total	1,752	2,120	2,574	3,519	1,034	2,984	1,054	319	1,260	1,203	1376	1917	1973	23085
Rolling Throughput per Hour	292	303	429	440	129	373	151	40	210	201	172	240	247	
Allocation	1,560	2,460	2,460	2,460	2,460	2,460	2,460	2,460	2,460	2,460	2460	2460	2460	31080
Transfer	500		300	2000		500		–2000				–300		
Net H1N1 Remaining	308	340	186	1,041	1,426	–24	1,406	141	1,200	1,257	1084	243	487	9095

(*continued*)

TABLE 27-1 *(Continued)*

	DOSES GIVEN a/o 16:00/10-24-09													
	Adv. Park	**Balboa Sports Center**	**Beach Cities Health Dist.**	**Herald Cmmty Center**	**Harvard Rec Center**	**Concourse Med Ctr**	**Chevy Chase Rec Ctr**	**Entrprse Park**	**Granada Hills Rec Ctr**	**Lincoln Park Center**	**Oakwood Rec Ctr**	**Wilmn. Rec Ctr**	**Wood HillsRec Ctr**	**TOTAL**
Waiting														
Adventure Park		Inc	900	200	150	150	100	20	0	0	0	0	0	
Balboa		Inc	360	250	91	50	20	20	0	0	0	0	0	
Beach Cities		Inc	1,000	1,000	0	0	900	-	0	0	0	0	0	
Herald Community		Inc	2,000	1,500	1,000	500	500	197	0	0	0	0	0	
Harvard Rec		Inc	80	1	20	20	16	10	0	0	0	0	0	
Concourse		Inc	1,000	1,400	625	0	50	50	0	0	0	0	0	
Chevy Chase		Inc	100	50	0	0	20	84	0	0	0	0	0	
Enterprise PK		20	0	0	0	20	10	10	0	0	0	0	0	
Granada Hills		Inc	300	200	200	100	10	–	0	0	0	0	0	
Lincoln Park		Inc	250	200	150	50	50	–	0	0	0	0	0	
Oakwood Rec Ctr		35	100	80	0	5	0	10	0	0	0	0	0	
Wilmington		Inc	300	300	0	40	75	100	0	0	0	0	0	
Woodland Hills		Inc	250	150	100	0	10	60	0	0	0	0	0	

Branch, a division of the Operations Section, provided direction and communication between the DOC and the POD Command Post to ensure that DOC directives were instituted and that the DOC had current situational awareness of every POD. The Intervention Branch provided direction to the POD incident commander, and if needed, would troubleshoot problems. Common issues included: inadequate or missing supplies, staffing issues, vaccine eligibility, weather problems, crowd control, and media presence. The Intervention Branch conducted daily briefings or "hot washes" with POD command staff via conference calls to identify problems or discrepancies in POD operations, and to help resolve issues and share lessons learned. The branch director then provided a summary report to the operations chief for the day.

At the conclusion of the POD campaign, an external evaluator conducted a formal hot wash and after action report (AAR). The evaluation team conducted individual hot washes with each AHO and program participant in the response. A separate hot wash also was conducted for the executive level staff and DOC personnel.

After the AAR took shape, an Improvement Plan was developed from the findings. This LAC DPH H1N1 AAR Improvement Plan was created to guide the Department's future actions and leadership. Its goals:

1. Review response gaps and areas of improvement from the H1N1 response;
2. Identify specific actions and activities necessary for improvement; and
3. Designate an executive team leader and respective departmental and programmatic subject matter experts (SMEs) to carry out specific improvement activities.

The plan addresses six thematic Improvement Areas, all adopted by the Director, Deputy Director and participating executive team members at an AAR Leadership Conference. They are:

1. ICS Structure and Processes
2. Operational Planning
3. Strategic Planning
4. Process Improvement
5. Information Management
6. Response Culture

The recommendations are being tracked as part of the department's quality improvement process (see Chapter 7).

■ IMPACT

By December 8, 2009, the DPH had administered 195,000 doses of vaccine at 109 POD events in 45 days. PODs ran on average, 18 to 20 times per week. Over the next five months, an additional 50,000 vaccines were administered through community outreach and at the 14 CHS Health Centers. The DPH provided vaccine to many of its most vulnerable residents who otherwise would not have been able to access it.

The DPH expanded its capacity to provide mass prophylaxis exponentially; 2 PODs in 2006, 10 PODs in 2008, and 109 PODs in 2009. The H1N1 POD campaign provided the first opportunity for the DPH to work across programs to plan and implement a response strategy requiring "all hands on deck." The H1N1 pandemic offered the first opportunity to engage the DOC and activate and sustain an ICS structure to support a year-long planning process. It became a singular learning opportunity for staff who had never participated in department emergency response activities or exercises, forcing all to learn through necessity.

The campaign gave participants opportunity to build new community partnerships while also threatening some extant ones due to the fallout from cancellation of some POD sites because of delayed vaccine delivery.

The AAR and improvement plan identified strengths and weaknesses within the department's emergency plans and operating procedures, and exposed ways to improve processes and performance. The experience allowed internal stakeholders to identify "best practice" strategies. Lessons learned from 2009 have strongly influenced how the Department will respond to future public health emergencies.

CONCLUSION

Among the key lessons learned are:

- Clear communication is critical at every level in the organization—within the division, in the field, throughout the ICS structure, across all jurisdictions. Information must be communicated effectively and accurately, every time, all the time.
- Appropriate staff delegation based on experience and skill improves process outcomes. Pre-event training and JITT are critical for all department staff.
- Policies and procedures should be current, relevant, and applicable to promote best practice. An emergency is not the time to be developing new policy, though new situations may necessitate modified policies.
- Public information needs to be carefully managed and coordinated. This is critically important, and can have serious consequences if not properly executed. It is essential to provide accurate information in the face of competing media forces, 24 hour news, social networks, blogs, and word of mouth.
- It is important to leverage community partners and resources and to sustain those relationships to improve community resilience and overall emergency response capacity. The DPH's relationship with partners in LAC's first responder community continues to be mutually supportive, particularly in cooperative planning for medical surge, mass care, and mass sheltering.
- Incorporating ICS principles into all appropriate situations improves emergency response capabilities. For the DPH, this has meant extensive internal planning to incorporate ICS methodology into scalable use, including large communicable disease outbreaks.
- H1N1 provided an unusual opportunity for extensive pre-need planning, since most disasters and emergencies are sudden and unannounced. Taking this into account, many of our extant community and cultural accommodations would not have been achievable as response to an immediate public health emergency.

REFERENCES

1. Point of Dispensing Field Operation Guide. Emergency Preparedness and Response Program. County of Los Angeles, Department of Public Health; 2008.

2. Hubert N, Wattson D. Weill Cornell bioterrorism and epidemic outbreak response model (BERM). Funded by U.S. DHHS (Agency for Healthcare Research and Quality [AHRQ], CDC, and NIH). 2005.
3. H1N1 POD Throughput Tool. Emergency Preparedness and Response Program. County of Los Angeles, Department of Public Health; 2009.

28 Real Time Information in Emergencies

Automating Medication Data Collection

SINAN KHAN AND DEE ANN BAGWELL

THE NATURE OF THE PROBLEM

In 1999 the U.S. Congress charged the Department of Health and Human Services (HHS) and the Centers for Disease Control and Prevention (CDC) with establishing a national pharmaceutical stockpile. The repository contains large quantities of essential medicine and medical supplies for use during a public health emergency (e.g., a terrorist attack, flu outbreak, or earthquake) (1). This repository is now known as the Strategic National Stockpile (SNS). The SNS is designed to supplement and resupply state and local public health agencies in the event of a national emergency within 12 hours of a federal decision to deploy, and contains enough medicine to assist whole populations of several large cities at the same time (2).

Following the anthrax attacks of September 2001, the emergence of SARS, and the spread of West Nile virus in the early 2000s, it became clear that after decades of eroding resources, state and local public health departments were poorly equipped to manage large-scale emergencies (3). The combined threats of bioterrorism and the reemergence of naturally occurring previously known and new diseases led to an unprecedented federal investment in state, local, territorial, and tribal health agencies to revitalize America's public health system. Los Angeles County (LAC) became a beneficiary of that investment, one of only four local jurisdictions identified by the CDC to receive direct funding (4).

In 2004, President George W. Bush signed Homeland Security Presidential Directive 10 to further strengthen the nation's ability to defend against biological and chemical agents. This increased the readiness of selected cities to make full and effective use of the SNS in the event of a catastrophic terrorist attack for which the SNS contained effective countermeasures (5). Under what became known as the Cities Readiness Initiative, the CDC provided funding through the Public Health Emergency Preparedness Cooperative Agreement and required all states and selected local health departments (LHDs) to devise comprehensive plans for providing life-saving medication and vaccines to the general population in the event of future terrorist attacks or natural disease outbreaks (6).

The CDC proposed dispensing these medications and vaccines at public sites called points of dispensing (PODs) (7). In addition to rapid access to the medications, PODs also reduce the expected surge on hospital and routine clinical care systems. PODs are typically held at non-clinical sites such as community centers, sport stadiums, and convention centers, thereby reducing excess demand on dedicated treatment centers so that they can continue treating their usual patients as well as anyone harmed in an emergency.

Public health emergencies, such as the apprearance of H1N1, demonstrated that information systems are critical to documenting who has received countermeasures, monitoring the available amount of each type and at every site, and reporting adverse events (8). However, in an emergency most local health departments would find it extremely difficult to collect, manage, analyze, and accurately report client data to decision makers in a timely way due to inefficient data collection, management, and processing tools.

Depending on the scale of an emergency, potentially thousands of client forms might be collected from dozens of sites. Simplifying data collection and streamlining analysis so that it is accurate and timely enough to support a response became major objectives of the LAC Department of Public Health (DPH). Developing a dual-purpose system—which functions both in daily activity and in an emergency—also became a focus.

■ CONTEXT

Each fall, the DPH for years has conducted a seasonal influenza vaccination campaign that includes clinics at various sites throughout the county to run PODs and to meet the need of vulnerable populations.

Mass vaccination data (e.g., client characteristics) were collected via "vaccine accountability" forms manually completed by clinic vaccination staff and forwarded to an Immunization Program Area Field Office for review and correction as needed. These forms were then forwarded to the Immunization Program's central office for data entry. Since client documentation and tracking relied on hand data entry, such a system did not provide time-critical information to decision makers on their outreach strategy effectiveness in emergent situations. Neither could it ensure that priority groups were reached efficiently. Delays in data reporting shrink the time available to decision makers to change their outreach strategy to contain an outbreak during a big public health emergency such as pandemic influenza.

■ APPROACH TO THE PROBLEM

In addition to LAC's residential population of some 10 million people (9), a large number commute from neighboring counties and LAC hosts many tourists from around the globe. Thus during a public health emergency requiring mass vaccination/prophylaxis, the DPH could need to provide countermeasures to as many as 12 million people, making data collection, management, analysis, and reporting a major challenge.

The DPH emergency planners focused on a solution that would accomplish three things:

- Significantly reduce data input and processing times;
- Provide for improved accuracy;
- Provide the ability to export data for in depth analysis.

The DPH first experimented with modifying the department's immunization registry to allow for client data to be entered manually into the registry. Although this approach provided DPH decision makers the ability to export data for analysis, it did not reduce data input time or improve accuracy. Consequently, the department explored scan-based technology using widely available scanning features to capture digital copies of forms, and to convert handwritten text into digital data as a part of its automated data collection system. The system was implemented in phases and tested during each year's influenza PODs exercises.

Several components of this data collection and management approach were already in use by other parts of the department: the tuberculosis and tobacco control programs had used this technology to scan survey results into databases for analysis. When debate traded off scan-based versus manual-entry data collection systems, the department evaluated each to assess data entry time and accuracy. The test showed superiority of a scan-based approach as it significantly saved time (2 days vs. 3 weeks, respectively) and improved accuracy. Due to the success of this primary testing, the department developed a business plan for rolling out the automated system.

IMPLEMENTATION OF SOLUTIONS

First, the DPH expanded use of the system and tested it again with 10 PODs. At the same time, the DPH brought in various department program leaders with responsibility for mass prophylaxis/vaccination activities to develop a strategy for full deployment. This encompassed all aspects of emergency data management—form development, remote form scanning, data verification, and data retrieval at the department's operation center (DOC). The strategy called for all stakeholders to jointly provide input on the form's development and in multiple languages (see Figure 28–1). In addition, the DPH pre-developed forms for Category A agents such as anthrax, plague, and tularemia.

Client forms are developed centrally by the department to assure uniformity in addressing all relevant countywide departmental activities. The forms are programmed to be scan readable and then translated into multiple languages. Clients are asked to hand fill their portion of a form when registering at a POD. Clients must fill out demographic and screening questions to be vaccinated. The clinical portion is completed by the nurse administering the countermeasure. On conclusion of the POD, health district staff scan all client forms from each local public health center to its own subfolder over a secure, preset server pathway. This decentralization of the scanning process saves a lot of time, reduces transportation costs, and significantly reduces the scanning burden. Once scanned, forms are automatically processed and any handwritten text is converted to digitally typed text and queued for evaluation of unrecognized fields due to omissions, bad handwriting or errant marks (which the system auto detects and highlights). Using a data cleaning software, multiple data cleaners can review the suspect fields and approve corrected fields. Once evaluated, the system places digitized text into designated fields of a searchable database.

Over the course of testing, DPH planners realized that the department lacked enough desktop software user licenses to facilitate data cleaning on significantly larger scale. In addition, procurement of more user licenses would not be cost-effective since all end users would not log onto the system at one time. DPH therefore revised its strategy to purchase the software and instead implemented a server-based system with shared licenses, which allows multiple end users to log into the system to clean data. The number of end users who can log onto the system at any one time equals the number of required licenses. This shared license strategy proved much more cost-effective and enabled data verification staff to do their work from

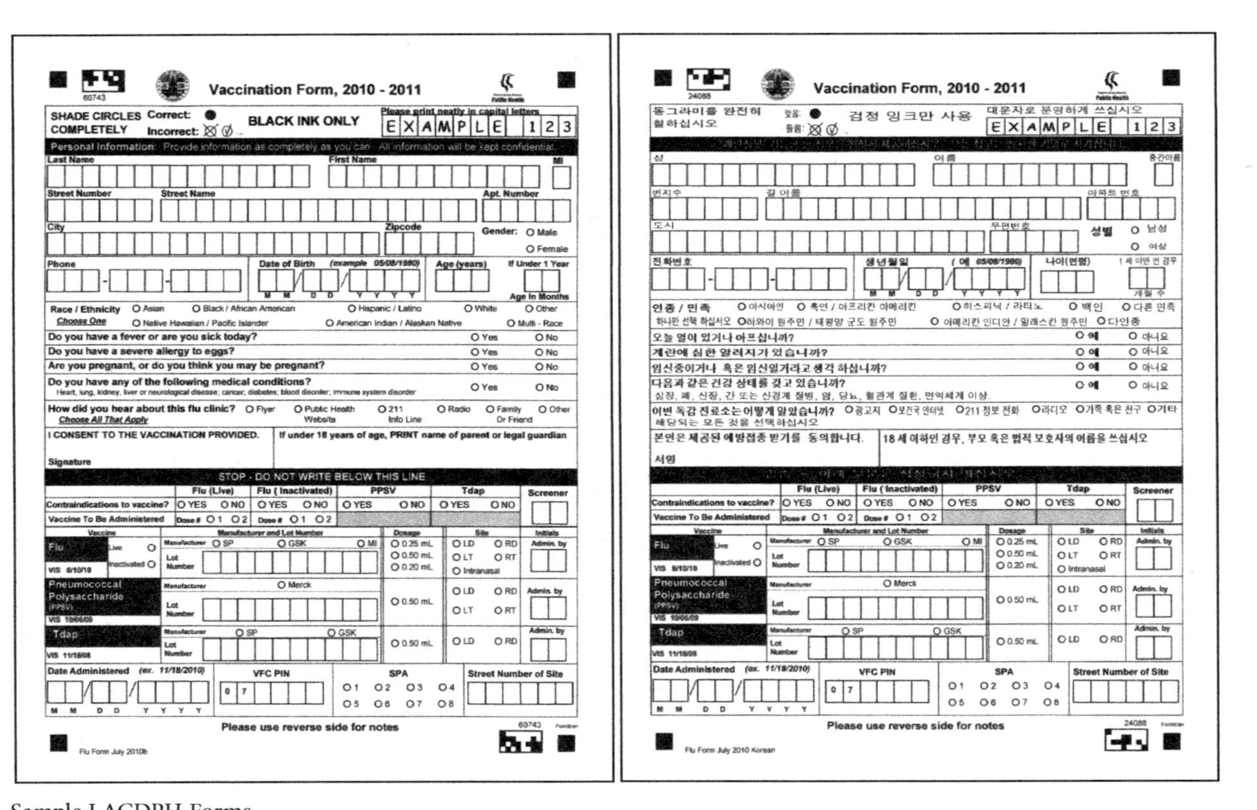

Vaccination Form, 2010 - 2011

60743

SHADE CIRCLES COMPLETELY Correct: ● Incorrect: ⊠ ⊘ BLACK INK ONLY

Please print neatly in capital letters E X A M P L E 1 2 3

Personal Information: Provide information as completely as you can. All information will be kept confidential.

Last Name | First Name | MI

Street Number | Street Name | Apt. Number

City | Zipcode | Gender: O Male O Female

Phone | Date of Birth (example 05/08/1980) M M D D Y Y Y Y | Age (years) | If Under 1 Year Age in Months

Race / Ethnicity *Choose One* O Asian O Black / African American O Hispanic / Latino O White O Other O Native Hawaiian / Pacific Islander O American Indian / Alaskan Native O Multi - Race

Do you have a fever or are you sick today? O Yes O No

Do you have a severe allergy to eggs? O Yes O No

Are you pregnant, or do you think you may be pregnant? O Yes O No

Do you have any of the following medical conditions? O Yes O No
Heart, lung, kidney, liver or neurological disease; cancer; diabetes; blood disorder; immune system disorder

How did you hear about this flu clinic? *Choose All That Apply* O Flyer O Public Health Website O 211 Info Line O Radio O Family Or Friend O Other

I CONSENT TO THE VACCINATION PROVIDED. | If under 18 years of age, PRINT name of parent or legal guardian

Signature

STOP - DO NOT WRITE BELOW THIS LINE

	Flu (Live)	Flu (Inactivated)	PPSV	Tdap	Screener
Contraindications to vaccine?	O YES O NO	O YES O NO	O YES O NO	O YES O NO	
Vaccine To Be Administered	Dose # O 1 O 2	Dose # O 1 O 2			

Vaccine	Manufacturer and Lot Number	Dosage	Site	Initials
Flu (Live O / Inactivated O) VIS 8/10/10	Manufacturer O SP O GSK O MI; Lot Number	O 0.25 mL O 0.50 mL O 0.20 mL	O LD O RD O LT O RT O Intranasal	Admin. by
Pneumococcal Polysaccharide (PPSV) VIS 10/06/09	Manufacturer O Merck; Lot Number	O 0.50 mL	O LD O RD O LT O RT	Admin. by
Tdap VIS 11/18/08	Manufacturer O SP O GSK; Lot Number	O 0.50 mL	O LD O RD	Admin. by

Date Administered (ex. 11/18/2010)	VFC PIN	SPA	Street Number of Site
M M D D Y Y Y Y	0 7	O 1 O 2 O 3 O 4 O 5 O 6 O 7 O 8	

Please use reverse side for notes

Flu Form July 2010b 60743

Vaccination Form, 2010 - 2011

24088

동그라미를 완전히 칠하십시오 맞음: ● 틀림: ⊠ ⊘ 검정 잉크만 사용

대문자로 분명하게 쓰십시오 E X A M P L E 1 2 3

성 | 이름 | 중간이름

번지수 | 길 이름 | 아파트 번호

도시 | 우편번호 | 성별 O 남성 O 여성

전화번호 | 생년월일 (예 05/08/1980) M M D D Y Y Y Y | 나이(연령) | 1세 미만인 경우 개월 수

인종 / 민족 O 아시아인 O 흑인 / 아프리칸 아메리칸 O 히스패닉 / 라티노 O 백인 O 다른 민족
하나만 선택 하십시오 O 하와이 원주민 / 태평양 군도 원주민 O 아메리칸 인디안 / 알래스칸 원주민 O 다인종

오늘 열이 있거나 아프십니까? O 예 O 아니오

계란에 심한 알레르지가 있습니까? O 예 O 아니오

임신중이거나 혹은 임신일거라고 생각 하십니까? O 예 O 아니오

다음과 같은 건강 상태를 갖고 있습니까? O 예 O 아니오

이번 독감 진료소는 어떻게 알았습니까? 해당되는 모든 것을 선택하십시오 O 광고지 O 보건국 웹사이트 O 211 정보 전화 O 라디오 O 가족 혹은 친구 O 기타

본인은 제공된 예방접종 받기를 동의합니다. | 18세 이하인 경우, 부모 혹은 법적 보호자의 이름을 쓰십시오

서명

	Flu (Live)	Flu (Inactivated)	PPSV	Tdap	Screener
Contraindications to vaccine?	O YES O NO	O YES O NO	O YES O NO	O YES O NO	
Vaccine To Be Administered	Dose # O 1 O 2	Dose # O 1 O 2			

Vaccine	Manufacturer and Lot Number	Dosage	Site	Initials
Flu (Live O / Inactivated O) VIS 8/10/10	Manufacturer O SP O GSK O MI; Lot Number	O 0.25 mL O 0.50 mL O 0.20 mL	O LD O RD O LT O RT O Intranasal	Admin. by
Pneumococcal Polysaccharide (PPSV) VIS 10/06/09	Manufacturer O Merck; Lot Number	O 0.50 mL	O LD O RD O LT O RT	Admin. by
Tdap VIS 11/18/08	Manufacturer O SP O GSK; Lot Number	O 0.50 mL	O LD O RD	Admin. by

Date Administered (ex. 11/18/2010)	VFC PIN	SPA	Street Number of Site
M M D D Y Y Y Y	0 7	O 1 O 2 O 3 O 4 O 5 O 6 O 7 O 8	

Please use reverse side for notes

Flu Form July 2010 Korean 24088

Figure 28–1 Sample LACDPH Forms.

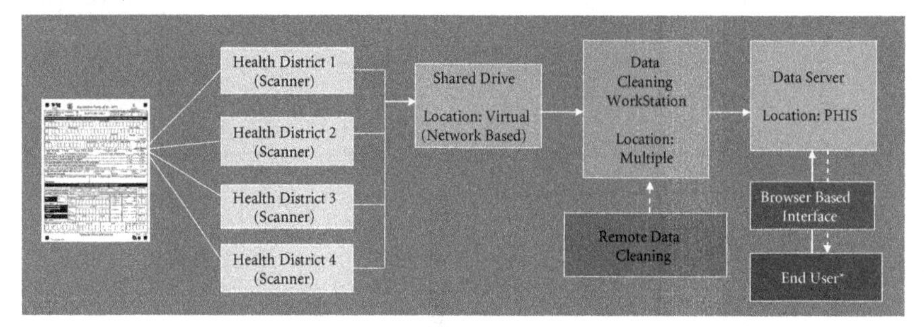

Figure 28–2 Overarching Structure of Los Angeles County OCR system.

their own workstations rather than designated desktops. End users (with database authorization via the public health directory) using a web browser now can search the database on any field or combination of fields on the form. This promptly provides decision makers any assortment of data. The database allows for data export for statistical analysis or for Geographic Information System based analysis (see Figure 28–2). It stores an archived PDF of the originally scanned client form, which can be retrieved with the touch of a button. The system is Health Insurance Portability and Accountability Act (HIPAA) compliant and requires user/workgroup verification against the Public Health Active Directory (a repository of LAC personnel contacts).

EVALUATION STRATEGY

Use of Client Data to Enhance Outreach Strategy During Pandemic Influenza 2009

As client forms were scanned and data became available, staff began conducting data analysis based on priority targets and vaccination rates among various ethnic groups. Since the data structure of the export file was predetermined and standardized, analysts were able to write the SAS analysis code prior to the POD activation. Data analysis determined that the African American community was grossly under-represented in vaccination (only 3% of POD clients, compared to 9% percent of the LAC population). Using these data LAC DPH developed a new outreach strategy tailored to the African American community (see Chapter 14).

Electronic Client Data in a Searchable Data Repository

Since LAC DPH anticipates large numbers of clients in a pandemic, an accompanying electronic client database was developed to house searchable client data from the scan-based system, and to link the data to a PDF copy of individual client forms. During the H1N1 pandemic, the DPH received 32 client form requests for Vaccine Adverse Events Reporting System (VAERS; a national vaccine safety surveillance program) reporting and client follow-up. DPH analysts searched the database and successfully retrieved the client form for follow up on 30 of these occasions. DPH analysts then conducted queries on client data for information requested by the County Board of Supervisors, department decision makers, and officials from the 86 cities in LAC.

Reporting to the CDC Countermeasures Response Administration (CRA) System

CRA is a federal tool that enables standardized local health data to go to the CDC. During H1N1, the CDC required all states and major cities to report aggregate data to CRA weekly. Given the many vaccinations given, with no automated data system DPH reports would be very difficult to fulfill. With automation, the DPH consistently sent aggregate data to the CDC in the mandatory reporting period.

Despite successes, improvements needed during the H1N1 pandemic caused forms to be changed after PODs had been activated. Lack of time to fully test related programming led to a greater error rate of scan-based forms. A Freedom of Information Act data request caused staff to prioritize the data fields being requested. And client form processing was delayed from use of unprogrammed draft versions and outdated forms inadvertently released to POD clients. Since they had not been programmed, the old forms lacked the number to tell the scan-based system how to proceed, causing further delays. A secondary non-scannable form was created and in most cases was stapled to the original. Later these had to be separated by hand—a further delay. Incorrect site numbers compounded the problem, making it impossible to trace the origin of a form once it left the POD.

The system was retested during the 2010 influenza exercises, when all POD forms (some 32,853) were scanned, thus making the system the operating standard for emergencies and routine activities.

The purpose for implementing the scan-based system in LAC was to provide DOC decision makers with real-time data in an emergency to ensure that their outreach strategy was effective in reaching target populations. Delays and form changes, logistics, and incorrect data entry now prompt the DPH to envision developing a completely electronic system.

This enhanced system would allow near real-time reporting if network access is available. POD clients will have the option of completing forms online with a 3-D barcode sent to their smart phones or printed. POD staff would scan barcodes and view all data on tablets/laptops, then would verify/update client responses and complete the clinical section. The nurse would then submit data to the server or save it to be synchronized with the server at the end of the day. The DPH will continue to provide paper forms to individuals who do not have web access or do not complete online forms.

■ IMPACT

During the H1N1 pandemic, the new system processed over 200,000 forms. It enabled the DPH to respond to the CDC-required data, and to process requests from the County Board of Supervisors, city council members, department executives, the incident commander, and the media. The system located forms for VAERS for CDC and clinician follow up, and provided copies to individuals. The DPH mapped client data to identify gaps in coverage (see Figure 28–3), and the system yielded data for presentations and publications.

The department's Emergency Preparedness and Response Program spent a year to gain stakeholder support in the system's business plan development phase. By giving decision makers timely vaccination information, scan-based data collection,

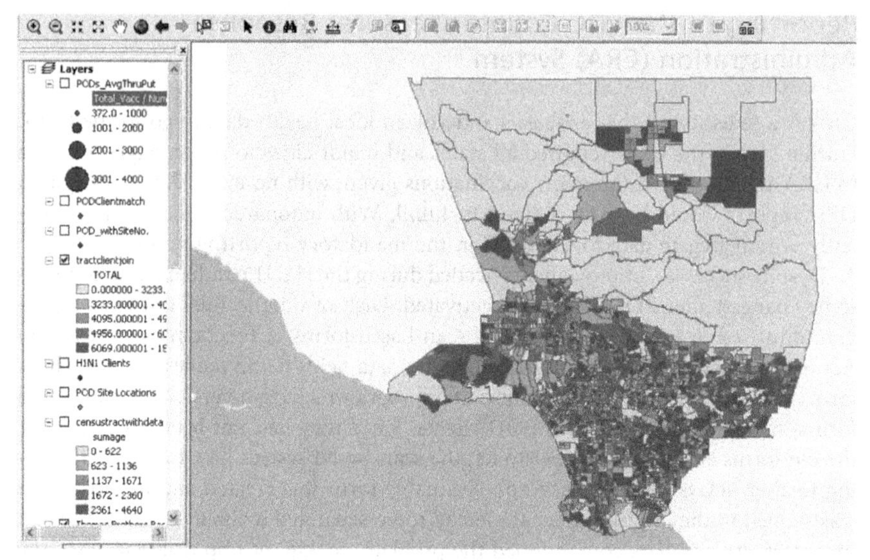

Figure 28–3 POD Client Data by Census Tracts.

management, and retrieval were universally accepted by emergency management stakeholders within LAC.

Now used for all influenza vaccination forms from PODs and other outreach programs, plans are in place to also use the system in public health emergencies due to anthrax, pneumonic plague, tularemia, hepatitis A, meningitis, or smallpox. All forms are available in the 10 foreign languages most commonly spoken in LAC.

■ CONCLUSIONS

The scan-based system allowed the DPH to:

- Use data to identify gaps and target outreach;
- Rapidly locate individual forms for individuals, physicians, and for VAERS;
- Obtain data and meet CDC and state report obligations in a timely manner;
- Fulfill data requests from various DPH programs and the Board of Supervisors, city officials, Incident Command staff, and media;
- Streamline data flow by creating a system to scan from multiple locations to a central repository; and
- Prepare data for presentations and publications.

Although the system worked well for the H1N1 pandemic, lessons emerged that could aid efficiency in the future:

- It is essential that forms be developed and tested before an emergency. During H1N1, form layout was finalized less than 10 days before the first POD. This left little time for programming, testing, and training POD clinical staffs. Although few issues arose on the form's client-completed section, the clinical portion became more complicated with respect to priority populations for immunizations. Several errors required additional cleaning and some led to data reporting deficiencies, for example several staff at various PODs entered incorrect site identification numbers. This resulted in extraneous data by site for cross tabs on shots given.

- It is essential that all stakeholders collaborate in developing new forms. It is also essential that form distribution be strictly controlled prior to finalization by the work group. The scan readable form processing was delayed by incorrect use of early inactivated draft versions at some sites and use of older forms.
- Faxed copies and poorly printed versions reproduced on colored paper complicated scanning; barcodes went undetected and had to be hand entered.
- Two-sided printing (English on one side, Spanish on the reverse) caused confusion in PODs. In several cases, DPH staff collected patient data on one side and clinical data on the other side of English/Spanish forms despite the clinical content on both sides being in English. Several forms bore adhered notes, or staff had crossed out sections, which required additional data cleaning.
- More confusion followed the presence of an additional screening form developed ad hoc. In several cases, this form was stapled to the OCR form, delaying data processing when staples and paper clips had to be removed before running forms through the high-speed scanner. Adding to the confusion, the additional screening forms were not developed to be scan-readable.
- The data (age, race, pregnant, contact with child less than six months, and prior qualifying medical condition) generated by the OCR system were exported to a CSV file. These data were analyzed using prewritten SAS code to determine the degree to which the CDC-defined target populations were being reached. DOC staff need to anticipate data requests and reporting requirements in advance of an emergency to assure that the data being collected can meet the needs. Similarly, a time line for reporting data needs to be established. During the H1N1 pandemic, deviation from time lines and generation of new reports required a significant diversion of resources. For example, the system reported "age by race" data and "age by 1st/2nd dose" data on a weekly basis for CRA reporting. While able to meet most routine data requests from the department director's office, incident commander, County Board of Supervisors, and city officials, some were onerous. Reports of vaccine use by type for the state's Vaccine for Children (VFC) program were not pre-planned and required data to be generated from lot numbers. A new algorithm had to be programmed and the lot number data cleaned before the report could be run, creating significant delays. To simplify processing, data such as date of birth, zip code, and lot number need to be transformed into easily machine-readable bubble fields rather than handwritten data fields.

REFERENCES

1. Pesik N, Gorman S, Williams W. The national pharmaceutical stockpile program: An overview and perspective for the Pacific Islands. *Pacific Health Dialog.* 2002;9(1):109–14.
2. Esbitt D. The Strategic National Stockpile: Roles and responsibilities of health care professionals for receiving the stockpile assets. *Disaster Management and Response.* 2003;1(3):68–70.

3. Agency for Healthcare Research and Quality. Mass prophylaxis: Building blocks for community preparedness. *Bioterrorism and Health System Preparedness.* 2006;10.
4. Pandemic and All-Hazards Preparedness Act of 2006 (P.L. 109–417).
5. Bush G. Homeland Security Presidential Directive #10. Biodefense for the 21st century. April 28, 2004.
6. Centers for Disease Control and Prevention. Key facts about the Cities Readiness Initiative Pilot Program. 2007.
7. Centers for Disease Control and Prevention. Receiving, distributing, and dispensing the National Pharmaceutical Stockpile: A Guide for planners. 2002.
8. PHIN CRA website. Available from: http://www.cdc.gov/phin/tools/cra/ (accessed June 19, 2012).
9. Census website. Available from: www.census.gov (accessed June 19, 2012).

PART FIVE
Service Delivery

29 Reducing Drug Use among Nonviolent Offenders

The Drug Court Program

JOHN VIERNES, JR. AND ANNA LONG

THE NATURE OF THE PROBLEM

Drug overdose is the fourth leading cause of premature death in Los Angeles County (LAC) (1). In 2007, drug overdose led to the premature deaths of 15,446 men and 5,495 women.

The adverse effects of drug use have an impact on both the individual and general public. Alcohol has been linked to digestive diseases, neuropsychiatric conditions, cancers, and premature death (2). Intoxication also endangers public health and safety by its role in high-risk sexual behavior, traffic accidents, and violent crimes (3). Alcohol alone is responsible for 2,500 deaths in LAC annually, causing 78,000 years of potential life lost to premature death (4).

Another problematic drug in LAC is methamphetamine, which is associated with psychotic behavior, brain and organ damage, stroke, and death (5). Users pose dangers to the public by engaging in high-risk sexual behavior, violence, and crime (6). In 2005, methamphetamine was the leading cause of admissions for substance abuse treatment in LAC, accounting for 30% of all admissions.

Historically, drug use causes significant impact on the criminal justice system and dramatic incarceration rates due to drug-related offenses. Between 1980 and 1997, a nationwide increase in incarcerations for drug-related crimes led to the tripling of nonviolent offenders committed to state prisons (7). Data from 1986 and 1996 showed California with the highest rate of incarceration for drug offenses in the United States. During this time, drug cases represented 38% of all LAC filed felony cases, and 70% of convicted drug offenders were incarcerated in already crowded LAC jails (8).

CONTEXT AND APPROACH TO THE PROBLEM

In May 1994, escalating criminal activity associated with substance abuse and overcrowded jails in LAC prompted the formation of a new type of court, "drug court," based on a criminal justice model used in other parts of the country (9).

The first U.S. drug court program was implemented in 1989 in Miami-Dade County, Florida, to divert nonviolent drug offenders with chronic substance use disorders (SUD) from the local jail and state prison systems into treatment. The Miami-Dade Drug Court soon became the model for subsequent drug courts (10). Support from national leaders and an infusion of federal funding facilitated its acceptance as an alternative to growing SUD-related incarceration rates (11).

The Violent Crime Control and Law Enforcement Act of 1994 permitted drug courts to be enhanced and expanded. Between 1995 and 1997, the U.S. Department of Justice provided $56 million to fund new and expand existing courts. Following the Miami-Dade County model, drug courts expanded nationwide (12). By June 2010, 2,559 such courts operated in all U.S. states and territories.

Research demonstrating the benefits of drug courts contributed to their rapid expansion. An evaluation of the Miami-Dade model compared drug offenders who did and did not participate in the Miami-Dade Drug Court (13). Researchers found that participating offenders had lower incarceration rates, less frequency of, and longer times between rearrests than non-participants (14).

The research on drug courts gave evidence that these specialized courts could reduce overcrowding and rearrest frequency, all with continued federal funding support. These factors encouraged the adoption of drug courts in LAC.

■ IMPLEMENTATION OF THE LOS ANGELES COUNTY DRUG COURT PROGRAM

In response to jail and prison overcrowding and high rearrest rates due to SUD, in 1994 LAC implemented drug courts to divert nonviolent offenders with chronic SUD out of local jails and state prisons into treatment. The mission of drug court is to provide integrated drug treatment with other rehabilitation services to promote long-term recovery, and to reduce social costs through collaborative efforts of multiple LAC individuals and agencies.

Formation and Development

The LAC Drug Court Program was established by collaboration among the county's criminal justice stakeholders and the Department of Public Health (DPH) Substance Abuse Prevention and Control, or–SAPC (previously known as the Department of Health Services, Alcohol and Drug Program Administration). Led by the Countywide Criminal Justice Coordination Committee (CCJCC), the DPH played a critical role in forming, coordinating, and implementing the LAC Drug Court Program (15). The community-based substance abuse treatment agencies at the program's core were and today still are funded and administered under contracts with DPH-SAPC.

The first two LAC courts were located in Downtown Los Angeles and in El Monte. These two pilot programs served as the genesis of local drug courts and began a shift in response to addiction and crime in LAC (16, 17).

In a study by Jonathan Fielding and colleagues, the efficacy of LAC Drug Court from 1994 to 1997 was evaluated, comparing participants against two separate groups (18). One group included those charged with felony possession who participated in the Penal Code (PC) 1000 diversion education program: these individuals could have their charges dismissed if they entered guilty pleas and completed a rehabilitation program. The other included felony defendants who went to trial and thus were not exposed to either program. Seventy-six percent of the drug court participants remained free from arrest after one year, the highest of three groups, compared to 63% of the PC 1000 participants and 49% of the felony defendants unexposed to either program. Offenders who completed their program had no arrests (80%) compared with those who did not (67%). Drug-related rearrests were significantly lower for drug court graduates (13%), compared to offenders who did not participate (30%).

To support and enhance the local drug court movement and those in other California counties, the state established the Drug Court Partnership (DCP) through the Drug Court Program Act of 1998 (SB 1587, Chapter 1007, Statutes of 1998) (19). Under the DCP Act, two state agencies, California Department of Alcohol and Drug Programs (ADP) and the Administrative Office of the Courts (AOC) were designated to assist and manage state drug courts. The ADP provides support, guidance, and is the funding source for the treatment system supporting all drug courts. The AOC, the policy-making body in California, provides the administrative support, standards, and guidance for California's drug courts.

The DCP Act also contained special appropriations of funds for 1998. After passing a grant awards application, 34 counties (including LAC) were awarded four-year grants to fund their drug court efforts. In 1999, the Comprehensive Drug Court Implementation (CDCI) Act established the CDCI Program that provided another major funding source for drug courts, which expanded capacity (20).

Overview

Success of LAC's pilot program and continued funding from the DCP and CDCI Acts allowed LAC to expand its program countywide. Today, 12 adult, two juvenile, and four specialized court programs are based on the 10 Key Elements of Drug Court (see Box 29–1).

These 10 elements are widely recognized as essential to the successful implementation and operation of the programs (21, 22).

Each drug court is headed by a designated bench officer and is served by a community-based treatment provider who works closely with the entire court team to provide substance abuse treatment services. Court teams require close collaboration among judicial officers, prosecution, defense, law enforcement, probation, and community-based treatment providers.

Procedure

Entry into the LAC drug court suspends any pending jail or state prison time while the offender is in the program; however, the offender must meet eligibility requirements, voluntarily participate, and fulfill court requirements. To be eligible, offenders must have a current felony drug possession or use charge, no history of serious or violent offenses, and a demonstrated substance use disorder (SUD). Eligible offenders are referred to drug court by the public defender and supported by the district attorney and are then screened for suitability by the treatment provider prior to admission.

As an incentive to drug court entry, those who meet all requirements will have their criminal drug charges dismissed. Although the bench officer and court team supervise drug court offenders, program participation is voluntary. Offenders who fail to adhere to drug court rules after admission may have to fulfill their initial jail or state prison sentences.

The program follows a treatment and recovery regimen based on assessment of each offender's addiction severity and treatment needs. Treatment providers continuously screen potential program candidates, create treatment and supervision plans, and monitor individuals through all program phases.

BOX 29–1 ■ 10 Key Elements of Drug Court Model

Element 1: ***Integration of treatment services with justice system case processing***
All court team members agree to and approve a treatment plan for participants.

Element 2: ***Non-adversarial approach***
The team functions as a collaborative body with the prosecutor, defense counsel, and bench officer working together to serve the best interests of public safety and the participants' treatment plans.

Element 3: ***Early identification and placement of eligible clients***
Both defense counsel and prosecution work to identify clients for drug courts. Early screening and assessment are key elements of the LAC DCP.

Element 4: ***Access to a continuum of alcohol, drug, and related treatment services***
All LAC treatment providers are required to offer a continuum of services for court clients based on their needs. All participants are assessed for addiction severity and then placed for appropriate treatment level.

Element 5: ***Frequent alcohol and drug testing***
A key element is accountability. Frequent and random drug testing is vital to the program. Frequent testing is determined by severity of addiction and is agreed upon by the court team.

Element 6: ***Coordinated strategy for responses to client compliance***
All LAC drug courts operate with specific procedures for reporting progress and client compliance with treatment plans. Treatment providers give regular progress reports to the court and swiftly notify the court team when a participant is non-compliant.

Element 7: ***Ongoing judicial interaction with each client***
One vital element is the role of the bench officer. Frequent court appearances are the hallmark of drug courts. Participants are required to appear before the judge to report their progress and discuss non-compliance issues. Bench officers provide guidance, encouragement, rewards, and sanctions when needed.

Element 8: ***Monitoring and evaluation measures***
Monitoring, oversight, and evaluation of the LAC drug courts are hallmarks of the program. CCJCC's Drug Court Oversight Subcommittee establishes standards and practices and regularly reviews operations and issues. LAC DPH—SAPC administers a contract for independent evaluation of the DCP.

Element 9: ***Continuing interdisciplinary education***
On-going training is essential. An annual training conference brings together drug court cross-discipline professionals to hear the latest research related to treatments. Specific training for providers is also held annually.

Element 10: ***Drug court partnerships***
Each LAC court is based on partnerships among all stakeholders in the criminal justice system and drug treatment network. These partnerships ensure that the courts operate efficiently and work effectively to assist offenders into recovery.

Completion requirements for a 12- to 18-month program consist of a two-week trial phase, and then three distinct phases of treatment and compliance with all court supervision requirements (see Box 29–2) (23).

Participants must complete specific criteria before advancing to the next phase. These criteria include having no positive drug results from at least 125 tests administered during the entire program, no unexcused absences, compliance with all treatment activities and court orders, adherence to treatment plans, employment or enrollment in an educational/vocational program, and regularly scheduled appearances before the bench officer.

To promote transition through the phases, bench officers typically motivate participants with incentives and praise in open court to foster confidence and to support program continuation. Participants struggling with program compliance may be subjected to a variety of court-ordered sanctions such as brief incarceration, community service, or an increased number of self-help meetings. Upon successful completion of the program, a graduation ceremony in court marks the dismissal of the various drug case offenses that were suspended upon admission into the drug court.

BOX 29–2 ■ Drug Court Phases

Trial Phase

The Trial Phase consists of frequent drug testing, mandatory group meetings, and counseling sessions. This phase is essential in assessing participants' commitment to treatment and level of motivation. The Trial Phase lasts approximately two weeks. Upon successful completion, participants formally transition into the program and begin Phase I.

Phase I

Phase I focuses on assessment, stabilization, and the start of an individualized treatment plan. Frequent counseling sessions, mandatory 12-step meetings, and mandatory drug testing. Emphasis is on initial treatment goals and objectives tailored to individual need.

Phase II

Phase II includes intensive treatment services, counseling focused on long-term recovery and socialization, mandatory 12-step meetings, and mandatory drug testing. The frequency of testing and meetings is less than Phase I and reflects a growing commitment to recovery by the participant. Emphasis is on pursuing individual employment and vocational/education goals.

Phase III

Phase III focuses on transition from intense treatment to long-term relapse prevention. Counseling sessions continue with a larger concentration on self-sufficiency. Mandatory 12-step meetings and drug testing continue, but on a less frequent basis than in Phase II. Phase III prepares participants for graduation from the program and for long-lasting recovery.

Types of Specialized, Collaborative Drug Courts

In addition to the Adult Drug Court, LAC established specialized drug courts serving populations of juveniles, sentenced offenders, family dependency, women's re-entry, and those with co-occurring disorders. Based on the traditional drug court model, each specialized court is adapted to better serve the specific population (see Box 29–3).

BOX 29–3 ■ Types of Specialized, Collaborative Drug Courts

Juvenile Drug Court

- Targets nonviolent juvenile offenders at greatest risk of becoming chronic, serious offenders
- Voluntary, though referrals are initiated by Public Defender's Office
- 12-month program includes individual, group, and family counseling, vocational training, and job placement (as needed)

Sentenced Offender Drug Court

- Targets convicted nonviolent felony offenders with long-term state prison sentences due to drug addiction and past criminal record
- Offers formal probation as an alternative to state prison
- Voluntary, though referrals are initiated by the Public Defender's Office, and must have support of District Attorney's Office
- Mandatory 90-day in-custody treatment component followed by 6–9 month program of supervision and outpatient care that includes frequent drug testing and formal probation supervision

Family Dependency Drug Court

- Targets parents of children in the child welfare system
- Assists parents in addressing substance abuse issues to allow continued family unity or reunification
- Voluntary, though referrals are initiated by the LAC Department of Children and Family Services
- 12-month program includes counseling and educational workshops

Women's Re-entry Program

- Targets female parolees with a new felony drug charge
- Voluntary, though referrals are made by the Public Defender, and both the District Attorney and California Department of Corrections & Rehabilitation must support program admission
- 18-month treatment program, with 6 months of residential services and 12 months of outpatient treatment
- Mental health and trauma counseling and employment assistance are made available

(*continued*)

BOX 29-3 (*Continued*)

Co-Occurring Disorders Court

- Targets criminal offenders who are clinically diagnosed with a severe and persistent mental illness and SUD
- Voluntary, though referrals are initiated by the Public Defender, and admission is granted after screening by Department of Mental Health
- 18-month integrated mental health and substance use treatment, with 6 months of residential services and 12 months of outpatient care

EVALUATION STRATEGY

In 2000, the Adult Drug Courts were linked to a comprehensive computer system known as the Drug Court Management Information System (DCMIS) (24). Grant funding secured by the CCJCC allowed LAC to develop the DCMIS as a sophisticated data collection and transmission system designed to accommodate reporting and statistical needs for LAC. The DCMIS is a browser-based, real-time application that supports the referral, treatment operations, and administrative requirements of the Drug Court Program. The system links community-based treatment providers with the courts to allow for timely electronic exchange of information. DCMIS captures statistical information required by ADP to support funding for pre-conviction and post-conviction court programs.

DCMIS evolves as needed with additional demographic and social outcome fields, and to identify offenders likely to be sent to state prison if they fail to complete drug court. The collaborative efforts of the CCJCC, DPH-SAPC, Internal Services Department (ISD), the LAC Superior Court, and treatment providers are essential in allowing this real-time database system to accurately track offenders.

The DCMIS is accessible to drug court team members, including judges, court officers, project coordinators, treatment staff, and program managers. For confidentiality, all DCMIS users are registered with specific access privileges. This classification ensures access only to authorized DCMIS users.

IMPACT

Program Successes

Since inception, 4,882 participants graduated from the traditional Adult Drug Court and the Sentenced Offenders Drug Court Program. As of January 2011, there were 1,175 active program participants.

From July 1, 2003, to June 30, 2009, 2,345 graduates demonstrated these social outcomes:

- 93% obtained employment while in the program;
- 100% enrolled in or completed an educational program;
- 94% of female graduates' babies were born drug-free;
- 86% of graduates with dependents were reunited with their families.

Additional social outcomes included completion of required community service hours, regular payment of court-ordered child support, and obtainment of valid driver's licenses. These outcomes support the overall quality of life and public safety for LAC communities and individuals.

Estimated Cost Savings

According to California Department of Corrections and Rehabilitation (CDCR), the average daily cost per prison inmate in FY 2008–2009 was $133 per day (25). During that time, 244,905 prison days were averted by participants in drug court, providing an estimated prison cost savings of $32,572,365. In FY 2009–2010 the daily prison cost was $122; drug court participation saved 278,564 prison days, resulting in an estimated cost savings of $33,984,808.

In addition to saving incarceration costs, drug court saved other costs, as shown in a study comparing outcome cost savings from El Monte Drug Court participants from 1998–1999. The study compared participants in the El Monte Drug Court for four years with a comparison group of PC 1000 and non–drug court participants with matched backgrounds (26). Each drug court participant had $6,958.26 less in outcome costs than each individual in the comparison group (see Table 29–1). In addition, Drug Court Partnership's examination of the cost of Sentenced Offender Drug Court effectiveness revealed less criminal activity and greater involvement in positive social and familial relations (27).

Drug courts save local and state money throughout the nation. Savings reported by the National Association of Drug Court Professionals (NADCP) indicate (28):

- Nationwide, for every $1.00 invested in drug court, taxpayers save as much as $3.36 in avoided criminal justice costs alone.
- Drug court cost savings range from $4,000 to $12,000 per client. These reflect reduced prison costs, victimization, and revolving-door arrests and trials.

Program Data

Table 29–2 shows annual new, continuing, and graduating participants between 2001 and 2009, when 16,582 new and continuing participants received SUD treatment. The decrease from 2,341 participants in FY 2001–2002 to the 1,588 participants in FY 2008–2009 reflects expansion in options for SUD offenders, due in part to Proposition 36.

Recidivism

Table 29–3 reports criminal recidivism rates among graduates from FY 2001–2002 through 2007–2008. Offenders are tracked for five years following graduation. Rates for intervening years reflect gradually reduced annual occurrences of recidivism, respectively. These compare favorably to rates for drug courts nationwide and demonstrate the effectiveness of the program. According to NADCP, 75% of court graduates nationwide remain arrest-free at least two years after leaving the program (29).

TABLE 29–1 *Average Criminal Justice Outcome Costs per Offender*

Transaction	Unit Cost	Avg. # of Transactions Drug Court Participants	Average Cost per Drug Cost Participant	Avg. # of Transactions Comparison	Average Cost per Comparison Individual	Percentage Change
Rearrests	$243.37	1.90	$462.40	1.96	$477.01	−3%
Police Bookings	$177.37	1.48	$262.51	1.78	$315.72	−17%
Court Cases (no-trial)	$1,868.73	.66	$1,233.36	.69	$1,289.42	−4%
Court Cases (trial)	$3,343.77	0	0	0	0	N/A
Jail Days	$73.79	42.51	$3,136.81	68.73	$5,071.59	−38%
Probation Days	$4.08	336	$1,370.88	331.37	$1,351.99	+1%
Victimizations—Personal Crimes	$40,698.60	.08	$3,255.89	.14	$5,697.80	−43%
Victimizations—Property Crimes	$12,563.35	.30	$3,769.01	.24	$3,015.20	+25%
Treatment Episodes	N/A	1.24	$718.79	.78	$576.53	+25%
Prison Days	$84.74	32.50	$2,754.05	72.30	$6,126.70	−55%
Total	N/A	N/A	**$16,963.70**	N/A	**$23,921.96**	−29%

TABLE 29-2 *New, Continuing, and Graduating Participants for FY 2001–2002 to FY 2008–2009*

Fiscal Year	New Participants	Continuing Participants	Graduated Participants
2008–2009	754	834	316
2007–2008	874	914	355
2006–2007	798	1075	447
2005–2006	1182	945	343
2004–2005	1068	995	433
2003–2004	1267	1128	451
2002–2003	1354	1053	452
2001–2002	1280	1061	585

Source: CCJCC, 2010

Program Challenges

Three substantive factors contributed to a steady decline in new participants referred into drug court. First, the Substance Abuse and Crime Prevention Act of 2000, known as Proposition 36, offered offenders new treatment options (30). Unlike drug court, Proposition 36 allowed nonviolent offenders treatment without the possibility of incarceration. Thus, most offenders chose the Proposition 36 treatment, leading to decreased enrollment in drug court. Second, Proposition 36–dedicated courtrooms began to be disbanded in FY 2009–2010, which also led to decreased drug court referrals. Historically, the main source of referrals into the program was Proposition 36 fallouts facing extensive prison time. By removal of dedicated courtrooms, Proposition 36 cases were supervised through over 200 courtrooms. Lastly, during FY 2008–2009, funding for the Proposition 36 program declined, and total

TABLE 29-3 *Recidivism Rates for Drug Court Graduates*

Fiscal Year	Graduated Participants	Number of Graduates Convicted of New Offense since Graduation	Recidivism Rates
2007–2008	355	45	12.68%
2006–2007	447	79	17.67%
2005–2006	343	88	25.66%
2004–2005	433	124	28.64%
2003–2004	451	145	32.15%
2002–2003	452	138	30.53%
2001–2002	585	182	31.11%

Source: CCJCC, 2010

program funding was eliminated during FY 2011–2012. This created a misperception that drug court funding had also been reduced or eliminated, resulting in a reduction in referrals into drug courts countywide.

By 2010, jail and prison overcrowding and the loss of some 4,500 jail beds due to budget cuts in the LAC Sheriff's Department resulted in early release of many nonviolent offenders. Some drug court partners attributed the current decline in drug court referrals to an increase in offenders refusing treatment in lieu of reduced jail sentences due to the to jail overcrowding.

Another potential challenge for drug court is the forthcoming health care reform. Although health care reform will require SUD treatment to be covered by Medicaid, it is unclear if court-supervised treatment will be a covered expense, or if federal and state funding for drug courts will continue.

CONCLUSIONS

The LAC Drug Court Program focuses on specific populations within the criminal justice system. The program targets nonviolent offenders with extensive histories of drug abuse and high risk for criminal recidivism. Drug court as an alternative to incarceration provides participants intensive SUD treatment needed to reduce criminal recidivism. Treatment of this population also reduces incarceration costs in both county and state facilities.

Lessons Learned

- The program demonstrates that providing treatment to repeat drug offenders offers opportunities for life changing behavior modifications. The 10 Key Elements of the Drug Court Model offer offenders a structured treatment regimen through a program that promotes ending the cycle of addiction and criminal activity.
- A success for the Drug Court Model is the provision and enforcement of sanctions for non-compliant participants. This motivates participants to take responsibility for their actions and to actively participate in maintaining their sobriety. Those deemed capable of completing the program are issued sanctions (e.g., brief incarceration) as a result of non-compliance, after which treatment resumes. Others may be dismissed from the program for non-compliance.
- The collaborative partnership between stakeholders in the criminal justice system and the SUD treatment provider network is essential to program success. This relationship ensures that drug courts operate efficiently and helps drug-dependent offenders into recovery.
- Drug use is a serious problem in LAC that not only affects the individual, but also the greater community. Ultimately, the decision to remain sober and free from criminal activity after completing a drug court program lies with the individual.
- Offering an alternative to incarceration for this target population helps LAC to support and encourage offenders to make positive choices and to experience reduced risks by eliminating substance abuse, which not only improves their health, but also benefits general public health.

REFERENCES

1. Substance Abuse Prevention and Control (SAPC). Substance abuse prevention and control. Fact sheet: Drug use and misuse in Los Angeles County. Los Angeles: Los Angeles County Department of Public Heath; 2010a. Available from http://publichealth.lacounty.gov/sapc/FactSheet/DrugUseFactSheet.pdf (accessed June 19, 2012).
2. Substance Abuse Prevention and Control (SAPC). Facts and figures: Alcohol in Los Angeles County. Los Angeles: Los Angeles County Department of Public Health; 2010b. Available from: http://publichealth.lacounty.gov/sapc/FactSheet/AlcoholFactSheet.pdf (accessed June 19, 2012).
3. SAPC & Office of Health Assessment Epidemiology (OHAE).Reducing alcohol-related harms in Los Angeles County. Los Angeles: Los Angeles County Department of Public Health; 2011.
4. SAPC & OHAE, 2011 (see number 3 above).
5. Office of Health Assessment and Epidemiology. Methamphetamine use in Los Angeles County adults. L.A. Health. 2006, December. Available from: http://publichealth.lacounty.gov/wwwfiles/ph/hae/ha/Meth05.pdf (accessed June 19, 2012).
6. OHAE, 2006 (see number 5 above).
7. Schiraldi V, Holman B, Beatty P. *Poor Prescription: The Costs of Imprisoning Drug Offenders in the United States.* Washington, DC: Justice Policy Institute; 2000. Available from: http://www.drugpolicy.org/docUploads/PoorPrescription.pdf (accessed June 19, 2012).
8. Petersilia J,Turner S.*Management of Criminal Justice Offenders in Los Angeles County: Final Report.* Los Angeles: Los Angeles County Community Based Punishment Planning Committee; 1996.
9. Fielding JE, Tye G, Ogawa PL, Imam IJ, Long AM. Los Angeles County drug court programs: Initial results. *J Subst Abuse Treat.* 2002;23:217–224. 10. Goldkamp JS, Weiland D. *Assessing the Impact of Dade County's Felony Drug Court.* Washington, DC: U.S. Department of Justice; 1993. Available from: http://www.ncjrs.gov/pdffiles1/nij/145302.pdf (accessed June 19, 2012).
11. Belenko S. Research on drug courts: A critical review. *National Drug Court Institute Review.* 1998;I(1):1–42. Available from: http://www.drugpolicy.org/docUploads/2001drugcourts.pdf (accessed June 19, 2012).
12. National Association of Drug Court Professionals (NADCP). Drug court history. 2011a. Available from: http://www.nadcp.org/learn/what-are-drug-courts/history (accessed June 19, 2012).
13. Goldkamp,Weiland, 1993 (see number 10 above).
14. Countywide Criminal Justice Coordination Committee (CCJCC). *Los Angeles County Drug Court Program: Bi-annual Report 2007–2008 and 2008–2009.* Los Angeles: Los Angeles County Department of Public Health; 2010. Available from: http://www.ccjcc.info/cms1_152516.pdf (accessed June 19, 2012).
15. Sugita W. Personal communication. 2011.
16. Fielding et al., 2002 (see number 9 above).
17. CCJCC, 2010 (see number 13 above).
18. Fielding et al., 2002 (see number 9 above).
19. California Department of Alcohol and Drug Programs (ADP) & Judicial Council of California, Administrative Office of the Courts (AOC). Drug Court Partnership Act of 1998, Chapter 1007, Statutes of 1998 Final Report. 2002. Available from: http://www.prop36.org/pdf/CAdrugcts2002legrept.pdf (accessed June 19, 2012).

20. California Department of Alcohol and Drug Programs. Comprehensive Drug Court Implementation Act of 1999. 2004. Available from: http://www.adp.ca.gov/DrugCourts/pdf/CDCI_InterimReportToLegislature_March2004.pdf (accessed June 19, 2012).
21. CCJCC, 2010 (see number 13 above).
22. National Association of Drug Court Professionals. *Defining Drug Components: The Key Components*. Washington, DC: U.S. Department of Justice; 2004. Available from: https://www.ncjrs.gov/pdffiles1/bja/205621.pdf (accessed June 19, 2012).
23. CCCJC, 2010 (see number 13 above).
24. Countywide Criminal Justice Coordination Committee. Drug court program: Management information system. Unpublished manuscript.
25. California Department of Corrections and Rehabilitation (CDCR). *Corrections: Moving Forward, Annual Report 2009*. CDCR Office of Public and Employee Communications. Available from: http://www.cdcr.ca.gov/News/Press_Release_Archive/2009_Press_Releases/Oct_01.html (accessed June 19, 2012).
26. Carey SM, Crumpton D, Waller M, Finigan M. California Drug Courts: A methodology for determining costs and benefits. Phase II: Testing the methodology, Superior Court of Los Angeles County, El Monte drug court site-specific report. 2005.
27. ADP & AOC, 2002 (see number 20 above).
28. National Association of Drug Court Professionals. Drug courts work. 2011b. Available from: http://www.nadcp.org/learn/drug-courts-work (accessed June 19, 2012).
29. National Association of Drug Court Professionals. Drugs and crime in America. 2011c. Available from: http://www.nadcp.org/learn/how-well-do-drug-courts-work/drugs-and-crime-america (accessed June 19, 2012).
30. CCJCC, 2010 (see number 13 above).

30 Preventing Opiate Overdose Deaths

Legal Challenges and Effectiveness of Prevention Education and Naloxone Distribution

ELAN SHULTZ

NATURE OF THE PROBLEM

Drug overdose, one of the primary causes of premature death in Los Angeles County (LAC), caused almost 700 deaths and almost 21,000 years of potential life lost in 2007 (1); over a half of these involved heroin and other opiates. Even non-fatal overdoses are harmful, and it is estimated that for every fatal overdose there are between 19 and 29 non-fatal heroin overdoses (2, 3).

A vast majority of opiate overdoses can be prevented, and those that do occur can be effectively reversed. However, studies have shown that overdose victims often do not receive the emergency medical attention they require, in part because witnesses, who are often drug users themselves, are afraid to call 911 (4). The LAC Department of Public Health's (DPH) Comprehensive Opiate Overdose Prevention Pilot Program attempted to address this problem.

CONTEXT

Since opiate fatalities are largely preventable, several communities throughout the country established overdose prevention projects (5, 6). These programs teach intravenous drug users (IDUs) how to avoid fatal overdoses and how to save the life of someone who is overdosing. The programs also assist clients who are ready to get sober by referring them to drug treatment services. One of the key components of these programs is training program clients in the safe administration of naloxone.

Naloxone (trade name: Narcan) is an opioid antagonist that has been used by medical professionals for decades to reverse the deadly effects of an opiate overdose. It is a non-addictive and inexpensive medication (less than $2 per dose) that counteracts the effects of opiates, allowing the victim's breathing to return to normal. The drug is available by prescription and only works if a person has opiates in his or her system—the medication has no effect if opiates are absent.

IDUs are often hesitant to contact emergency medical services while witnessing a drug overdose. However, these same IDUs say that they would be willing to administer naloxone if they witnessed someone overdosing (7, 8). Since many overdose victims do not receive emergency medical services, some overdose prevention programs distributed naloxone in pre-filled syringes to IDUs and trained them to administer the medication to people who are overdosing.

Preliminary program results suggest that they are effective in getting naloxone into the hands of people who can administer it to overdose victims who may not otherwise receive medical attention (9). Anecdotal evidence suggests that the programs are preventing fatal overdoses and that some IDUs whose overdoses have been reversed with naloxone have been motivated to enter rehabilitation after the incident (10). By 2006 the DPH decided that enough evidence had accumulated to warrant establishing a pilot naloxone distribution program in LAC.

During this same period, the DPH became aware that local community-based agencies that provided needle exchange services wanted to establish naloxone distribution programs. In June 2006, attendees at the Los Angeles Overdose Prevention Summit discussed the need to address the large number of opiate overdoses in LAC and to establish comprehensive overdose prevention and naloxone distribution programs. Subsequently, the DPH began drafting a plan to establish a local program similar to those that had already been implemented in other cities.

■ APPROACH TO THE PROBLEM

Attempting to Find a Locally Replicable Intervention Model

Opiate overdose programs have been in existence in various forms for over a decade in other cities in the United States (11). The DPH investigated several of them and found that programs in Chicago, New York, and San Francisco seemed most suitable for replication in LAC (see Table 30–1).

Obstacles to Replicating Models from Other Cities: Liability and Lack of Funding

While all three of these programs have been effective in distributing naloxone and training IDUs in overdose prevention and response, none was directly replicable in LAC because of liability concerns and lack of funding.

Unlike the Chicago Recovery Alliance, which operated its program without assistance from the local health authority, the harm reduction agencies and needle exchange providers in LAC needed assistance from the DPH. The local providers could not find clinicians who were willing to write prescriptions for naloxone due to liability concerns.

The liability concerns centered on the ways in which the prescriptions are provided. In California, clinicians must assess a patient's need for a particular medication prior to prescribing it. However, in the programs described above, the clinician often does not know the eventual recipient of the naloxone. Since it would be difficult, if not impossible, for an IDU to self-inject the naloxone during an opiate overdose, most programs provide the medication with the understanding that it will likely be administered to someone other than the client. Consequently, there may be some measure of physician liability since the person administered the medication may not be the same person for whom the clinician wrote the prescription.

A second liability concern is the state law that prohibits the practice of medicine without a license. Some clinicians were concerned that they would be found to have assisted the person actually administering the naloxone to an overdose

TABLE 30–1 *Characteristics of Overdose Programs in Chicago, New York City, and San Francisco*

City	Lead Agency	Service Site	Affiliation with Local Health Officer	Prescribing Agency	Training Agency
Chicago	Chicago Recovery Alliance	Mobile clinic street stops; storefront clinic	None	Chicago Recovery Alliance	Chicago Recovery Alliance
New York City	Partnership: New York Department of Health and Mental Health and SKOOP (Skills and Knowledge on Opiate Overdose Prevention) Project	Partner agency sites	Strong partnership	New York Department of Health and Mental Health	SKOOP and other partner agencies
San Francisco	San Francisco DOPE (Drug Overdose Prevention Education) Project	San Francisco Department of Public Health clinic; homeless shelters; jails; SRO hotels	Strong partnership	San Francisco Department of Public Health	DOPE Project

victim to practice medicine without an appropriate license. Furthermore, some community-based organizations (CBOs) reported hearing that people who witnessed opiate overdoses were hesitant to administer naloxone to someone who was overdosing due to liability concerns. Other states, including New York, New Mexico, and Connecticut, had enacted legislation that provides specific immunities to health care providers and third persons who are involved in the distribution and/or injection of the naloxone. However, California had no such law.

These same liability concerns also existed for the DPH. Although the department had a physician who was willing to prescribe naloxone for IDU clients, County Counsel (the county's lawyers) advised the department that some measure of liability existed in any program model in which county staff were involved in writing prescriptions for or distributing naloxone. Since the county self-insures for medical malpractice, it has to pay any legal costs in their entirety, and must make a policy decision about when it wants to take on new risks. While the DPH could advocate for the establishment of a naloxone distribution program, and County Counsel could advise about the possible liabilities, the ultimate arbiter is the county's Board of Supervisors. The Board comprised five members (3 Democrats and 2 Republicans), but on contentious issues such as a needle exchange program, there were no guaranteed supporting votes.

Since local CBOs were not able to replicate the Chicago model without solutions to the liability issues and the DPH was not able to replicate the San Francisco or

New York models without support from the Board to assume the associated liabilities, another approach was needed. Further complicating the issues, the CBOs were also having trouble finding funds to support an overdose prevention program.

■ IMPLEMENTATION OF SOLUTIONS

To develop solutions to both the liability and funding problems, the DPH teamed up with the Los Angeles Overdose Prevention Task Force and the Northern California–based DOPE (Drug Overdose Prevention Education) Project. The DOPE Project had collaborated with the San Francisco Department of Public Health's (SFDPH) overdose prevention program and was the most experienced provider of overdose prevention training programs in California. The LAC DPH reached out to local CBOs and advocates from the Task Force, and using the programmatic expertise of the DOPE Project, formed an informal partnership ("Partnership") to solve the liability and funding obstacles.

The CBOs had already realized that there were very few funders who were interested in funding a program that might not be sustainable as long as the liability concerns persisted. Once the liability threats were eliminated, the CBOs would have an easier time fund-raising to support an overdose prevention program. DPH staff, along with local CBOs, the Task Force members, and the DOPE Project, recognized that they needed to solve the liability problems before they could address the lack of funding.

By September 2006, the DPH had developed a plan of action and sent it to the Board of Supervisors for its approval. The plan addressed both the liability and the funding problems while proposing a pilot overdose prevention program that was substantially different from any of the models used in other cities. Under the department's proposed pilot program, the DPH planned to fund CBOs that were already providing needle exchange and/or drug treatment services to incorporate distribution of naloxone into their service offerings. CBO agency staff would provide on-site training to clients about preventing narcotics overdose, administration of naloxone, and assistance with rescue breathing. Naloxone would be distributed in pre-prepared syringes under the direction of agency physicians. Program clients would also receive information about available treatment services and other resources. The CBOs would assist the DPH in evaluating the effectiveness of the pilot program. To minimize any potential liability to the county, the DPH agreed that no county staff would be involved in direct client care or distribution of the naloxone. The DPH also requested authorization from the Board to fund the 12-month pilot project within its current budget.

The DPH also recommended that the Board seek state legislation to limit the civil and criminal liability for prescribing and distributing naloxone for all parties involved in the pilot program. The Partnership reasoned that they could capitalize on the strengths of the Partnership's various members to achieve legislative success. The department could leverage the county's experience and substantial influence in the state capitol to ensure that the Partnership's arguments would receive full consideration by legislators. The DPH provided background data and spoke with scientific authority about the scope of the overdose problem that the legislation would address. The DOPE Project and the Harm Reduction Coalition provided technical expertise and answered legislators' questions. The DOPE Project also discussed the track record of overdose prevention programs in San Francisco and other smaller Californian communities and explained why this legislation was necessary to expand these programs elsewhere in the state. The members of the Task Force put a face on the problem, as several of the Task Force members had lost loved ones to opiate overdoses.

DPH presented its proposal to the Board at a public meeting. The department discussed how naloxone was already widely used by emergency responders in the county to reverse opiate overdoses and carefully explained the benefits and risks of its plan. Task Force members spoke with great passion about the need to provide emergency overdose interventions to all those at risk. Local CBOs explained how a successful overdose reversal offers users another chance to enter into treatment and get sober. After hearing the moving testimony from Task Force members, as well as the scientific argument supporting overdose prevention programs, the Board approved the DPH's two-pronged approach.

Pursuing Legislation

For controversial bills that are destined for legislative battles, it is critical to identify a champion for the bill who will shepherd it through the legislative process. Fortunately, the Harm Reduction Coalition had already located a willing author, a state senator from Los Angeles, Mark Ridley-Thomas. Working closely with the Senator's office, the Partnership suggested draft language that would provide liability protection for medical providers who prescribed and/or distributed naloxone within a carefully defined comprehensive overdose prevention program.

The Senator introduced Senate Bill 767, titled "Drug overdose treatment: liability." Testifying before the Senate Judiciary Committee, he explained that the overdose prevention programs that were saving lives in New York and New Mexico could not be established in California without the protections offered by SB 767. He also discussed the safety of naloxone and how its use is similar to the use of an Epi-Pen® on someone with a life-threatening allergic reaction. Once again, a Task Force member's personal testimony about her daughter's death due to an opiate overdose, and her plea to the Committee to approve SB 767 so that others could avoid her daughter's fate, were extremely compelling.

Although no organization went on record as opposing SB 767, several professional associations had concerns. After several weeks of discussions with the staff of the Senate Judiciary Committee, the bill was amended to address some of those concerns. To limit the liability protections to only those parties for whom the protection was absolutely necessary, language protecting third parties administering naloxone was withdrawn. The bill was also amended to include a three-year sunset date, and the bill's provisions were limited to several counties rather than the entire state. The amended version of the bill also required participating counties to collect data on the opiate overdose prevention programs and to report their findings to the Senate and Assembly Judiciary Committees. Despite these changes, the bill succeeded in its original mission—to protect the licensed providers in LAC who prescribed naloxone to people as part of a comprehensive opiate overdose prevention and intervention training program. On October 11, 2007, the Governor signed SB 767 and the bill officially became state law.

DPH Pilot Project Overview

With the Board of Supervisors' approval to implement the pilot program, DPH solicited applications from interested providers. In response to the requirements of the new law, applicants were required to include: comprehensive overdose prevention education; naloxone distribution and overdose reversal education, including the importance of calling 911, how to perform rescue breathing, and how to properly administer naloxone; referrals for treatment services; and setting up a process for clients to report the outcomes of naloxone administration episodes.

DPH selected four CBOs to participate in the pilot program: one that provided services to homeless people; another that specialized in services for people living with HIV and AIDS; and two that provided a wide range of substance abuse treatment services. Each received funding for 13 months. Due to the small size of the pilot, services were delivered at needle exchange sites in select areas of LAC. One provider also implemented the program at some of its treatment sites.

■ EVALUATION STRATEGY

To meet the legal requirements established by SB 767, the DPH collected data from the four local providers, including the number of clients trained, the number of naloxone doses distributed, and information about where the clients were served. The programs also reported the number of times that clients reported administering naloxone, the number of successful overdose reversals, and any adverse effects of naloxone administration. Both DPH and the providers understood that clients' reporting of the outcomes of episodes of naloxone administration was likely to be suboptimal. Although clients who returned to one of the participating CBOs to refill their naloxone prescription had to report the outcomes of prior naloxone use, program managers knew that some clients would not return to do so. Unfortunately, no better reporting alternative emerged. Results were sent to the Senate and Assembly Judiciary Committees as required.

Programs also reported obstacles that they encountered, information that will be used to modify the programs if they are expanded in the future.

■ IMPACT

The first success was passage of SB 767. With liability protection in place, local community-based agencies could implement programs, and the DPH was able to fund four agencies to provide the overdose prevention training and naloxone distribution services.

By the end of the 13-month pilot, 369 clients had been trained in overdose prevention, 818 doses of naloxone had been distributed to program participants (two doses per client plus some refills), and 39 successful overdose reversals had been reported. One overdose reversal attempt was unsuccessful. Men comprised 68% of the clients.

The program had limited but promising results. The DPH's Substance Abuse Prevention and Control (SAPC) program recommended expanding the pilot project and funding an evaluator to determine the impact of the pilot (and naloxone distribution in particular). However, before the project can be expanded, some problems need to be addressed. For example, even with the liability protections, one agency still had difficulty finding program staff, and others experienced problems dispelling myths about utilizing naloxone to reverse opiate overdoses, recruiting clients, and reducing the number of clients who attended the training sessions intoxicated.

Although the pilot project yielded promising results, it is unclear what will happen to overdose prevention training and naloxone distribution programs in LAC. In 2010, the original sunset date of SB 767 was extended to the end of 2015. However, the DPH has not been able to continue funding the community agencies since the pilot ended. To the extent that local CBOs are able to secure funding to support their programs, they still have liability protection. The question that the DPH and local community providers face is: in light of shrinking budgets, where does an overdose prevention training and naloxone distribution program fall on a list of funding priorities? Only time will tell.

LESSONS LEARNED

After realizing that exact replication of a program implemented in another jurisdiction was not possible, the DPH sought alternatives. The DPH attempted to adopt elements of program models that had been successful in other jurisdictions to the local environment. In the end, the DPH's two-pronged approach to pursue state legislation that would offer liability protection and to request authorization from the Board of Supervisors to fund a local pilot project that would be operated by community-based agencies proved successful.

One of the major keys to the DPH's success in garnering support from both the Board and state legislators was the framing of naloxone distribution as a medical intervention for opiate overdoses, and not simply as a harm reduction measure. By keeping naloxone distribution out of the murky political realm of harm reduction and framing it as an emergency medical intervention, the DPH avoided some of the political controversy that often hampers harm reduction services such as needle exchange services.

The strong partnership between the DPH and local advocates proved critical to passage of SB 767. The impact of the Task Force members' testimony before various legislative committees cannot be overstated. Their personal stories of losing loved ones to opiate overdoses ensured that the legislators as well as the Board of Supervisors could not easily ignore the problem.

Perhaps the greatest lesson was that even though the DPH was not able to directly provide the services that the community needed, it could still play an important role in changing the policy environment so that other agencies were able to provide services. While the DPH could not write the prescriptions, it could leverage its credibility and expertise with the Board of Supervisors to pursue legislation that ultimately allowed the CBOs to offer naloxone.

REFERENCES

1. Los Angeles County Department of Public Health, Office of Health Assessment and Epidemiology. *Mortality in Los Angeles County 2007: Leading Causes of Death and Premature Death with Trends for 1998–2007.* June 2010.
2. Warner-Smith M, Darke S, Day C. Morbidity associated with non-fatal heroin overdose. *Addiction.* 2002;97:963–7.

3. Darke S, Mattick R, Degenhardt L. The ratio of non-fatal to fatal heroin overdose. *Addiction.* 2003:98:1169–72.
4. Baca C, Grant K. Take home naloxone to reduce heroin death. *Addiction.* 2005:100:1823–31.
5. Seal K, Thawley R, Gee L, et al. Naloxone distribution and cardiopulmonary resuscitation training for injection drug users to prevention heroin overdose death: A pilot intervention study. *J Urban Health.* 2005;82:303–11.
6. Galea S, Worthington N, Piper T, et al. Provision of naloxone to injection drug users as an overdose prevention strategy: Early evidence from a pilot study in New York City. *Addictive Behaviors.* 2006;31:907–12.
7. Seal K, Downing M, Kral A. Attitudes about prescribing take-home naloxone to injection drug users for the management of heroin overdose: a survey of street-recruited injectors in the San Francisco Bay Area. *J Urban Health.* 2003;80:291–301.
8. Lagu T, Anderson B, Stein M. Overdoses among friends: Drug users are willing to administer naloxone to others. *J Subst Abuse Treat.* 2006;30:129–33.
9. Sporer K, Kral A. Prescription naloxone: A novel approach to heroin overdose prevention. *Annals Emerg Med.* 2007;49(2):172–7.
10. Seal K, Thawley R, Gee L, et al. Naloxone distribution and cardiopulmonary resuscitation training for injection drug users to prevention heroin overdose death: A pilot intervention study. *J Urban Health.* 2005;82:303–11.
11. Sporer K, Kral A. Prescription naloxone: a novel approach to heroin overdose prevention. *Annals Emerg Med.* 2007;49(2):172–7.

31 Increasing Accountability among Substance Abuse Treatment Providers

Development of a Performance Management System

DESIREE CREVECOEUR, RACHEL GONZALES, RICHARD A. RAWSON, JONATHAN E. FIELDING, AND JOHN VIERNES, JR.

OVERVIEW

National policy, research and evaluation discussions inform and improve the measured accountability and effectiveness of treatment services for substance abuse[a] (1). Locally, the Los Angeles County (LAC) Department of Public Health (DPH) made a strategic priority to improve organizational effectiveness, as reflected in its 2008–2011 Strategic Plan. Objective 4.2.3 states the intention to "[d]evelop and implement performance measures department wide, review progress on a regular basis, and ensure that interventions are based on best evidence." The push for improved accountability underlies the long-term goal of implementing performance-based contracting. This overview of system-level efforts taking place in the LAC DPH reveals our efforts to improve the quality and performance of substance abuse treatment programs. The goal is to show how understanding performance challenges associated with substance use disorders can improve system level responses.

THE NATURE OF THE PROBLEM

Substance use disorders in the United States have been a long-standing public health issue, having great impact on health care, educational, and legal systems. According to the LAC Participant Reporting System, an online tracker of admissions and discharges into publicly funded substance abuse treatment programs, in Fiscal Year 2009–2010, 60,629 LAC residents were admitted to publicly funded treatment programs. The most frequently reported drugs for which clients received treatment were marijuana/hashish (27.2%), alcohol (35.6%), methamphetamine (18.1%), and cocaine/crack (13.0%). Ettner et al.(2) found that substance abuse treatment costs about $1,583 and produces a benefit of $11,487 per individual treated, mainly due to reduced crime and increased employment. An analysis of LAC admission and discharge data found that treatment resulted in savings to both primary and mental health care of over $10 million for the 2007–2008 fiscal year, based on average costs (3). A top priority in the health care system as a whole is delivering high-quality treatment for a range of medical and mental health conditions, including substance

TABLE 31-1 *Performance Measurement*

	Measures
Initiation and Engagement	Initiation is defined as having received services at two treatment visits within 14 days of the date that a client was enrolled in treatment; whereas engagement is defined as initiation plus having received services at two additional visits between 15 and 30 days from the admission date (18, 19).
Retention	This measure has been defined differently depending on treatment context; however, for the most part, retention is defined as length of treatment that a client is retained in treatment (20).
Care Continuity	Linkage of detoxification and substance use disorders plan services within 14 days (21).

use disorders (4). As a result, treatment for substance use disorders has been under intense pressure to not only achieve successful client outcomes, but also to more systematically measure and monitor the "performance" of treatment programs. A nationwide emphasis on state and county agency accountability for performance has led to the DPH, Substance Abuse Prevention and Control (SAPC) Department's decision to begin to measure and monitor the effectiveness of treatment programs (5).

Performance and outcome measurement differ. Outcome measures are used at the client level to examine changes in substance use behaviors and psychosocial functioning areas that are expected to be positively influenced by treatment (6). Performance measures are used at the program level to evaluate how a program is doing in conforming to standards of quality (7). Performance measures can help identify where service problems exist, which programs are meeting or exceeding expectations of treatment quality, and what, if any, changes should be made to improve service delivery (8). Overall, distinguishing features of these two types of measurement are 1) for performance data to inform quality improvement strategies aimed at changing clinical practices and organizational cost management; and 2) for outcome measures to be used to understand the effectiveness of treatment services in improving substance use and related functioning of individuals who have received treatment (9).

■ CONTEXT

Improved performance measurement efforts in substance abuse treatment programs have been gaining momentum throughout the United States (10). Health care reform focuses on this, as does an increased emphasis on accountability and improving the cost effectiveness of health care services. Performance measures show promise for evaluating a treatment program's initiation and engagement (11, 12), treatment retention (13–15), and care continuity (16). These measures (see Table 31-1) have been promoted by the Washington Circle, a multidisciplinary group of service providers, researchers, managed care representatives, and policy makers, to establish a set of performance measures for substance abuse treatment (17).

The development of performance measures for substance abuse treatment is novel—with the possible exception of initiation/engagement and retention, much of the published literature on such measures has been published since 2009. Although improvement in a performance measure is expected to lead to improved client outcomes, little information exists regarding the specific impact of each measure on client outcomes.

Key Elements of the Performance Measurement Framework

Performance measurement is often described as problematic. As straightforward as this may appear, several variables can make the use of performance measures extremely difficult. These include: 1) *Focus*: ensuring that measures reflect important clinical or program dimensions related to improving client outcomes; 2) *Operationalization*: clearly defining the measures to ensure understanding across programs; 3) *Availability of data*: determining the feasibility of collecting data at the program level or identifying the means to collect data without adding a data collection burden to a program; and 4) *Reliability/Validity*: assessing the competencies of individuals tasked with collecting the measures/data to ensure consistent use of the same definitions across programs. Finally, assurance is needed that measures have empirical validation with improved outcomes.

Program Performance and Client Outcomes

Research on treatment effectiveness interventions in the United States suggests that factors related to improved client outcomes include longer retention in treatment (22, 23). However, the use of evidence-based practices and approaches, including appropriate medications (24); receiving complementary services for medical, psychiatric and/or family problems (25); and promoting the participation in mutual self-help groups (26) has led to a quest for determining the extent to which improved program performance leads to long-term effectiveness of client outcomes. To date, only a few studies have been conducted to show such associations (27, 28). For example, a positive relationship exists between increased program engagement rates (measured by number of treatment encounters in the initial month of treatment) and self-reported client outcomes of decreased criminal involvement (27). An increase in continuity of care, as measured by a successful transfer of a patient from one level of care to another prescribed level of care (within a 2-week period), is associated with self-reported reductions in substance use/relapse. Overall, these measures are being pilot tested in a variety of settings to determine issues of measurement feasibility and of implementation within existing state and local treatment infrastructures.

■ APPROACH TO THE PROBLEM

The development of performance and outcome measures for a system as large as LAC proved challenging. Substance use disorder treatment in LAC is largely based on the social model. According to Wright (29), treatment based on the social model has several traits and characteristics wherein the basis of authority is new experiential knowledge as a way to recovery. The primary therapeutic relationship is between the person and the program, rather than between the person and an individual therapist. Everyone involved both gives and receives help. In social model programs, staff often say that they are there as much for the support of their own sobriety as to help others. All residents, using the social model recovery home as their context, are expected to make some contribution toward program operations. It is notable that the basic principles and dynamics of Alcoholics Anonymous (AA) create the fundamental framework for social model programs. AA values, such as honesty, tolerance, willingness to try, and the emphasis on helping other substance abusers, form the fundamental basis for social model program operation. A fifth trait is requirement for a positive sober environment as a crucial part of the program operation. Alcoholism is viewed as centered in the reciprocal relationship between the individual and his or her surrounding social unit, rather than centered on the individual. Thus, alcohol and drug abuse issues are considered to be not only individual problems, but problems of families, communities, and society. Contract providers operate most treatment programs, and many are operated by small agencies with limited budgets and nominal staffing. Some programs employ prior clients as paraprofessionals to lead group counseling sessions and assist in the administrative duties. At some sites, prior clients have worked their way through the ranks and are employed as program managers or directors. This is important to note because many people, even those with advanced degrees, have a limited understanding of data collection and evaluation procedures. This lack of skills for the work required to implement dashboard and site reports had to be addressed, especially in light of the fact that pay for performance is a relatively new concept for engaging treatment providers, and the development and implementation of dashboard and site reports was being met with discomfort, to say the least. The unease occurred in the SAPC context, where performance improvement and pay-for-performance were parts of the same process.

In 1999, SAPC (formerly known as the Alcohol and Drug Program Administration) contracted with the University of California, Los Angeles (UCLA) to create an evaluation system for its adult alcohol and drug treatment programs to improve service and outcomes. The goals were focused on client-, program-, and system-level evaluations, the provision of training, tailored reports, and other means of information dissemination. Reports given to providers proved to be invaluable tools in educating providers on the importance of data and how data can be used to improve treatment.

Prior to the implementation of the site reports or the dashboards, providers were not engaged in any form of systematic performance management. SAPC contract monitors included some measures of performance; however, these dealt mostly with contract compliance (e.g., expenditure of funds, with pertinent laws, and adherence to the scope of work). Annual reports also were created, based on the client-level information from providers on rates of completion and employment, and abstinence at discharge. However, neither abstinence nor completion of treatment had been defined consistently across programs or even within programs—counselors within the same program may define these terms differently. Some programs had the infrastructure and contacts to provide employment and housing services, but typically these services depend on economic variables; even programs with expertly trained staff who faithfully use evidence-based practices and have ample community contacts face problems placing clients in jobs or housing when the economy is depressed.

Some programs' internal systems of performance management examined these measures (e.g., completion, employment, abstinence). The review of performance measures by other programs often took a back seat to more pressing, fiscal concerns until SAPC required programs to meet specific benchmarks. In other words, a significant proportion of providers did not measure, or even monitor, their performance consistently. Regardless, there is evidence that programs made positive impacts on clients by reductions in reported substance use between admission and discharge and in additional follow-up studies with clients treated in LAC (30–36).

Development and Implementation of Site Reports

Site reports were developed to provide treatment programs with information concerning key outcomes gleaned from data already collected at admission to and discharge from treatment. To determine what information should be included in such reports, a thorough review of the already collected data was conducted at meetings with SAPC and UCLA staff, as well as with some two dozen provider organizations representing the spectrum of contracted service providers. The later included large providers capable of administering a broad range of services and mid-size and smaller providers that frequently tailored or specialized services for hard-to-reach populations. At each meeting, the admission and discharge information collected through the data system was reviewed and discussed as potential content for the site report. Each question asked of the client was a potential data point to be considered for inclusion in the report. In the end, the site reports featured several outcome measures: days of substance use, days of injected drug use, homelessness at admission and at discharge, participation in social support activities and employment-related activities (education or job training as well as part-time or full-time employment).

In addition to the outcome measures, SAPC and UCLA considered including a comparison for treatment providers to use as an informal standard of their program's performance. For example, if the mean length of stay at one program were 100 days, it was unclear if that was representative of what was going on countywide. To address this, the report cited means or percentages for certain measures, calculated by examining all programs of that same type. This allowed a program to compare its individual results with the county mean (or percentage—as appropriate). During these meetings, the providers reviewed examples of draft site reports, and discussions were held to determine ways to increase the reliability, validity, and usefulness of the admission and discharge data. Much of the information collected at admission and discharge was included in the site report. In addition, the instructional manual that detailed the questions asked at admission and discharge was edited and revised to increase question clarification.

Given the size of the treatment system—over 100 agencies providing services in approximately 500 programs at over 300 locations—the site reports needed sufficient specificity to give agencies enough information to determine which program was being detailed and relevant comparators. The decision was made to create site reports that provided data for a single program type (e.g., residential, outpatient, day care habilitative, or narcotic treatment) at each location. This resulted in about 350 site reports. Because providers needed to view the reports on regular bases, the reports are created on quarterly and annual schedules for large providers (at least 80 admissions in the prior year) and annually for small providers (less than 80 admissions in the prior year). To complete some 1,000 quarterly and annual reports every year, the data analysis and writing system was automated.

The first batch of site reports was created about 18 months after initial discussions and was posted online, where agencies submitted their admission and discharge data. At the same time, SAPC and UCLA held over a dozen regional meetings with all the contracted service providers to discuss the purpose of the site reports. These meetings conveyed key information and fostered buy-in from the community organizations. The agencies were assured that the purpose of the site reports was to provide them with information about their clients' outcomes. The service providers also received clarification on the origins of information pertaining to admissions and discharges. Emphasis during these trainings pointed to the importance of submitting accurate and timely data and ways that inaccurate data ultimately reflect inaccurate outcomes. And the meetings were used to allay fears that the site reports would be used as evidence to cancel contracts. In fact, they were not developed with that purpose. The site reports are still posted quarterly (and annually), and many providers review them to determine the accuracy of data submitted to SAPC and to verify that they are meeting their internal goals regarding client outcomes.

The site reports have provided effective tools to get treatment agencies to pay closer attention to the data that they collect and submit to SAPC; however, the reports did not provide any benchmarks. Benchmarks can be used in evaluation as a "goal" or "ideal" level of performance toward which agencies should work. With the site reports, providers whose outcomes or performance was significantly above or below the LAC average were not required to improve their performance or make changes to their program's process; but they were encouraged to make pertinent changes or to examine their program practices to improve their data. UCLA provided training to several hundred providers on standardized assessment tools like the Addiction Severity Index and evidence-based practices such as cognitive behavioral treatment, motivational interviewing, and contingency management. SAPC and UCLA also worked together to provide training opportunities for agencies to improve program performance through the use of process improvement techniques. Since the site reports were only informational tools, not used to formally monitor program performance, discussions then began around the development of a performance management tool.

Development and Implementation of Performance Measures and Dashboards

At the time of the development of the performance measures, substance use treatment providers had been receiving site reports for a few years, yet the reports did not set performance benchmarks or report on whether a program had met the benchmark. Further, the federal government and the State of California discussed the need to learn how well various treatments worked. This, coupled with research from the Washington Circle, the Substance Abuse and Mental Health Services Administration, and other organizations, was the impetus to develop and implement performance measures.

The first set of performance measures considered included engagement (four sessions in first month of treatment) as well as retention (services for at least 90 days). The number and type of services were to be examined to ascertain if there were an optimal "dose" of treatment and whether four services (e.g., individual counseling, group counseling, case management, and drug testing) within the first 30 days was sufficient to "engage" the LAC substance use disorder treatment population. Twenty-two outpatient treatment

TABLE 31–2 *Performance Measure Logic Model*

Performance Measures:		Impact/Short-term changes		Impact/Long-term changes
Initiation (first 14 days)	→	Greater rapport developed between client and clinician.	→	Reduction of early dropouts—better engagement.
Engagement (first 30 days)	→	Greater rapport, more initial contact between client and counselor.	→	Reduction of early dropouts—longer lengths of stay.
Increased Retention	→	Increased client behavioral and cognitive changes.	→	Reductions in substance use, greater likelihood of abstinence, improved client outcomes in other areas.
Use of Evidence-Based Practices		Clients learn ways to deal effectively with triggers, cravings, and other tools for relapse prevention.		Increased likelihood of clients maintaining abstinence.
Use of Medication-Assisted Treatment	→	Address withdrawal and cravings at the biological level.	→	Increase client's ability to be "present" in treatment.
Continuity of Care	→	Move clients through system of care in a way that addresses their needs.	→	Ensures clients receive the appropriate levels of services needed.

programs participated in two pilot studies. The data from these pilots indicated that four sessions in the first 30 days were not sufficient to keep the client motivated to remain in treatment beyond the first month. In fact, it appeared that 12–16 sessions were required for full client engagement (eight group sessions—two per week, four individual counseling sessions, one per week, and one or two case management and or drug tests in the first month). This level of treatment "front loading" yielded the best outcomes (longer lengths of stay, greater reductions in substance use, greater likelihood of abstinence at discharge) for those clients who participated in the pilot (37). The second pilot revealed that limitations to the web-based system providers use to submit data did not permit mandating or even monitoring the number and type of services provided. Therefore, performance measures were proposed that did not require tracking of services to individual clients (see Table 31–2). The following measures were considered:

- Reducing early drop outs (discharged in less than 30 days);
- Retaining clients for at least 90 days;
- Using evidence-based practices with fidelity;
- Using medically assisted treatment;
- Including continuing care in treatment planning for all clients.

CHALLENGES AND OPPORTUNITIES

SAPC and UCLA continued meeting with a group of providers to evaluate potential performance measures. The meetings involved intense discussions concerning the need to measure and hold providers accountable for performance. Some resistance to the process arose, and agencies expressed concerns about the administrative burden and how performance measures could somehow be used against them. Unfortunately, in 2009 a significant economic downturn slowed necessary funding, and providers reported increased difficulty in fund-raising to support those in LAC who requested or required treatment. The DPH first argued that the timing, while inconvenient, gave no good reason to wait. And the DPH indicated that no program would be penalized immediately. It became clear that an expanded system could take months or more than a year to develop and should begin immediately. Once providers accepted that the system was going to be developed, discussions began concerning performance measures.

Extensive dialogue raised a few new issues. First, given the economic crunch and budget reductions, and the requirement that treatment agencies provide non-reimbursed services (e.g., continuing care or drug tests for all clients), participants argued that the additional burden of data collection was unreasonable. It was agreed that such a burden would be substantial. So, it was decided that performance measures should be based on client data already collected by SAPC. This would allow SAPC to review the data and use data from prior years to develop the benchmarks, and would not add to the administrative burden of provider agencies. New data would require changes to the current data system and require additional time for programming, troubleshooting, and training. In addition, consensus emerged that performance measures could differ for each program type (i.e., residential treatment versus outpatient), but even in those instances when the performance measures did not differ, the benchmarks would. Concern also arose about the possibility of selective admission of clients that was likely to adversely influence an agency's data. Before benchmarks could be finalized, providers requested an examination of the data to determine if a case mix adjustment should be made. A UCLA statistician did the job and found that the captured system demographics predicted less than one tenth of one percent of the variance in the outcomes, evidence that there was no selective referral of clients (unemployed, mentally ill, homeless, high use, long history of use, or otherwise) and a case mix adjustment would not be warranted.

Current outstanding issues include possible inaccuracies and late submission of data. SAPC and UCLA are working to determine the best ways to address these. One solution could combine multiple data systems; for example, the joining of billing and the admission/discharge data systems. While this does not eliminate all data inaccuracies, it does provide an extra check and balance.

As the discussions ended, a decision was made to focus on performance benchmarks in outpatient counseling. Three performance measures were decided upon, and a fourth is under development. These include: 30-Day Engagement, 90-Day Retention, and completed exit interviews.

Defining Measures and Developing Benchmarks

The 30-day engagement performance measure assesses how many clients leave treatment within a month. Engagement is calculated by examining the date of admission and comparing it to the date of the last face-to-face encounter (discharge). In addition to engagement, retention was also selected as a performance measure. Retention is calculated using the same formula as engagement, but instead of looking at 30 days in treatment, retention assesses those in treatment for at least 90 days. Engagement is typically defined as including at least four encounters in a month's time. Despite the limitations of the LAC data collection system in examining services at the individual client level, the requirement of four encounters in the first

30 days should be met under most circumstances (e.g., an intake, an assessment, and two group/individual counseling sessions).

The final performance measure is more of an administrative measure and considers those programs that are able to collect discharge information from clients. When a client is discharged, questions similar to those asked at admission are asked in an exit interview to measure behavioral changes that occurred during treatment. However, a significant number of clients and programs did not collect this information for a variety of reasons (e.g., client departure against program advice, client leaving treatment and not returning, or providers not prioritizing the collection of discharge information). This data is of particular importance because without it, client outcomes cannot be calculated.

Once performance measures were finalized, discussion began on where to set the benchmarks. Data on the three performance measures were examined over a three-year period, including only the 110 programs with at least 20 discharges in any given year. For the 30-Day Engagement performance measure, 79% of the clients remained in treatment at least 30 days. For the 90-Day Retention measure, about 67% remained in treatment, and about half of the clients were completing an exit interview. Given these data, about half of the providers would be performing above mean and half below; this appeared to be a good starting point for establishing performance benchmarks since developers understood that the benchmarks could be adjusted in the future. The final accepted benchmarks were these:

- At least 80% of the clients discharged must remain in treatment 30 days or more (Engagement benchmark);
- At least 65% of the clients discharged must remain in treatment 90 days or more (Retention benchmark);
- At least 50% of the clients discharged must have completed exit interviews.

Table 31–3 shows the actual results at baseline, suggesting that some far exceeded and some substantially underperformed the benchmarks.

When performance measures and benchmarks were finalized, work began on designing the reports that would inform providers of the measures, benchmarks, and performance of each provider. In addition, providers who fell short of the benchmarks would be offered technical assistance, training, and other help to improve their performance. In order not to overload providers, SAPC and UCLA staff focused the initial technical assistance project on the 30-Day Engagement measure.

TABLE 31–3 *Performance Measures—Agencies Below the Benchmarks at Baseline*

Performance Measure	Benchmark	Number (Percent) of Agencies Below Benchmark at Baseline (Out Of 110)
Participants in treatment at least 30 days	80%	57 (52%)
Participants in treatment at least 90 days	65%	77 (70%)
Participants with exit interviews	50%	37 (34%)

Implementation

The development and implementation of the performance measures and benchmark reports followed a similar trajectory to the site reports. Meetings were held to discuss the format and content and reports were automated. Once design was finalized, the reports (now referred to as dashboards) were posted to the same system where providers enter data and view site reports (see Table 31–4).

SAPC continued to work with contracted providers to ensure that their computer software and hardware met minimal requirements for obtaining dashboards and reporting program participant data. Many problems were avoided through these collaborative efforts and ongoing communication between the county and providers.

SAPC informs its contracted providers monthly on their progress toward meeting measures on the SAPC Performance Dashboard. The Dashboard is available to contracted providers through an automated web-based system to which only designated staff members at each individual agency have access.

For the first six months after implementation, SAPC held numerous meetings to educate adult outpatient treatment providers about using the performance measures and benchmarks and also made clear that all performance measures and benchmarks will be included in every adult outpatient treatment contract. They know that the integrated SAPC billing and data collection system will be developed and implemented for measuring contractor performance. Such measures also will be included in new agreements resulting from the competitive re-solicitation process. In addition, SAPC, in conjunction with UCLA, plan to continue offering technical assistance to low-performing agencies on an as-needed basis.

Several strategies were implemented to improve treatment. First, trainings were provided to programs on motivational interviewing, medication-assisted treatment, cognitive behavioral therapy, and contingency management (38). Process improvement trainings were also held with two dozen programs prior to the implementation of dashboards to let providers know how minor changes to program processes can have big impacts in client engagement and retention. Programs that participated in these process improvement activities showed significant improvements over the course of the project, including 28%–93% decreases in no-shows, as well as doubling of the rates of engagement (39). Providers who participated in process improvement

TABLE 31–4 *Performance Measures—Progress of Agencies Who Started Below the Benchmark*

Performance Measure	Benchmark	Initial Number of Agencies Below the Benchmark	Of These Agencies, Number (percent) Now Above the Benchmark
Participants in treatment at least 30 days	80%	57	14 (25%)
Participants in treatment at least 90 days	65%	77	26 (34%)
Participants with exit interviews	50%	37	18 (49%)

evaluations reported that they learned specific steps to improve performance (e.g., use of appointment cards, changed policies) and that most had already implemented programmatic changes to make process improvement a part of their program's culture (40). Process improvement worked so well that a focused improvement project was begun for those providers whose engagement numbers fell more than 20% below the benchmark—Process Improvement Technical Assistance (PITA).

■ EVALUATION OF THE IMPLEMENTATION STRATEGY

Process Improvement Technical Assistance (PITA)

Given where benchmarks were set (at the mean), a number of providers fell below the standards. However, less than a quarter of 110 outpatient service providers fell significantly lower (more than 20%) than the benchmark.

To inform all program managers, SAPC and UCLA created three different versions of the performance benchmark reports. The first addressed those programs that met or exceeded all three benchmarks. It consisted of a single-page document listing the measures, the program's current quarter performance, cumulative year performance, and the benchmark for each performance measure. Definitions of each performance measure were also included in the report.

A second addressed programs that fell 1–19% below on any single benchmark. This version of the dashboard includes the same information as the first report plus information and resources to help providers develop ways to improve performance on their own.

A third was for program managers whose performance was 20% or more below the benchmark. This included all of the information from the first report, but it also suggested intermediate (monthly) goals for the provider to meet until they reach the benchmark. The intermediate goals were set at no more than 10% above their current performance. To assist the two dozen providers who fell below the benchmark for engagement in reaching intermediate goals, SAPC and UCLA offered technical assistance. Of those, about half a dozen worked with SAPC and UCLA on various strategies to improve client engagement. All but one program that participated in PITA showed improvements in their engagement numbers by the second or third quarter.

Although it is not known what, if anything, the providers who chose not to receive technical assistance at this time are doing to improve their performance, the programs whose performance falls short of the benchmark for the 2010–2011 fiscal year will be offered technical assistance similar to that offered as part of the PITA. The Addiction Technology Transfer Center (ATTC) also will offer training.

■ IMPACT

Standardizing outcomes to improve delivery of substance abuse treatment services is a complex process. Standardization allows service providers to effectively gauge their performance and gain knowledge to support modifications to their protocols that can improve their performance.

The most significant impact of standardization is that providers become accustomed to collecting and examining previously overlooked data. SAPC and UCLA have worked with providers for years to improve the reliability and validity of data through trainings and through provision of regular reports. The resulting data accuracy has improved dramatically. In the early days of the site reports, several providers would call to note the problems in their data. Currently, less than a half dozen providers contact SAPC quarterly or annually about site report inaccuracies.

Although a plan is in place to review this process and make appropriate changes, it is early to say what additional impacts dashboards have had on the system. It is the expectation that because the use of dashboards requires a certain level of knowledge of the programs' performance, providers will seek out opportunities to improve their performance, especially given that the related benchmarks are (or will be) included in all forthcoming contracts and requests for proposals. Use of the dashboards should also help providers who do not meet the benchmarks because without mastery of dashboard guidelines, some agencies are likely to be ineligible to apply for new contracts or submit proposals. Providers have been informed that due to funding restrictions, no additional financial incentives will be available to encourage their performance; however, good performance will help to secure the future of their programs in upcoming contract bidding cycles. Because the information collected by providers is also typically asked of other organizations that fund treatment (NIDA, SAMHSA, and insurance companies), providers also can use these site reports and dashboards to secure funding from these sources.

■ CONCLUSION

SAPC and UCLA found the development and implementation of performance benchmarks and dashboards to be worthwhile activities. Key lessons learned:

- By working with treatment providers toward the determination of benchmarks, key factors for the evaluation of program performance are determined and scored through the dashboard. Likewise, the information received from the dashboard determines whether treatment providers are in need of technical assistance.
- Implementation of a data collection and performance management system presents challenges that can be addressed through a continuous improvement process.
- Developing performance measures is sometimes fraught with disagreements and compromises. Issues that emerged during this process include provider discontent with the development of measures, possible inaccuracies and late submissions of data, and concern over the selective referral of clients. SAPC and UCLA provided trainings to improve the accuracy of data submitted and will continue to monitor data to inhibit selective client admission.
- Involving the providers from the start of the process is integral to obtaining provider and other stake holder buy-in. The fact that the providers were given several opportunities to voice their concerns and have their concerns addressed helped move the development and implementation along. It took about nine months from the first memo announcing the plan to implement performance measures to the implementation of the dashboards—not a lengthy timeline given the size of the county system.
- The ongoing meetings between SAPC and UCLA were key to developing the major data collection tools and related reports. Face-to-face discussions also helped LACPRS system providers learn how to monitor their data. All of this was necessary for effectively improving provider accountability and client outcomes and program performance measures.

NOTES

[a] The term *substance use disorders* will be used interchangeably with *abuse* and *dependence* as these terms are represented by the *Diagnostic and Statistical Manual of Mental Disorders, Fourth Edition – DSM-IV* (American Psychiatric Association, 1994).

REFERENCES

1. Capoccia VA, Cotter F, Gustafson DH, Cassidy EF, Ford JH II, Madden L, et al. Making "stone soup": Improvements in clinic access and retention in addiction treatment. *Joint Comm J Qual Patient Safety.* 2007;33(2):95–103.
2. Ettner SL, Huang D, Evans E, Ash DR, Hardy M, Jourabchi M, Hser YI. Benefit-cost in the California Treatment Outcome Project: Does substance abuse treatment "pay for itself"? *HSR: Health Serv Res.* 2006;41(1):192–213.
3. Crèvecoeur-MacPhail D. Costs savings for treatment populations based on LACPRS admission and discharge data. Unpublished report. 2009.
4. Institute of Medicine. *Improving the Quality of Mental Health and Substance Use Conditions.* Washington, DC: IOM; 2006.
5. U.S. Department of Health and Human Services, Substance Abuse and Mental Health Services Administration, Knowledge Application Program. Treatment improvement protocols 14 developing state outcomes monitoring systems for alcohol and other drug abuse treatment. Available from: http://www.kap.samhsa.gov/products/manuals/tips/14.htm (accessed June 6, 2011).
6. McLellan AT, Chalk M, and Bartlett J. Outcomes, performance, and quality: What's the difference? *J Subst Abuse Treat.* 2007;32:331–40.
7. Garnick DW, Hodgkin D, Horgan CM. Selecting data sources for substance abuse services research. *J Subst Abuse Treat.* 2002;22:11–22.
8. Garnick DW, Lee M, Chalk M, Gastfriend D, Horgan CM, McCorry F, McLellan AT, Merrick EL. Establishing the feasibility of performance measures for alcohol and other drugs. *J Subst Abuse Treat.* 2002;45:124–31.
9. McLellan AT, Chalk M, Bartlett J. Outcomes, performance, and quality: What's the difference? *J Subst Abuse Treat.* 2007;32:331–40.
10. McCorry F, Garnick DW, Bartlett J, Cotter F, Chalk M. Developing performance measures for alcohol and other drug services in managed care plans. *Joint Comm J Quality Improv.* 2000;26:633–43.
11. Garnick DW, Lee M, Chalk M, Gastfriend D, Horgan CM, McCorry F, McLellan AT, Merrick EL. Establishing the feasibility of performance measures for alcohol and other drugs. *J Subst Abuse Treat.* 2002;45:124–31.
12. McCarty D, Gustafson DH, Wisdom JP, Ford J, Choi D, Molfenter T, et al. The Network for the Improvement of Addiction Treatment (NIATx): Enhancing access and retention. *Drug and Alcohol Depend.* 2007;88:138–45.
13. Hubbard RL, Craddock SG, Anderson J. Overview of 5-year follow-up outcomes in the Drug Abuse Treatment Outcome Studies (DATOS). *J Subst Abuse Treat.* 2003;25:125–34.
14. Simpson DD. A conceptual framework for drug treatment process and outcomes. *J Subst Abuse Treat.* 2004;27:99–121.
15. Simpson DD, Joe GW, Rowan-Szal GA. Linking the elements of change: Program and client responses to innovation. *J Subst Abuse Treat.* 2007;33:201–9.
16. Garnick DW, Lee MT, Horgan CM, Acevedo A, Washington Circle Public Sector Workgroup. Adapting Washington Circle performance measures for public sector substance abuse treatment systems. *J Subst Abuse Treat.* 2009;36(3):265–77.

17. McCorry F, Garnick DW, Bartlett J, Cotter F, Chalk M. Developing performance measures for alcohol and other drug services in managed care plans. *Joint Comm J Qual Improv*. 2000;26:633–43.
18. Garnick DW, Hodgkin D, Horgan CM. Selecting data sources for substance abuse services research. *J Subst Abuse Treat*. 2002;22:11–22.
19. Garnick DW, Lee M, Chalk M, Gastfriend D, Horgan CM, McCorry F, McLellan AT, Merrick EL. Establishing the feasibility of performance measures for alcohol and other drugs. *J Subst Abuse Treat*. 2002;45:124–31.
20. Galloway GP, Marinelli-Casey P, Stalcup J, Lord RH, Christian D, Cohen J, Reiber C, Vandersloot D. Treatment-as-usual in the Methamphetamine Treatment Project. *J Psychoactive Drugs*. 2000;32:165–75.
21. Garnick DW, Lee MT, Horgan CM, Acevedo A, Washington Circle Public Sector Workgroup. Adapting Washington Circle performance measures for public sector substance abuse treatment systems. *J Subst Abuse Treat*. 2009;36(3):265–77.
22. Hubbard RL, Craddock SG, Anderson J. Overview of 5-year follow-up outcomes in the Drug Abuse Treatment Outcome Studies (DATOS). *J Subst Abuse Treat*. 2003;25:125–34.
23. Simpson DD. A conceptual framework for drug treatment process and outcomes. *J Subst Abuse Treat*. 2004;27:99–121.
24. National Quality Forum. Evidence-based practices to treat substance use conditions. 2007. Available from: http://www.qualityforum.org/pdf/projects/sud/lsENTIRE-DRAFT1-22-07.pdf (accessed April 22, 2011).
25. McLellan AT, Skipper GS, Campbell M, DuPont RL. Five year outcomes in a cohort study of physicians treated for substance use disorders in the United States. *British Med J*. 2008;337:a2038.
26. McKay JR. Is there a case for extended interventions for alcohol and drug use disorders? *Addiction*. 2005;100:1594–610.
27. Garnick DW, Horgan CM, Lee MT, Panas L, Ritter GA, Davis S, et al. Are Washington Circle performance measures associated with decreased criminal activity following treatment? *J Subst Abuse Treat*. 2007;33:341–52.
28. Garnick DW, Lee MT, Horgan CM, Acevedo A, Washington Circle Public Sector Workgroup. Adapting Washington Circle performance measures for public sector substance abuse treatment systems. *J Subst Abuse Treat*. 2009;36(3):265–77.
29. Wright A. What is social model? In: Shaw S, Borkman T, editors. *Social Model Alcohol Recovery*. Burbank, CA: Bridge Focus, Inc.; 1990. p. 7–10.
30. Anglin DM, Conner BT, Annon J, Longshore D. Longitudinal effects of LAAM and methadone maintenance on heroin addict behavior. *J Behav Health Serv & Res*. 2009;36:267–82.
31. Anglin MD, Urada D, Brecht ML, Hawken A, Rawson R, Longshore D. Criminal justice treatment admissions for methamphetamine use in California: A focus on Proposition 36. *J Psychoactive Drugs*. 2007;Suppl. 4:367–81.
32. Brecht ML, Anglin MD, Dylan M. Coerced treatment for methamphetamine abuse: differential patient characteristics and outcomes. *Am J Drug and Alcohol Abuse*. 2005;31:337–56.
33. Evans E, Longshore D, Prendergast M, Urada D. Evaluation of the Substance Abuse and Crime Prevention Act: Client characteristics, treatment completion and re-offending three years after implementation. *J Psychoactive Drugs*. 2006;SARC Suppl. 3:357–67.
34. Hser YI, Evans E, Huang D. Treatment outcomes among women and men methamphetamine abusers in California. *J Subst Abuse Treat*. 2005;28:77–85.

35. Grella CE, Stein JA. Impact of program services on treatment outcomes of patients with comorbid mental and substance use disorders. *Psychiatric Services.* 2006;57:1007–15.
36. Anglin DM, Conner BT, Annon J, Longshore D. Longitudinal effects of LAAM and methadone maintenance on heroin addict behavior. *J Behav Health Serv& Res.* 2009;36:267–82.
37. Crèvecoeur-MacPhail D, Ransom L, Myers AC, Rawson R. Inside the black box: Measuring addiction treatment services and their relation to outcomes. *J Psych Drugs.* 2010; SARC Suppl 6:269–76.
38. Higgins ST, Petry NM. Contingency management incentives for sobriety. *Alcohol Res & Health.* 1999;23(2):122–7.
39. Rutkowski B, Gallon S, Rawson RA, Freese TE, Bruehl A, Crèvecoeur-MacPhail D, Sugita W, Molfenter T, Cotter F. Improving client engagement and retention in treatment: The Los Angeles County experience. *J Subst Abuse Treat.* 2010;39:78–86.
40. Crèvecoeur-MacPhail D, Bellows A, Rutkowski B, Ransom L, Myers AC, Rawson R. I've been NIATxed: participants' experience with process improvement. *J Psychoactive Drugs.* 2010; SARC Suppl 6:249–6.

32 Preconception Health

A Life Course Perspective for Maternal and Child Health

CYNTHIA HARDING, DIANA RAMOS, GIANNINA DONATONI, SHIN MARGARET CHAO, AND JEANNE SMART

THE NATURE OF THE PROBLEM: NEED FOR NEW STRATEGIES TO IMPROVE BIRTH OUTCOMES

Encouraging early prenatal care was the key strategy to improve birth outcomes during most of the twentieth century when infant mortality rates steadily declined (1). Between 2000 and 2005, rates plateaued (6.8–6.9 deaths/1,000 live births) causing local public health officials to seek new solutions to optimize infant health. In addition, disparities in birth outcomes persist. African American babies die at more than twice the rate of other race/ethnicities (see Figure 32–1) (2).

Public health practitioners, clinicians and researchers increasingly emphasize that many important determinants of poor birth outcomes are social/environmental, not medical (3–5). Frick & Lantz state:

> Focusing on prenatal care in our public health policy prescriptions ignores the socioeconomic contexts in which women live, medicalizes a problem that is socially and historically complex, and contributes to the illusion that there is a "medical policy bullet" that can provide a comprehensive and efficacious solution. (6)

Today, in the United States and in Los Angeles County (LAC), half of all births are unintended (7). Planned pregnancies are associated with lower rates of preterm births. In LAC in 2007, 40% of women with a recent infant loss reported their pregnancy as unintended (8). Women who have had prior adverse birth outcomes are at increased risk for repeated problems in subsequent pregnancies. The risk of recurrence can be reduced with appropriate follow-up during the interconception period (9). Table 32–1 indicates conditions prior to pregnancy that correlate with poor birth outcomes, including lack of health insurance before pregnancy, poverty, low educational attainment, and perception of living in an unsafe neighborhood.

Clearly, poor birth outcomes cannot be alleviated through prenatal care alone, and a broader focus on the social and physical conditions that contribute to those outcomes is needed. Thus a life course framework that explains and addresses health and disease patterns across population groups is now being adopted by federal, state, and local Maternal Child Health (MCH) programs to address health disparities (10). It embraces social determinants as major factors underlying health and focuses on

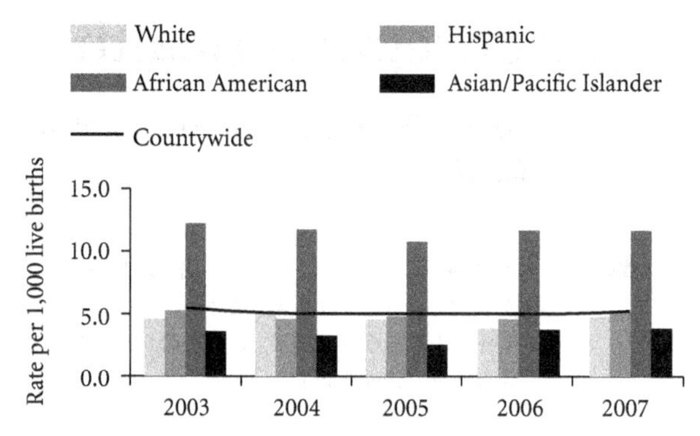

Figure 32–1 Infant mortality by race/ethnicity, Los Angeles County, 2003–2007.
Source: California Department of Public Health, Center for Health Statistics, OHIR Vital Statistics Section, 2003–2007

four key concepts as described in Table 32–2: timeline, timing, environment, and equity (11).

The life course approach draws on two concepts: first, specific health risks and determinants vary during a lifetime; second, health and disease result from their cumulative effects, creating a life course health "trajectory." Typically, the trajectory "rises" during childhood, adolescence, and early adulthood, then plateaus during middle age, and declines with advancing age. Trajectories can be improved by reducing risk factors and promoting protective factors through individual and societal/population-level actions, particularly during early childhood (12–17). Evidence suggests that these factors are not immutable but can be positively influenced later in life (12, 15).

Personal behaviors, social, psychological, and environmental exposures shape the life-course model (16) and broaden the work of MCH to identify preconception

TABLE 32–1 *Barriers to Favorable Birth Outcomes Risk Characteristics of Women Who Delivered Low Birth Weight (LBW) and Preterm (PT) Infants, Los Angeles Mommy and Baby Survey, 2007*

Measure	LBW or PT (Percent)	LAC Birth, 2007 Excluding LBW/PT (Percent)
No health insurance before pregnancy	38.2	36.5
Poverty (<$20,000/yr.)	46.5	40.9
Low education level (< 12 years)	36.1	30.9
Perceiving neighborhood as unsafe	18.1	16.2
Entered prenatal care after 1st trimester	12.2	9.8
Unintended pregnancy/mistimed	54.9	53.1
Overweight/Obese before pregnancy	38.7	38.2
Smoked in the 6 months before pregnancy	10.2	9.5

TABLE 32–2 *Key Life Course Theory Concepts*

Timeline Health is cumulative and longitudinal, shaped by exposures to risk and protective factors.
Timing Risk and protective factors have impact during critical or sensitive periods of the life course.
Environment The broader environment (biological, social, physical, and economic) affects health and development.
Equity Genetics and personal choice do not fully explain severe, ongoing health inequities.

Adapted from Fine A, Kotelchuck M. Rethinking MCH: The life course model as an organizing framework. Concept Paper. U.S. Department of Health and Human Services. Health Resources and Services Administration. Maternal and Child Health Bureau. November 2010.

factors as well as manage medical conditions that could pose risks to women, their pregnancies and their new babies.

■ CONTEXT: PRECONCEPTION HEALTH

Prior to 2006, LAC'S Maternal, Child, and Adolescent Health (MCAH) primarily oversaw interventions to improve access to early prenatal care, employed traditional surveillance of infant and maternal mortality, and provided case management for high risk individuals. Little effort went beyond traditional public health interventions. That year CDC published "Recommendations to Improve Preconception Health and Health Care" to improve pregnancy outcomes (18). Its eighth recommendation is Public Health Programs and Strategies:"Integrate components of preconception health into existing local public health and related programs, including emphasis on interconception interventions for women with previous adverse outcomes." CDC and City **MatCH,** the national organization of local urban Maternal and Child Health Directors, selected the MCAH program as part of a national effort to integrate preconception health into public health practice. This triggered the MCAH program's new focus on the life course.

■ APPROACH TO THE PROBLEM

In 2006, the LAC Preconception Health Collaborative (PHC) was formed to improve preconception health by integrating the efforts of multiple county and community agencies concerned with MCH and improving lifelong health outcomes. The PHC incorporates preconception health promotion into public health and clinical practice, educates the public about preconception health, strives to reduce disparities in maternal and infant morbidity and mortality, and monitors progress in achieving improved preconception health for all women of reproductive age in LAC (18). MCAH convenes the quarterly meetings. A website (19) shares information on activities focused on preconception and interconception health.

The PHC adopted five strategies. Projects were led by individual members and collaboratively. Regular Collaborative meetings refined the work, provided feedback and technical assistance, and planned and evaluated it. Table 32–3 lists PHC's key activities.

TABLE 32-3 *Five Preconception Health Strategies—Implemented by the Los Angeles County Preconception Health Collaborative*

Strategy	Description
Preconception Health Indicators	The Collaborative selected key indicators of preconception health that could be tracked over time. A Preconception Health Brief (22) developed by DPH focused on preconception health indicators representing data from three local sources: the Los Angeles County Health Survey (LACHS) - a sample of all women of reproductive age; the Los Angeles Mommy and Baby Project (LAMB) - women who had recently delivered a live baby; and the Los Angeles Overview of a Pregnancy Event (LA HOPE) - women who had experienced fetal or infant loss. [See Chapter 9]. LAC indicators were compared with the Healthy People 2010 recommendations.
Workforce Development	Two trainings for health care providers and DPH workforce were developed as a joint collaborative activity. Evidence-based education models were utilized in order to motivate change in practice. The initial training, **"The ABCDE's to Envisioning a Healthy Future,"** defined preconception health for public health employees and gave them a curriculum they could present to community partners and the public (23). [See Text Box 1.] The second training entitled, **"The Preconception Health Update,"** focused more specifically on recommendations for integrating preconception health promotion into daily practice for health providers. It combined presentations and panel discussions with agency administrators, nurses, physicians, and community outreach workers, providing 'nuts and bolts' strategies on how to successfully integrate preconception health into daily practice. Local data on preconception health indicators was used to focus action on activities that could have the biggest impact for particular geographic areas of the county. For example, in a geographic area that had the highest rate of overweight and obesity among women of reproductive age, strategies to address healthy weight were discussed. In another geographic area that had the highest rate of binge drinking in women of reproductive age, strategies on reducing alcohol consumption were discussed (24).
Consumer Education	The March of Dimes developed materials and media campaigns to promote folic acid and raise awareness of preconception health. Bilingual consumer materials written at a 5th- to 7th-grade literacy level on preconception health, pregnancy, preterm birth, baby care, genetics and birth defects were shared with collaborative partners throughout LAC.
Innovative Program Models	Two innovative program models were developed by collaborative partners: WIC Offers Wellness ("WOW") - The Special Supplemental Nutrition Program for Women, Infants and Children (WIC) is a federally funded food and nutrition education program for pregnant, breastfeeding, and postpartum women, infants and children under the age of five who are low to moderate income and at nutritional risk. While WIC is primarily a nutrition education and referral program, PHFE-WIC, the largest WIC provider in the nation, is in the unique position of being a primary point for the underserved and hard to reach women of reproductive age in LAC. The WOW Program, funded by the March of Dimes, is a prematurity prevention demonstration project that provides screening, health promotion and psychosocial intervention services to low-income mothers who have recently delivered a preterm and/or low-birth-weight baby.

(*continued*)

TABLE 32–3 *(Continued)*

Strategy	Description
	Integration with Family Planning – The California Family Health Council (CFHC) developed a curriculum to integrate preconception health promotion in family planning clinics throughout California, known as the Preconception Integration Project. Providers integrated brief preconception messages within family planning visits.
Quality of Care Improvement	Key efforts were undertaken to improve the quality of care for women by increasing awareness and integration of pre/interconception care among prenatal care providers. The Comprehensive Perinatal Services Program (CPSP), is a Medicaid perinatal health care program that provides enhanced nutrition, psychosocial and clinical health care to pregnant women on Medicaid. There are over 425 CPSP providers in Los Angeles County. Providers are educated on what pre/interconception care is and how they may be reimbursed for services. As part of the training sessions, baseline knowledge and assessments are compared with post-training evaluations. A follow up visit with the participating provider is made to assess adoption of the recommended pre/interconception suggestions. Efforts to impact the quality care delivered by CPSP that will also impact a life-course trajectory of the patients include programs to increase breastfeeding and depression screening. These subject areas were selected because they have some of the highest impact on maternal and child health outcomes throughout the life course.

IMPLEMENTATION OF SOLUTIONS: INTEGRATING A LIFE COURSE PERSPECTIVE BEYOND PRECONCEPTION HEALTH PROMOTION

The work in preconception health provided a framework for MCAH to move beyond preconception health to adopt a life course perspective which included:

1. Using local data to identify key points in the life trajectory that can be influenced by MCAH programs;
2. Identifying how program resources influence life-course trajectories;
3. Educating MCAH staff on the Life Course Framework;
4. Developing new partnerships to address issues that impact MCAH populations but are beyond our scope of practice.

Three issues—perinatal depression, breastfeeding promotion, and maternal stress—illustrate this (see Boxes 32–2, 32–3, and 32–4). Using LAC data, MCAH staff identified strategies to address these issues using local program resources. Training on the life course framework helped staff learn the importance of physical and social environments to the long-term health of mothers and children and the role of MCAH programs in shaping those environments. New partnerships with community providers, gang prevention agencies, family resource centers, community empowerment agencies, and neighborhood revitalization groups were formed to address malleable factors in the social environments where MCAH programs add value (see Figure 32–2).

BOX 32–1 ■ The ABCDEs to Envisioning a Healthy Future

A buse—Alcohol, Cigarettes, Illicit Drugs, Domestic Violence
B ehavioral—Mental Illness
C hronic Disease—Overweight/Obesity, Hypertension, Diabetes, Epilepsy, Deep Vein Thrombosis, Asthma
D iet, Drugs, & Dads—Nutrition and Exercise, Pharmaceuticals, and the Role of Men
E nvironmental Exposures—Occupational, Household, Food
S TIs (sexually transmitted infections), Shots, Screening

BOX 32–2 ■ Maternal Depression

Depression during pregnancy is common and treatable, but is often not diagnosed due to stigma, lack of screening, and lack of treatment resources. In LAC, one in three mothers reported feeling depressed during their pregnancy, yet only 11% of women suffering from it are diagnosed. Left untreated, maternal depression increases the risk of long-term depression in the mother, a lack of emotional availability for the baby, and negative development outcomes for infant and child. The benefits of prevention and treatment to public health are enormous and can avoid negative outcomes for mother and child that can result in entanglement in the dependency, delinquency, and adult criminal justice systems. Screening for perinatal depression should be a routine part of prenatal and postpartum care. Studies suggest that 50% of women experiencing postpartum depression are never treated (24–26). Barriers to screening among medical providers include lack of training on validated tools, lack of resources for referrals, and lack of reimbursement.

BOX 32–3 ■ Breastfeeding

Breastfeeding is one of the earliest and most impactful interventions available to prevent disease and improve health outcomes for infants and children, while also improving the health of mothers (27). Abundant evidence exists as to the benefits of breastfeeding for both the mother and infant. Maternal benefits include a lower rate of breast cancer, ovarian cancer, and type 2 diabetes. Women who breastfed longer than 12 or more months throughout their life had lower rates of hypertension, hypercholesterolemia, and cardiovascular disease (28–32).

According to the Agency for Healthcare Research and Quality (AHRQ), breastfeeding is a means of optimizing a child's ability to reach his or her full potential. Recent meta-analyses demonstrate that breastfeeding can provide short-term benefits for infants in terms of common illnesses such as ear infections, vomiting and diarrhea, as well as lowering the incidence of sudden infant death syndrome (SIDS). Those benefits extend into childhood and adulthood. Rates of eczema, childhood leukemias, obesity, and diabetes are lower in breastfed infants (27).

BOX 32-4 ■ Maternal Stress

Psychosocial stress, defined as stressful life events, daily hassles, and general anxiety, is negatively associated with preterm and low-birth-weight deliveries (30–32). Recent research points to racism as an additional stressor for racial minorities (30). Cumulative lifetime experiences of racial discrimination are associated with poor birth outcomes, such as preterm and low-birth-weight babies, that further contribute to black-white disparities in perinatal outcomes (32, 33).

Examples follow of projects MCAH programs initiated that showcase adoption of a life course perspective:

a. **Comprehensive Perinatal Services Program (CPSP).** Breastfeeding and perinatal depression curricula were developed for CPSP providers, and all clinic staff, not just medical providers, were trained. This cross-training from providers' offices assures that patients receive consistent recommendations. Community partners, such as Women's, Infants and Children (WIC), refer patients for breastfeeding support and additional resources.
b. **Integration with Home Visitation Services.** MCAH's Nurse Family Partnership (NFP) uses David Old's national model of nurse home visitation. The program

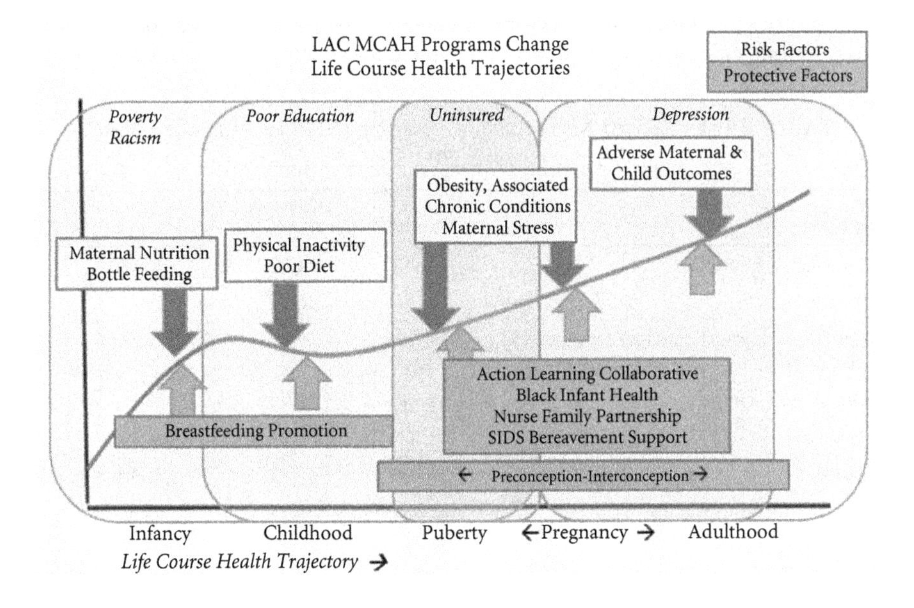

Figure 32-2 Los Angeles County Maternal, Child, and Adolescent Health Programs change life course health trajectories.
Adapted from Lu MC, Halfon N. Racial and ethnic disparities in birth outcomes: a life-course perspective. *Maternal and Child Health Journal* 2003;7:13–30.

provides home visitation case management services by public health nurses to high-risk first-time mothers who live in poverty, and serves primarily teens. Women receive guidance for their current pregnancy, and recommendations that can modify their lifelong health and that of their children. Local program data show consistent improvement in women's receipt of prenatal care, reduction in subsequent pregnancies, increased paternal involvement, increase in women's employment, reduction of families on welfare and food stamps, decrease in child abuse, and increase in children's school readiness (see Table 32–4). Topics covered include contraception, birth spacing, nutrition, and parenting. Because of high rates of depression, NFP staff screen for depression and offer referrals for mental health treatment. To increase clients' low breastfeeding rates, staff nurses were trained as certified lactation consultants to coach clients. Since a number of pregnant teens belonged to gangs or lived in neighborhoods with prevalent gang and drug activities, NFP partnered with HomeBoy Industries, a gang rehabilitation and job training program, to reach out to pregnant teens and to learn how to keep or get these young women out of gangs, or to better serve them while in gangs. Expanding these efforts, the NFP partnered with family resource centers and neighborhood revitalization efforts to improve the economic and physical environments in which their clients live.

c. **The Black Infant Health (BIH) Program.** California's BIH Program, created in 1989, works with pregnant and parenting African American clients to address alarming disparities in infant mortality between African Americans and other race/ethnicities (see Chapter 33). In LAC, BIH initiatives focus on healthy lifestyles and avoiding high-risk behaviors. Services are delivered through street outreach to link clients to resources including Medi-Cal and prenatal care; and through a peer support curriculum entitled Social Support and Empowerment,

TABLE 32–4 *Selected Nurse-Family Partnership (NFP) Program Data—LAC, July 2011*

Category	LAC- NFP	California NFP	National NFP
Cumulative # enrolled	2,754	11,585	128,801
Average age	17	20	19
Enrolled in high school/GED (at 6 months post partum)	69.95%	50.4%	40.7%
Use of food stamps	31.6%	10%	22.5%
MediCaid	85.35%	51.9%	56.6%
Latina	54.45%	45.5%	21.4%
Primary Spanish speaking	22.2%	15.3%	9.3%
African American	21.4%	8.2%	22.9%
Relative change in experience of violence during pregnancy (reduction/escalation of domestic violence)	−66.8%	−44%	−37%
Premature births	7.8%	7.8%	9.3%
Low birth weight births	6.7%	7.1%	8.8%

which teaches clients to advocate for their health and well-being and the future health needs of their babies.

d. **Racism and Birth Outcomes.** The Partnership to Eliminate Disparities in Infant Mortality (PEDIM) resulted from a national effort led by City MatCH, the Association of Maternal and Child Health Professionals (AMCHP) and the National Healthy Start Association. MCAH formed a team of 20 community-based organizations serving LAC African American women and their families to reduce racism and create a more equitable and health-promoting environment by educating providers on how racial discrimination can impact patient care and health outcomes.

e. **Grief Support.** The Sudden Infant Death Syndrome Program holds monthly peer support group meetings to help parents process their grief and addresses issues that could affect their next pregnancy outcome. Discussion topics include interconception health, safe sleeping, and overall health and wellness.

EVALUATION STRATEGY

Multiple evaluation strategies assess the impact of this work.

PHC, a logic model, was developed by selecting indicators representing collaborative performance over time (see Figure 32–3). Indicators were based on ongoing initiatives, available data, and Healthy People objectives to compare local progress against national benchmarks.

Provider Training Evaluation, pre- and post-birth questionnaires, evaluated workforce development courses. The Preconception Health Workforce Development course, entitled ABCDE's to Envisioning a Healthy Future (see Table 32–3), demonstrated that 99% of participants could identify aspects of preconception health. However, only 20% could identify optimal ways to address preconception health, and 16% could not determine how to incorporate preconception health into their work. These data informed the development of the second preconception health training, the Preconception Health Update (see Table 32–3). Attendees at the second training completed commitment cards to show at least one step that they would take to apply what they had learned. Follow-up data confirmed 97% of attendees as able to define preconception care, and 83% knew who in their community could provide it. Commitment cards showed attendees' focus on: breastfeeding (70%); folic acid promotion (63%); contraception (69%); healthy weight (72%); and use of online preconception health resources (72%).

Follow-up visits to provider sites and chart reviews were used to evaluate changes in use of training concepts. Patients were asked about peripartum depression and their attitudes about providers asking them about it. Almost all (95%) said they liked their providers asking about depression and providing related information. Eighty percent of providers trained now routinely use a validated tool for depression screening, compared to 27% who did so at baseline.

WIC Offers Wellness (WOW) (see Table 32–3) collected data on increasing intake of folic acid, birth spacing, attendance at the six-week postpartum medical visit, attainment of a healthy weight, and depression screening, and made program changes in response. Following WOW's folic acid campaign, participants increased their daily multivitamin consumption by 80%. The Preconception Integration Project of the California Family Health Council (CFHC) assessed participants' recall of

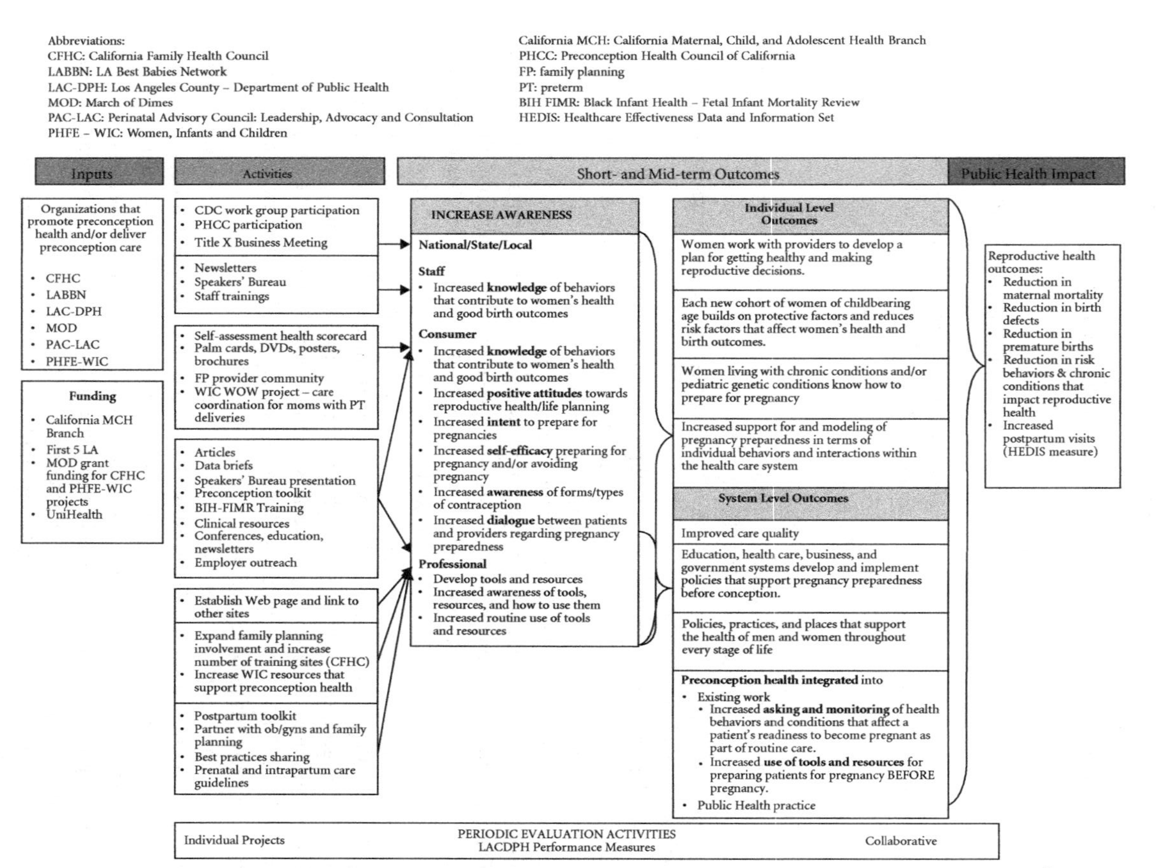

Figure 32–3 Los Angeles County Preconception Health Collaborative logic model, 2008–2011.

intervention messages and interest in making preconception health behavior changes. Evaluation revealed that 97% of women were very receptive to preconception messages and interested in making behavioral changes. Clinicians also encouraged integration of brief (1–3 minutes) preconception counseling in family planning visits (34).

MCAH program interventions incorporating a life course approach are just beginning to be evaluated for impact. Table 32–4 compares the NFP client outcomes with California and national programs. NFP uses these data for quality improvement as it aims to meet Healthy People 2020 benchmarks. BIH program clients were less likely than African American women on Medi-Cal to have preterm infants.

IMPACT

Significant changes in practice have resulted from work with health care providers, WIC, and family planning clinics, particularly, practice changes reflecting a life course framework. Long-term impacts will be assessed through future population surveys (see Chapters 2 and 9), and birth and infant death records. Another measure is the adoption of the LAC MCAH life course approach by others. Pertinent training and program materials have been adopted in other counties and organizations. Our website features abstracts and publications on pre/interconception health and MCAH Life Course work (23). The ABCDE's curriculum was distributed to all the MCH directors in California. A report from the Health Resources and Services Administration's MCH Bureau on implementing a life course framework highlighted LAC's success (35). The PHC appears in a compendium of national activities developed for the New York State Department of Health's Division of Family Health, as a best practice on the website for the Urban Initiative on Reproductive Health, and in an article published in *Pulse*, AMCHP's national newsletter (36).

CONCLUSIONS

Successful implementation of a life course framework in MCH requires collaboration and a common vision among stakeholders. Four lessons from refocusing MCAH programs to a life course framework are:

1. Data are critical to identify gaps at crucial periods in the life trajectory; know where to intervene, spot actions with the best return on investment, and monitor progress to inform program improvements.
2. Workforce education is needed to translate the science base into actionable steps for daily practice.
3. New partnerships are needed to connect MCAH programs with community stakeholders and to improve the physical and social environments and the quality of clinical care. Racism and socioeconomic and environmental determinants perpetuate inequalities in disease prevalence, and are best addressed in collaborative partnerships.
4. Promoting health before and between pregnancies allows MCAH to embrace a life course framework and increases focus on primary prevention.

REFERENCES

1. Pies C, et al. (2011) Integrating the life course perspective into a local maternal and child health program. *Maternal Child Health Journal*, published online June 1, 2011.

Available from: http://www.aap.org/commpeds/htpcp/Training/Life_Course_Handout-2.pdf (accessed June 20, 2012).
2. National Center for Health Statistics. *Health, United States, 2004 with Chartbook on Trends in the Health of Americans*. Washington, DC: US Government Printing Office; 2004.
3. Wise P. The anatomy of a disparity in infant mortality. *Annu Rev Publ Health*. 2003;24:341–62.
4. Anachebe NF, Sutton MY. Racial disparities in reproductive health outcomes. *Am J Obstet Gynecol*. 2003;188(4):S37–42.
5. David RJ, Collins JW. Differing birth weight among infants of U.S.-born Black, African-born Blacks and U.S.-born Whites. *NE J Med*. 1997;227:1209–14.
6. Frick KD, Lantz PM. Selection bias and prenatal care utilization: Linking economic and health services research. *Med Care Res & Rev*. 1996;53:371–96.
7. Finer L, Henshaw S. Disparities in rates of unintended pregnancy in the United States, 1994 and 2001. *Perspect Sex Repro H*. 2006;38(2):90–6.
8. Los Angeles Health Survey of a Pregnancy Event, Data 2006.
9. Centers for Disease Control and Prevention. Preconception health and care, 2006 at a glance. National Center on Birth Defects and Developmental Disabilities, CDC 2006. Available from: http://www.cdc.gov/ncbddd/preconception/documents/At-a-glance-4-11-06.pdf (accessed July 6, 2011).
10. The California Pregnancy-Associated Mortality Review Report from 2002 and 2003. Maternal death reviews, April 2011. Available from: http://www.cdph.ca.gov/data/statistics/Documents/MO-CA-PAMR-MaternalDeathReview-2002–03.pdf (accessed July 27, 2011).
11. Fine, A Kotelchuck, M. Rethinking MCH: The life course model as an organizing framework concept. U.S. Department of Health and Human Services Health Resources and Services Administration Maternal and Child Health Bureau. November 2010. Version 1.1. Available from: http://www.hrsa.gov/ourstories/mchb75th/images/rethinkingmch.pdf (accessed June 1, 2011).
12. Kuh D, Ben-Sholmo Y, Lynch J, Hallqvist J, Power C. Life course epidemiology. *J Epidemiol & Comm H*. 2003;57(10):778–83.
13. Halfon N, Horchstein M. Life course health development: An integrated framework for developing health policy and research. *The Milbank Quarterly*. 2002;80(3):433–79.
14. IOM. *Leading Health Indicators for Healthy People 2010: Final Report*. Washington, DC: Institute of Medicine; 1999.
15. Wise P. The anatomy of a disparity in infant mortality. *Annu Rev Publ Health*. 2003;24:341–62.
16. Halfon N. Life course health development: A new approach for addressing upstream determinants of health and spending. *Expert Voices*. Washington, DC: NIHCM Foundation; 2009.
17. Fielding J, Teutsch S. An opportunity map for societal investment in health. *JAMA*. 2011;305(20):2110–2111.
18. Centers for Disease Control and Prevention. Recommendations to improved preconception health and health care-United States/A Report of the CDCCIASTDR Preconception Care Workgroup and the Select Panel on Preconception Care. *MMWR* 2006:55 (No. RR-6).
19. Los Angeles County Department of Public Health, Maternal Child and Adolescent Health website. www.publichealth.lacounty.gov/mch/index.htm (accessed June 20, 2012).
20. Los Angeles County Department of Public Health, Office of Health Assessment and Epidemiologly. Healthy women, healthy children: Preconception health in LA County. LA Health, March 2010.
21. The training and resources are available from the Los Angeles County Department of Public Health; Maternal, Child, and Adolescent Health Programs. Call 213–639–6400 or FAX your request to 213–427–6160.

22. Presentations from the Preconception Health Update are available at the Los Angeles County Preconception Health website: http://publichealth.lacounty.gov/mch/ReproductiveHealth/PreconceptionHealth/PCH_Resources.htm.
23. Maternal, Child and Adolescent Health posters http://www.publichealth.lacounty.gov/mch/MCAHPosters_1108/MCAHPoster_Pres.htm (accessed June 20, 2012).
24. Maternal depression. Making a difference through community action: A planning guide (n.d.). Mental Health America, Substance Abuse and Mental Health Services Administration (SAMHSA). Available from: http://www.mentalhealthamerica.net/go/maternal-depression (accessed Mar. 4, 2009).
25. Ramsay R. Postnatal depression. *Lancet.* 1993;314:1358.
26. Pagel MD, Smilkstein G, Regen H, Montano D. Psychosocial influences on newborn outcomes: A controlled prospective study. *Social Sci Med.* 1990;30:597604.
27. Meyers D. Breastfeeding and health outcomes. *Breastfeed Med.* 2009 October;4(s1):S13–15.
28. Kjos SL, Henry O, Lee RM, Buchanan TA, Mishell DR. The effect of lactation on glucose and lipid metabolism in women with recent gestational diabetes. . *Am J Obstet Gynecol.* 1993;82:451–5.
29. Bimla E, Schwarz MD, et al. Duration of lactation and risk factors for maternal cardiovascular disease. *Am J Obstet Gynecol.* 2009;13:974–82.
30. Parker Dominguez T, Dunkel-Schetter C, Mancuso R, Rini CM, Hobel C. Stress in African American pregnancies: Testing the roles of various stress concepts in prediction of birth outcomes. *Ann Behav Med.* 2005;29:12–21.
31. Institute of Medicine. *Preterm Birth: Causes, Consequences, and Prevention.* Washington, DC: National Academies Press; 2006.
32. Myers HF, Lewis TT, Parker Dominguez T. Stress, coping, and minority health: Biopsychosocial perspectives on ethnic health disparities. In: Bernal G, Trimble J, Burlew K, Leong FTL, editors. *Handbook of Racial and Ethnic Minority Psychology.* Thousand Oaks, CA: Sage; 2003. pp. 377–400.
33. Mustillo S, Krieger N, Gunderson EP, Sidney S, McCreath H, Kiefe CI. Self-reported experiences of racial discrimination and Black-White differences in preterm and low-birthweight deliveries: The CARDIA Study. *Am J Publ Health.* 2004 Dec;94(12):2125.
34. Unpublished article from California Family Health Council—Preconception care and family planning—exploring the potential for integration.
35. Koshel J. Promising practices to improve birth outcomes: What can we learn from the West Coast? MCHB Technical Assistance Report, June 2011.
36. Translating MCH data into policy: An integrated approach to improve preconception health and birth outcomes in Los Angeles County. *Pulse.* July 2008: 9.

33 Narrowing the Infant Mortality Gap

Data Tools and Strategies for Improved Birth Outcomes

SHIN MARGARET CHAO, GIANNINA DONATONI, ANGEL HOPSON, DEBORAH DAVENPORT, AND CYNTHIA A. HARDING

THE NATURE OF THE PROBLEM

Infant mortality is a sentinel measure for community health. Tracking it is an essential surveillance function of local public health departments. Between 2000 and 2005, infant mortality in the Los Angeles County (LAC) plateaued between 5.2 and 5.3 deaths per 1,000 live births. The halted decline in infant mortality is a local concern. Most striking is the disparity between rates for African Americans and other racial/ethnic groups. Though infant mortality rates for African Americans (AAs) and whites decreased in LAC, the AA rate remained nearly twice the rate for whites. Figure 33–1 illustrates the high AA infant mortality rates and points to the need for new ways to address this persistent and unjust problem.

This chapter focuses on the efforts of the LAC Department of Public Health (DPH) to reduce racially disparate infant mortality rates in birth outcomes in one community, the Antelope Valley (AV). Since 2000, AV has had the highest infant mortality rate in LAC. Figure 33–2 compares infant mortality rates between AV and the rest of LAC. Although AV represented 6% of infant deaths reported in 2002, that rate measurably surpassed all other LAC areas. AV experienced an increased infant mortality rate of 112% between 1999 and 2002. As Figure 33–2 shows, AA rates in AV dramatically increased from 1999 through 2002, while rates for Asian/Pacific Islanders, Hispanics, and whites rose only slightly during the same period.

CONTEXT

Causes of infant death are multifactorial and complex. Studies suggest that some potential risk factors include: prematurity and disorders related to short gestation, low birth weight, congenital anomalies, young maternal age, low maternal education level, substance abuse, poor maternal nutrition, inadequate prenatal care, unintended pregnancy, maternal psychosocial problems including stress, existing medical conditions during pregnancy and delivery, pregnancy complications, short inter-pregnancy interval, injury (including domestic violence), infections, respiratory distress syndrome, and a lack of breastfeeding (1–4).

The 2002 infant mortality data in AV showed that of the 52 deaths, 37 (71%) occurred during the neonatal period (less than 28 days), and 15 (29%) occurred in

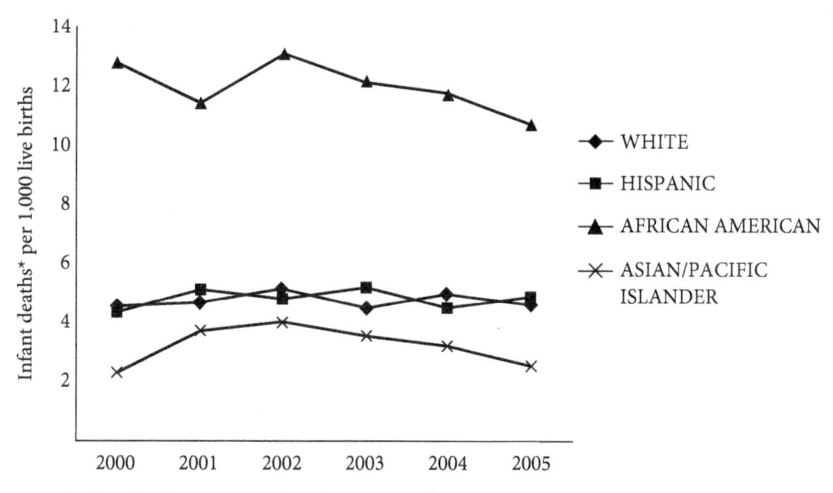

Figure 33–1 Infant Mortality by Race/Ethnicity, Los Angeles County 2000–2005. *Source:* California Department of Public Health, Center for Health Statistics, OHIR Vital Statistics Section, 2000–2005.

infants during the post neonatal period (28–364 days). Death certificate data provided limited answers. Analysis of the neonatal deaths indicated that maternal health, birth trauma, low birth weight or extreme prematurity, and fatal congenital conditions were factors. Among the older infants, respiratory disorders, including pneumonia and sudden infant death syndrome (SIDS), were prevalent. That analysis did not yield clues about maternal risk behaviors or other areas for prevention that could be addressed to improve infant mortality rates.

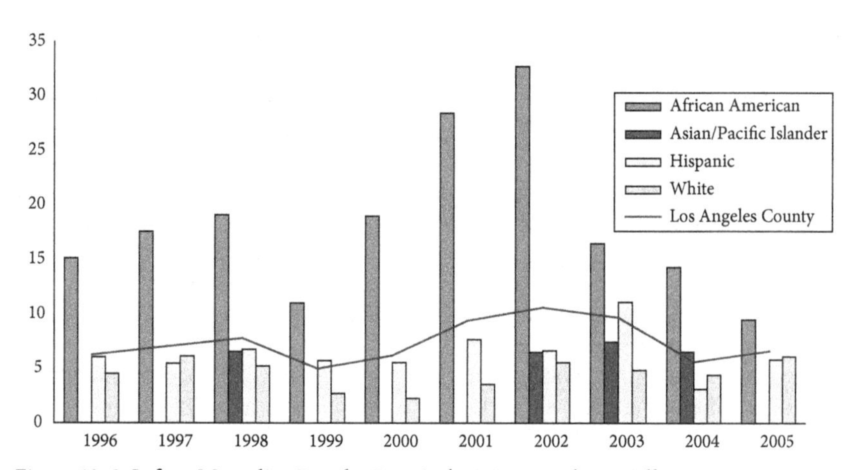

Figure 32–2 Infant Mortality Rate by Race/Ethnicity, Antelope Valley 1996–2005. *Source:* California Department of Public Health, Center for Health Statistics, OHIR Vital Statistics Section, 1996–2005.

TABLE 33–1 *Demographic Comparisons Antelope Valley vs. Los Angeles County, 2003*

	Antelope Valley	Los Angeles County
African American	13.2%	9.3%
Asian Pacific Islander	3.6%	12.8%
Hispanic	31.5%	46.8%
White	51.0%	30.8%
Native American	0.7%	0.3%
Total Population	328,334	10,035,419

Source: July 1, [2003] Population Estimates prepared by Walter R. McDonald & Associates, Inc. (WRMA) for Urban Research, LA County CAO released May 25, 2005.

The AV is the most geographically isolated, sparsely populated region of LAC, its 2,200 square miles located in LAC's northeast region and the southeast region of neighboring Kern County. Table 33–1 shows the region's demographics and indicates a higher proportion of AAs compared to the rest of LAC. Affordable middle-income housing attracted many new, young families to the area, and the population grew 32% from 1990 to 2003. One city, Palmdale, was among the fastest growing cities in California. Nearly one-third of workers had daily commutes of three or four hours, which increased stress and meant less time with families at home (5). New residents also experienced disrupted health care while changing to local health care providers.

Several health care organizations provide care in AV, where most adults had health insurance, but there still were difficulties in obtaining health care services (6), possibly due to overcrowded emergency facilities and high demand as new families began to populate the region. Three obstetrics providers served through the Comprehensive Perinatal Services Program, offering enhanced services to Medi-Cal eligible women. Uninsured women and Medi-Cal clients reported limited access to prenatal care and difficulty obtaining Medi-Cal coverage.

■ APPROACH TO THE PROBLEM

A sentinel event that triggered attention to the high infant mortality rates in AV was the release of a DPH publication, *The Key Indicators of Health* (7), which provides information about disease and health in each LAC Service Planning Area. The report's documentation of high infant mortality rates among AAs caught the media's attention and that of the Board of Supervisors and concerned community stakeholders such as the AV Partners in Health (AVPH). The DPH responded to community outrage by facilitating a community participatory approach and introducing new data tools to engage stakeholders to develop solutions.

A community collaborative was formed to define priorities for intervention, identify solutions, and sustain ongoing work. DPH worked closely with AVPH as the core task force. Its members included faith-based organizations, medical care providers, key perinatal stakeholders, and governmental agencies. The DPH Area Health Officer (AHO), who had an established working relationship with the AVPH, connected the DPH, local providers, politicians, and the media. The DPH provided data to help stakeholders better understand the problem and focus resources and interventions for the best return on investment. Focus groups with local women who had recently given birth further clarified the experiences and concerns of the families most directly affected by infant deaths and provided essential information to tailor the use of new data tools and the development of solutions. Finally, the DPH shared findings with stakeholders at community meetings where actions for change were adopted.

The DPH used both new and standard tools to investigate the problem during the initial months of the initiative. These included Perinatal Periods of Risk (PPOR) (8), traditional Fetal Infant Mortality Review (FIMR), a population-based survey of AV women who had recently delivered a live birth, and focus groups with women and providers. Each of these tools are described below.

Perinatal Periods of Risk (PPOR) has been widely used to examine fetal and infant deaths by age at death and birth weight. It is a powerful tool because it is easily understood by community members, focuses attention on a community's gaps where reductions in infant mortality are possible, targets resources to the best prevention strategies, and mobilizes a community to action. A PPOR analysis groups age at death and birth weight into four categories to identify areas which suggest the primary preventive strategy for preventing deaths in that group: 1) maternal health/prematurity; 2) maternal care; 3) newborn care; and 4) infant health (see Figure 33–3). A comparison group is selected to estimate the excess or preventable deaths for these periods of risk, periods with the highest excess or preventable deaths and thus greatest opportunities for intervention. Figure 33–4 illustrates how the PPOR analysis identifies areas in which to intervene.

The DPH used birth cohort data (9) to calculate overall fetal/infant death rates for AV mothers and compared that against a reference group with one of the lowest rates in LAC (non-Hispanic white mothers, with 12 years or more education, over 20 years of age, residing in LAC outside AV). This reference group was chosen to show the community how low a rate could be attained in LAC and, reflecting social justice, the rate that should be the goal in AV. This analysis is described in Figure 33–5, showing maternal health and infant health as two areas where babies of AV women experienced excess mortality compared to the reference group. To improve AV's infant mortality rates, these were the two obvious areas for action.

The second MCAH data tool was a traditional Fetal Infant Mortality Review (FIMR). It evaluated the medical and social histories associated with the 53 AV infant deaths. Trained public health nurses conducted FIMR investigations over a six-month period using the FIMR protocols approved by the State of California (10).

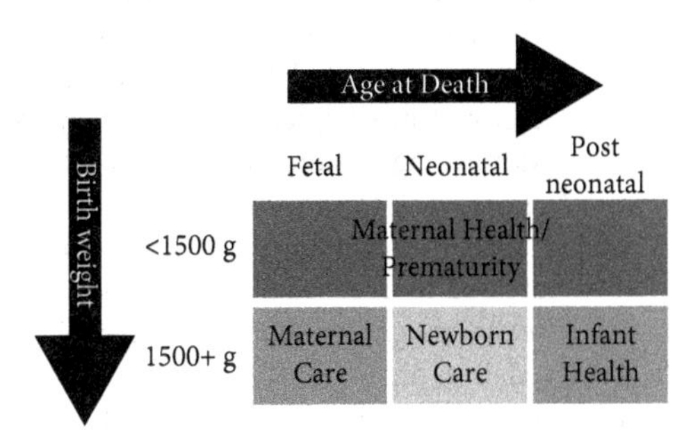

Figure 33–3 Perinatal Periods of Risk (PPOR).

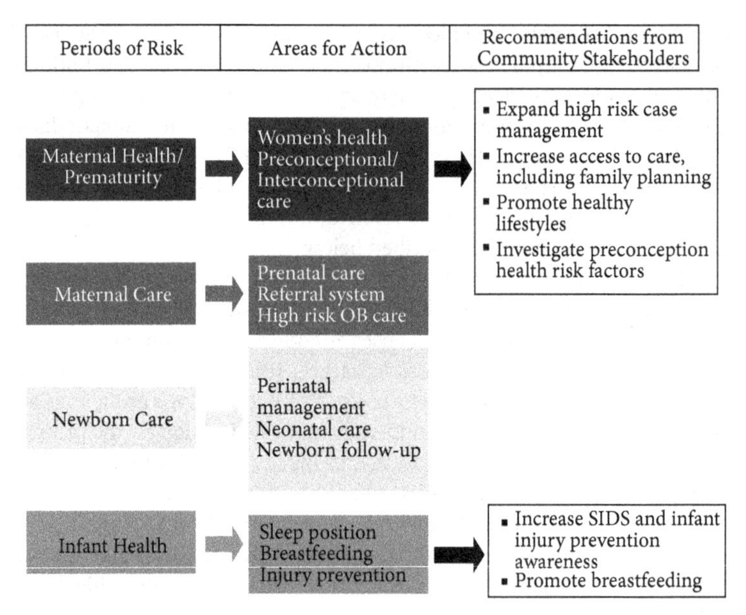

Figure 33–4 Perinatal Periods of Risk (PPOR): Periods of Risk for Fetal and Infant Death and Corresponding Areas for Action.

A salient finding was the lack of social support networks for women who had lost infants. Many of the women interviewed reported that this was not their first experience with infant loss, and yet there had been no medical or social support interventions to prepare them for their next pregnancy. PPOR and FIMR used together gave the task force a clearer picture of the causes of infant mortality in AV. The 53 deaths were divided into the PPOR areas of risk so that FIMR findings could then be used to more fully explain the factors underlying fetal and infant deaths that fell in the two priority intervention areas: maternal health and infant health.

While PPOR and FIMR yielded useful information, analyses were still limited by the data found in patients' charts and vital records, and by the difficulty in locating clients. The task force recommended collecting additional information to understand the underlying risk factors that could not be ascertained from medical records. Consequently, MCAH implemented a third data tool, the Los Angeles Mommy and Baby (LAMB) project (described in Chapter 9). The survey followed the CDC Pregnancy Risk Assessment Monitoring System (PRAMS) protocol to collect data (11). LAMB findings in AV clearly pointed to women's health prior to pregnancy (preconception health) and quality of prenatal care as having impacts on birth outcomes, each needing to be addressed to improve infant mortality rate.

MCAH also conducted three focus groups with AA, Hispanic, and white mothers who had recently delivered live births in AV. We learned that women faced transportation barriers to keeping prenatal care appointments. AA women felt that their health concerns were not taken seriously by providers, and many felt that they were treated as single welfare moms regardless of their marital or economic status. Clinicians shared concerns about women entering prenatal care late, the number

Antelope Valley

Birthweight	Fetal	Neonatal	Post-Neonatal
	Age Group		
<1500 g	Maternal Health/Prematurity 9.7 (N=48)		
1500+ g	Maternal Care 2.8 (N=14)	Newborn Care 1.8 (N=9)	Infant Health 2.6 (N=13)

Total fetal/infant mortality rate: 17.0/1,000 (N=84)
(Total live births + fetal deaths = 4934)

Reference Group*

Birthweight	Fetal	Neonatal	Post-Neonatal
	Age Group		
<1500 g	Maternal Health/Prematurity 4.1 (N=82)		
1500+ g	Maternal Care 1.2 (N=25)	Newborn Care 0.8 (N=17)	Infant Health 0.6 (N=12)

Total fetal/infant mortality rate: 6.8/1,000 (N=136)
(Total live births + fetal deaths = 20,139)

Excess Fetal/Infant Mortality Rates

Birthweight	Fetal	Neonatal	Post-Neonatal
	Age Group		
<1500 g	Maternal Health/Prematurity 5.6		
1500+ g	Maternal Care 1.6	Newborn Care 1.0	Infant Health 2.0

Total Excess Rate: 10.2/1,000

This PPOR analysis compares fetal-infant mortality rates between the AV and a reference group. The difference between the rates is the AV "excess" rate. The overall 2002 fetal-infant mortality rate in the AV was 17 deaths per 1,000 live births plus fetal deaths. Compared to the reference group rate of 6.8 deaths per 1,000 live births plus fetal deaths, the AV excess rate was 10.2 deaths per 1,000 plus fetal deaths. The highest rate of excess fetal and infant deaths was among very low birth weight (VLBW) infants (5.6 deaths per 1,000 live births plus fetal deaths). The next highest rate of excess deaths was among post-neonatal infants who were not VLBW (2.0 deaths per 1,000 live births plus fetal deaths).

*Reference group: LA County non-Hispanic white residents aged 20 and above with more than 12 years of education who gave birth or had a fetal death.
Data Sources:
1.Birth, Fetal Death, and Death data, California Department of Health Services, Center for Health Statistics, Vital Statistics, 2002.
2.Birth Cohort data, California Department of Health Services, Center for Health Statistics, Vital Statistics, 2002

Chao SM, Donatoni G, Bemis C, Donovan K, Harding C, Davenport D, Kasehagen L, Gilbert G, Kasehagen L, Peck M. Integrated approaches to improve birth outcomes: Perinatal Periods of Risk, Infant Mortality Review, and the Los Angeles Mommy and Baby Project. Matern Child Health J, 2010 Nov;14(6):827–37.

Figure 33–5 Perinatal Periods of Risk (PPOR): Analysis of Fetal and Infant Deaths Antelope Valley, Los Angeles County, 2002.

of health issues that could not be solved in nine months of prenatal care, and the difficulty in getting their patients access to high risk obstetrical care. Providers also shared concern about high rates of infant mortality and their commitment to working with mothers on solutions.

Throughout the process, the DPH involved community stakeholders in reviewing data, assisting with the selection of solutions, and providing input into the analysis.

Findings from the PPOR/FIMR and focus groups were shared at a community forum. The task force focused on strategies for prevention and intervention that addressed the two areas of excess mortality: maternal health and infant health. The audience broke into small groups and brainstormed to identify strategies that could be implemented with existing resources using the new information to inform their discussion (see Figure 33–6).

■ IMPLEMENTATION OF SOLUTIONS: USING DATA TO DRIVE COMMUNITY ACTION

Together, the PPOR, FIMR, LAMB, and focus group findings gave community members information on the periods of risk when deaths occurred, potential causes, and factors that placed women at risk of poor birth outcomes. Information was presented on evidence-based interventions for reducing infant mortality found effective with AA women, their infants, and their families. Five recommendations were developed to guide community action:

1. Increase capacity and target access to high-risk family support programs for AA women and their families.
2. Decrease barriers to accessing care by increasing the number of women and infants with medical insurance.
3. Collaborate with and educate local health care providers to ensure higher quality care for AA women and their infants.

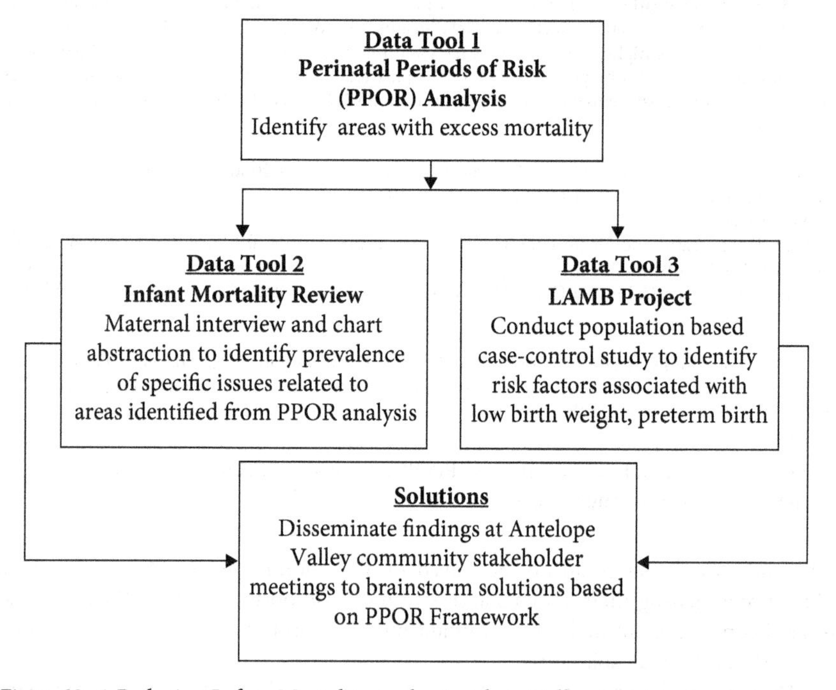

Figure 33–6 Reducing Infant Mortality in the Antelope Valley, Los Angeles County: Use of New and Standard Data Tools to Reach Community Solutions.

4. Conduct a healthy life practices education and outreach/marketing campaign aimed at AA women and the local community
5. Conduct research to determine the causes of infant mortality in AV

Within these five recommendations, community consensus yielded several actions (see Figure 33–4). Over 40 local agencies, health care providers, the faith community, residents, the AV Area Health Office, MCAH program staff, and staff from the LA Best Babies Network formed a local collaborative, the AV Best Babies Collaborative, to continue promoting healthy births in AV and to carry out the recommendations (5). The results are described in the Impact section and are listed in Table 33–2.

Throughout the process, local media and state and local politicians remained engaged. A reporter from the AV press attended meetings and reported task force progress. Local and state politicians sponsored health fairs to increase awareness of the issue and to connect AV residents with resources to support healthy pregnancies. Public funders and philanthropic organizations became aware of the issues and committed resources to fund new programs and educational campaigns.

Community involvement was crucial to drive actions with long-lasting impact on infant mortality. A collective sense of urgency motivated community stakeholders to review data and take ownership of the problem. Working group meetings were open and inclusive. With the support of political leaders and public and private funders, the community demonstrated a tremendous ability to take action based on the new recommendations.

■ EVALUATION

The DPH and the AV community helped to reduce the AV infant mortality rate and also narrowed disparities between AAs and other groups. Three integrated factors played a role: data collection and analysis, community engagement, and an infusion of funding for targeted community prevention programs. Evaluation of the community approach included measuring the project's overall impact on infant mortality, assessing the quality of data collected through FIMR and LAMB, and noting the project's resulting impact of services added or expanded.

DPH analysis of infant mortality data pointed out significant, long-term reduction of AV infant mortality. Between 2002 and 2003, the infant mortality rate among AAs dropped from 32.7 deaths per 1,000 live births to 16 per 1,000 live births and continued to decline from 2004 to 2005 (see Figure 33–2).

■ IMPACT

The three data tools—PPOR, FIMR, and LAMB—provided valuable information in infant deaths that were previously unavailable. LAMB collected data unavailable through chart review and increased understanding of the health and social issues impacting infant mortality. As a result, DPH replaced the traditional FIMR approach with LA HOPE (see Chapter 9). Information from these sources convinced medical providers of a serious problem, and gained their commitment to be part of the solution.

LAMB and LA HOPE have been expanded countywide. The PPOR framework is used in other service planning throughout LAC in partnership with community stakeholders to effectively address infant mortality. And several funders have

TABLE 33–2 *Recommendations to Improve Birth Outcomes in the Antelope Valley and Community Actions*

Recommendation	Community Action
1. Increase capacity and target access to high-risk family support programs for African American women and their families	First 5 LA invested $1 million in the AV Best Babies Collaborative. Title X dollars were targeted to the Black Infant Health Program to link African American women to family planning services in AV. DPH Public Health Nurses supported the Black Infant Health Program in conducting initial home assessments of clients. DPH submitted grant applications to secure additional funding.
2. Decrease the barriers to accessing care by increasing the number of women and infants that have medical insurance	Childrens' Health Outreach Initiatives (see Chapter 34) raised awareness of the issue of infant mortality among their contractors who conduct outreach activities to enroll families in health insurance. In addition to enrolling families in health insurance, contractors follow up to encourage families to use their benefits for preventive care and to assist families in retaining their health benefits over time. Local faith-based organizations offered vans for transportation to and from medical appointments and to job training programs.
3. Collaborate with and educate local health care providers to ensure quality care for African American women and their infants	DPH partnered with local health care providers to review infant mortality data and make recommendations regarding issues impacting access to, and quality of care. DPH trained home visitor staff to be certified lactation educators to promote breastfeeding. AV Hospital committed to enhancing information on SIDS and infant injury prevention as part of their discharge procedures. UCLA has been working to expand access to high-risk OB care in the AV.
4. Conduct an education and outreach marketing campaign aimed at African American women and the local community regarding healthy life practices	Engaged the local faith community to take a lead in community support and mentoring for women and families at risk. Developed a community health messaging program to address healthy births in collaboration with the Los Angeles Best Babies Collaborative. March of Dimes funded the AV Black Infant Health program to develop a preconception health curriculum that could be implemented through local churches. Local politicians hosted health fairs. DPH worked with community agencies to develop a referral guide for resources and services. DPH staff developed a presentation on improving birth outcomes that was presented at several local meetings and made available for distribution.
5. Conduct research to determine the causes of infant mortality in the Antelope Valley	LAMB was implemented in the AV and subsequently countywide (see Chapter 9).

modified their grant processes to require data generated from these new tools. DPH staff have presented related findings from AV at national conferences and have given technical assistance to communities across the United States.

CONCLUSION

Since 1980, declines in infant mortality slowed or stagnated nationally, even as racial disparities widened. When confronted in 2002 with a rise in the AV rate, the DPH recognized the need for new data tools and ways of involving community stakeholders. The community approach achieved and sustained reductions in infant mortality and racial disparities. Key lessons learned were:

- Building upon existing collaboratives gained the participation of key stakeholders in the project's ongoing activities.
- Involving local politicians and the print media brought publicity to the problem, political support for the project, and funding for increased services.
- Developing new ways of analyzing and presenting data at community stakeholder meetings helped participants understand the issues and identify areas where interventions would produce the greatest impact.
- Community ownership of the problem encouraged the adoption of solutions that continue to be implemented.
- The combined use of new (PPOR and LAMB) and traditional (FIMR and focus groups) instruments for conducting infant mortality reviews helped us to address social and environmental factors along with traditional medical issues.

REFERENCES

1. National Center for Health Statistics. Vital statistics of the United States, 1993, vol II: mortality, part A. Hyattsville, MD: National Center for Health Statistics; 2002.
2. Fiscella K. Racial disparity in infant and maternal mortality: confluence of infection and microvascular dysfunction. Matern Child Health J. 2004;8:45–54.
3. Hogan VK, Njoroge T, Durant TM, Ferre CD. Eliminating disparities in perinatal outcomes—lessons learned. Matern Child Health J. 2001;5:135–40.
4. Geronimus AT. Black/white differences in the relationship of maternal age to birthweight: a population-based test of the weathering hypothesis. Soc Sci Med. 1996;42:589–97.
5. Davenport D, Harding C. Infant mortality in the Antelope Valley: Follow-up report to the Board of Supervisors. Los Angeles County Department of Public Health, 2005 May. Available from: http://publichealth.lacounty.gov/mch/reports/Infant%20Mortality%20in%20the%20Antelope%20Valley.pdf (accessed Jun 22, 2012).
6. Los Angeles County Department of Public Health, Office of Health Assessment and Epidemiology. Los Angeles county profiles, 1997: Results of the 1997 LA County Health Survey by Service Planning Area. Available from: http://www.lapublichealth.org/ha/reports/haspaprf/spaprof.htm (accessed Jun 22, 2012).
7. Los Angeles County Department of Public Health, Office of Health Assessment and Epidemiology. Key indicators of health by Service Planning Area. 2003. Available from: http://lapublichealth.org/wwwfiles/ph/hae/ha/keyhealth.pdf (accessed Jun 22, 2012).

8. Peck MG, Sappenfield BM, Skala J. Perinatal periods of risk: a community approach for using data to improve women and infants' health. Matern Child Health J. 2010 Nov;14(6):864–74.
9. California Birth Cohort data, California Department of Health Services, Center for Health Statistics, Vital Statistics, 2002.
10. California Department of Public Health. Fetal Infant Mortality Review (FIMR) Program. FIMR Policies and Procedures. Available from: http://www.cdph.ca.gov/services/funding/mcah/Pages/ProgramandFiscalPoliciesProcedures-FY2010-2011.aspx (accessed Jun 22, 2012).
11. Pregnancy Risk Assessment Monitoring System. U.S. Department of Health and Human Services, Centers for Disease Control and Prevention, National Center for Chronic Disease Prevention and Health Promotion, Division of Reproductive Health; 2003 May 22. Available from: http://www.cdc.gov/prams/ (accessed Jun 22, 2012).
12. Davenport D, Harding C. Infant mortality in the Antelope Valley: Follow-up report to the Board of Supervisors. Los Angeles County Department of Public Health, 2005 May. Available from: http://publichealth.lacounty.gov/mch/reports/Infant%20Mortality%20in%20the%20Antelope%20Valley.pdf.

34 Assuring Medical Coverage

An Effective Outreach Initiative for Children and Families

WENDY K. SCHIFFER, SUZANNE BOSTWICK, CHANDRA HIGGINS, AND CYNTHIA A. HARDING

THE NATURE OF THE PROBLEM

In the late 1990s, more than one-third of Los Angeles County's 9.5 million residents lacked health insurance coverage. While the percentage was much lower among children, about 382,000 children were uninsured. Uninsured children from low-income families experience higher levels of unmet health care needs than other children in Los Angeles County (LAC). Six of every 10 low-income families with uninsured children reported difficulty accessing needed medical care for their children. Almost one-third were unable to visit a doctor for a medical checkup, and 30% were unable see a doctor for illness because of cost concerns. A fourth of these children did not receive prescription drugs and over half went without dental care because of cost (1). A focus group conducted in 2009 by the Urban Institute with Healthy Kids parents found that health insurance increased the likelihood that children received preventive care by 27% (1).

It is troubling that many of these uninsured children were eligible for coverage. Most uninsured children are from low-income families with household incomes below 133% of federal poverty level (FPL). In California, almost all low-income, uninsured children are eligible for Medi-Cal (California's Medicaid program) or Healthy Families (California's Statewide Children's Health Insurance Program known as SCHIP) (see Figure 34–1). Complex eligibility rules make it difficult for families to know the public programs to which they are entitled. For example, Medi-Cal eligibility is based on income and age, wherein the income qualification for a young child's family is higher than for an older child's family. This leads to mixed-status families, for example, a young child eligible for Medi-Cal, an older sibling eligible for Healthy Families, and an undocumented family member ineligible for any public assistance program. Concerns of undocumented residents about the effect of using of public benefits on their immigration status compound the confusion. In the face of such complexity, not surprisingly, many eligible children remain uninsured.

Quantitative and qualitative studies by the Urban Institute have found that parents with insured children have demonstrably improved access to and use of clinical care, are less concerned about obtaining care for their children, and enjoy improved health status of their enrolled children (1). A 2009 survey found that parents with Healthy Kids coverage perceived that their children's health status was improved and had not had medical problems in the month prior to the survey (1). However, to achieve these gains, access to health insurance alone is insufficient. Significant outreach and enrollment efforts are critical to sign up and retain participants, and to educate participants about appropriately accessing care.

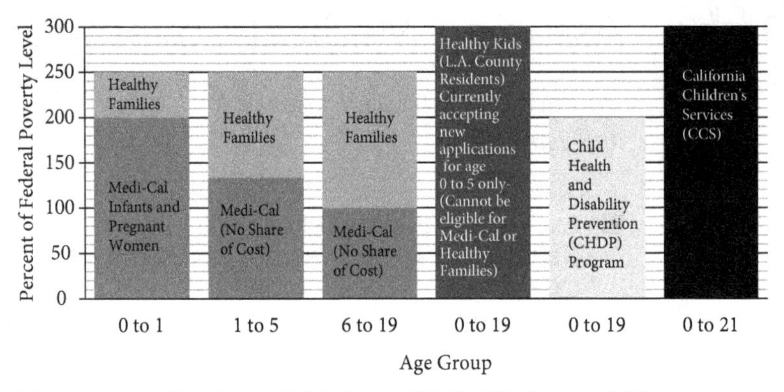

Information extrapolated from Maternal Child Health Access (MCHA) – 2009. All program eligibility requirements are based on age, income, citizenship documentation status and/or county residency.

Figure 34–1 Health Insurance—Income Guidelines.

■ CONTEXT

Passage in 1996 of the Personal Responsibility and Work Opportunity Reconciliation Act created confusion about eligibility for Medi-Cal and welfare. The law's changes to the safety net system "de-linked" Medi-Cal eligibility from welfare eligibility. Thus families losing welfare benefits still remained eligible for Medi-Cal. To allay some families' confusion, implementation of welfare reform in LAC included funding for community-based outreach and Medi-Cal enrollment.

In 1997, California created its SCHIP program, Healthy Families, which provided greater health insurance opportunities, but also added to families' confusion about their eligibility for the array of health programs. (SCHIP, enacted in the Balanced Budget Act of 1997, established a state-administered national program of medical coverage for children whose family incomes are too high to qualify for Medicaid.) With creation of the new coverage, California families often did not understand which program they were eligible for or how to qualify. To promote Healthy Families enrollment, the state funded community-based outreach and enrollment. The state also offered a $50.00 incentive fee to trained local certified application assistants (CAAs) per Healthy Families enrollment. But this incentive was only for Healthy Families enrollment and did not encourage a comprehensive approach to determine eligibility for all public health insurance programs available to children and their families. In many cases, children eligible for Medi-Cal were not assisted—particularly problematic since most uninsured children are Medi-Cal eligible.

Enrollment efforts for California's public programs traditionally have been impeded by insufficient funding for outreach (3). While several sources have supported community-based outreach and enrollment efforts, funding has been inconsistent (3). In one case, the state budget included locally administered outreach and enrollment services; but no sooner did the LAC Department of Public Health (DPH) conduct a competitive solicitation process and execute contracts with community-based agencies than the state retroactively eliminated the program.

Spurred by support from an LAC supervisor, First 5 LA, the local agency that administers LAC's Proposition 10 tobacco tax funding for services targeted to children aged 0–5, created an opportunity for universal coverage for that group. This initiative, called Healthy Kids, and modeled after similar initiatives in Northern California counties, included health insurance for children ineligible for Medi-Cal or Healthy Families because of family incomes that were too high or due to immigration status. Several issues had to be navigated in developing Healthy Kids. First 5 LA funding, by law, targets children 0–5, but advocates felt that the broader initiative was needed to reach out to other family members and siblings over the age of five. Also, immigration status had to be carefully finessed because of the politically tenuous support for providing health insurance to undocumented residents.

Given the challenge of enrolling participants in a new program, First 5 LA included substantial funding for comprehensive, community-based outreach and enrollment in the Healthy Kids initiative. Because of its past experience in administering community-based outreach and enrollment programs, First 5 LA selected the DPH to administer this funding and to manage community-based outreach and enrollment.

■ APPROACH TO THE PROBLEM

First 5 LA worked with DPH and L.A. Care Health Plan—the managed care organization that would administer the Healthy Kids insurance product—to draft a model for the broad Healthy Kids initiative to include health insurance for children 0–5 who were ineligible for Medi-Cal and Healthy Families and outreach and enrollment for young children and their families. The working group consulted with other health jurisdictions in the state that had implemented similar programs.

From the start, Healthy Kids was perceived as more than another stand-alone insurance product contributing to the patchwork of children's health programs. The ideal of the broader Healthy Kids initiative was to assure every child of coverage. To that end, a high-level coalition was formed in May 2003, called the Children's Health Initiative of Greater Los Angeles. The coalition was co-chaired by the directors of L.A. Care Health Plan, The California Endowment, and the LAC Department of Health Services (prior to 2006, the DPH was a division under the Department of Health Services). It had three main goals: 1) to identify funding to expand Healthy Kids to children above age five; 2) to recommend system changes to make it easier for children to enroll and remain enrolled in the low- or no-cost coverage programs for which they qualify; and 3) to effect statewide or national policy change to yield more sustainable solutions to medical coverage for all children. The Coalition formed workgroups for each of these three goals. The DPH chaired the Program Integration Workgroup, which focused on system changes for easier enrollment and retention.

The Children's Health Initiative coalition attracted high-level participation, enabling it to better meet its goals. More than 50 organizations participated, representing medical care providers, health insurance plans, the business community, advocacy organizations, foundations, labor unions, education, and the public health community. Principals generally attended coalition meetings, and managers with operational or client experience participated in the workgroups.

In addition to chairing the Program Integration Workgroup, the DPH administered the outreach, enrollment, retention, and utilization component of Healthy Kids. The DPH contracted with school districts, clinics, hospitals, community-based organizations with experience in working with the uninsured population, and with two training agencies. DPH required all contracted staff to attend intensive training on all available low- and no-cost medical coverage programs and eligibility rules. Training was also made widely available to all interested clinical care providers and CAAs in LAC. The DPH held monthly meetings with contracted agencies to share information and assure coordination and consistent practice. The DPH extended information sharing beyond the contractor network by holding CAA conferences and establishing a CAA LISTSERV to share, update and disseminate information about outreach and enrollment practices, plus changes to medical coverage programs.

DPH outreach and enrollment contractors were trusted by clients and understood local programs and safety-net opportunities. They tailored their approaches to meet clients' needs. They conducted outreach where children and families congregated—at schools, WIC sites, community clinics, and events. Community-based organizations were perceived as non-threatening and provided potential clients accurate information about immigration status and medical coverage, helping counter clients' fears that signing up for government benefits such as Medi-Cal would affect their immigration status or force them to pay for medical services received. Contractors also lacked the negative stigma of "welfare" offices and so could recruit clients who might have avoided applying for benefits at government offices.

The DPH developed a standard scope of work for contractors, for quality assurance as well as evaluation purposes. The approach included:

- **All programs, all family members**—Contractors took a holistic approach to assessing family needs. They assumed that parents would enroll their children if they could enroll other family members as well, so they assisted with applications for all family members who qualified for low or no-cost health insurance. Family members unable to qualify were referred to "safety net" medical providers and other social services such as Cal Fresh (California's Food Stamp program) and the Earned Income Tax Credit.
- **Retention and service use**—Enrollment in health insurance is only useful if services are received. One-on-one outreach and enrollment helps to promote program retention and appropriate use of medical benefits. Contractors help clients choose a health care plan and a primary care provider, explain how to use their benefits, and troubleshoot problems preventing access to care. Contractors also were required to check on clients at three months after completion of the application to confirm successful enrollment and receipt of insurance cards; at six months to assess whether families need help using their benefits; and at 11 months to offer renewal assistance. An annual retention study by DPH contractors identified the main reason that clients lost their coverage as failure to return required paperwork, but retention rates for families re-contacted by DPH contractors still exceeds 78% for all coverage programs (4).
- **Data system**—Contractors entered client-level data into a centralized system to determine follow-up needs, enabling DPH to run summary reports on contractor performance.
- **Federal Medicaid matching funds**—The First 5 LA funding was eligible for Medi-Cal Administrative Activities (MAA) matching funds. Contractors documented the activities performed to outreach and enroll individuals into Medi-Cal. MAA funds were then reinvested into the program.

IMPLEMENTATION OF SOLUTIONS

Healthy Kids insurance for children aged 0–5 and the accompanying outreach and enrollment services became available in July 2003. The CHI coalition succeeded in raising funds to expand Healthy Kids to children ages 6–18 in 2004, largely from private foundations. The DPH and its contractor network were instrumental in developing Healthy Kids as user-friendly, with easy client enrollment and retention. The initiative benefited from participation by several DPH contractors, including trainers, in the Program Integration Workgroup that the DPH chaired. Contractors contributed their firsthand experience assisting clients with Medi-Cal and Healthy Families enrollment and retention, and avoided some of the barriers in those programs. Common barriers include: inadequate income documentation (e.g., pay stubs) leading to enrollment delays; no pre-screening to determine eligibility, leading to denials for one program and reapplication to another; and clients with existing open Medi-Cal cases, where families reapply for coverage rather than "fixing" current problems (e.g., wrongful terminations, failing to turn in mandated reports). Addressing these barriers shortened Healthy Kids enrollment processing time and simplified the renewal process, which contributes to Healthy Kids' high retention rate.

The Program Integration Workgroup took systemic approaches to outreach and enrollment. DPH worked with the Department of Public Social Services offices (DPSS), the agency that administers Medi-Cal in LAC, to identify all children aged 0–5 who received emergency Medi-Cal, since they are, by definition, eligible for Healthy Kids. Families were sent a targeted mailing explaining that their child was provisionally eligible for Healthy Kids and that if they verified and returned the information on the mailing to L.A. Care Health Plan, their child could be enrolled. These mailings are now routine, as the number of applications increased after the mailing. The DPH and L.A. Care are tracking this trend.

Healthy Kids enrollment was highly successful, and enrollment quickly reached maximum capacity of 30,000 children. Since funding for older children was limited, new Healthy Kids enrollment for 6- to 18-year-olds was frozen in 2006 to avoid having to disenroll currently enrolled children. The enrollment freeze did not affect children aged 0–5, since First 5 LA funding remained stable.

The Healthy Kids enrollment freeze for 6- to 18-year-olds challenged outreach and enrollment contractors, as options were limited for this population. Contractors kept an "interest list" of those aged 6–18 who would qualify for Healthy Kids if not for the freeze, for later contact if additional funding were procured. The Program Integration Workgroup and L.A. Care developed criteria implementing the freeze and prioritized coverage for children close to age five, so they would not "age out" or lose coverage once they turned five.

The advantage of a well-trained outreach and enrollment contractor network is their familiarity with lesser known programs such as emergency Medi-Cal, the Child Health and Disability Prevention (CHDP) Gateway, CaliforniaKids, Healthy Way LA, and Kaiser Permanente Child Health Plan, and the ability to help clients access safety net medical care. These programs became the only options for those aged 6–18 who could no longer enroll in Healthy Kids. Contractors also focus on retention, so clients do not lose Healthy Kids coverage and then become unable to reenroll.

The complexity of health care options and enrollment procedures for children suggested electronic application submissions, preferably a system that could automatically route an application to the correct program for which a child is eligible. Local experts, including the DPH, DHS, DPSS, and selected outreach and enrollment contractors, helped develop and test such new systems, including One-e-App (which routed applications to the State's Single Point of Entry that processes Medi-Cal and Healthy Families applications, and to L.A. Care for Healthy Kids); also, Express Enrollment—Health e-app (in which a school lunch application doubles as a Medi-Cal application), and DPSS's online Medi-Cal application. The DPH also developed a local data system for contractors to enter client-level data for case management and reporting requirements. Previously, contractors had to hand-tally outreach contacts, applications they had assisted, demographic data of families helped, types of applications, and problems encountered. The DPH/Children's Health Outreach Initiatives "CHOI" data system now allows contractors to enter client-level data and receive reminders for follow-up. The DPH can view agency-level summary data about all the objectives in the contractors' scope of work and demographic data and enrollment problems.

EVALUATION STRATEGY

The CHOI data system proved invaluable for program evaluation. DPH can access encrypted agency-level summary reports on a wide range of data elements for all family members assisted since July 2003 and can assess overall performance management. Figure 34–2 is an example report.

The system also tracks contractor performance and the value they provide to families. Reports of the number of family members assisted help DPH ascertain whether agencies are being comprehensive. Examination of the enrollment among programs helps assess whether contractors "cherry-pick" the easy clients or help clients enroll in lesser-known programs. The DPH reviews these reports with contractors individually and as a group. Having real-time data helps with project management and improves service quality.

The Urban Institute and the University of Southern California (USC) conducted an external evaluation of the Healthy Kids initiative that included interviews with outreach and enrollment contractors, parent focus groups, and review of CHOI enrollment trend data (discussed below). Their evaluation found the Healthy Kids outreach

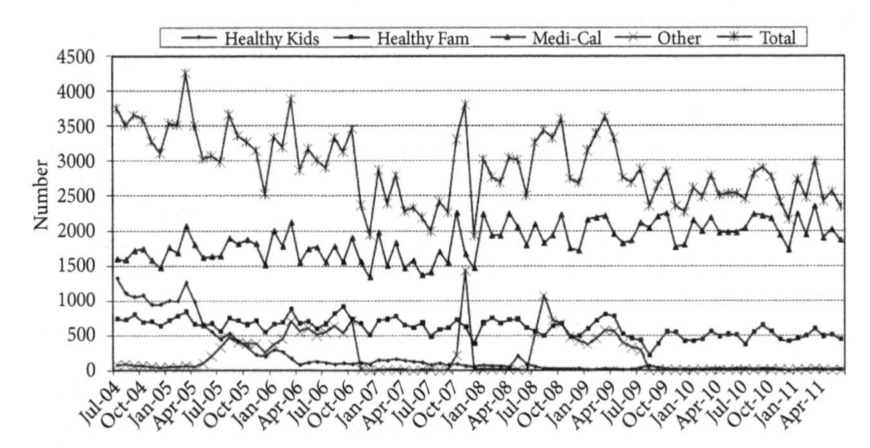

Figure 34–2 Total Applications Submitted by Contracted Agencies in Los Angeles County by Month and Program, July 1, 2004–June 30, 2011 (n = 280, 221).

and enrollment strategies successful in finding, enrolling, and retaining children who previously were uninsured (5).

IMPACT

The Healthy Kids outreach and enrollment project has been highly successful. More than 30,000 applications are submitted annually, and 84% are successfully enrolled (4). In the past fiscal year, 86% of Healthy Families applications were verified as enrolled, compared to a statewide success rate of 63% for Healthy Families applications submitted without assistance. A 14-month post-enrollment survey found that 78% of the individuals initially assisted are still enrolled in a health coverage program (4). Other California counties have requested information about the CHOI data system, particularly its ability to track local data for CAA enrollment trends and as a case management tool.

Another measure of success is that contractors are enrolling clients into a variety of programs. In fiscal year 2009/2010, 71% of applications for children aged 0–18 were for Medi-Cal; 27% for Healthy Families; and 2% for Healthy Kids and other health programs. This indicates that they are focusing on the lowest income families. Consistent with the comprehensive approach to families, more than 10,000 Medi-Cal applications were submitted for adults over age 19, most of whom (63%) were pregnant women (4).

As intended, families are entering the system through contacts made in the community at schools, WIC sites, and local neighborhood events, rather than traditional routes such as at DPSS or medical provider offices; without the assistance of CHOI contractors, these children could have remained uninsured.

National health care reform will increase the need for outreach and enrollment efforts. Once reform is fully implemented, children may either be eligible for Medi-Cal, Healthy Families, the state-managed insurance exchanges, or employer-sponsored plans. Families may not understand whether their employer is required to offer medical insurance or what level of subsidy they might receive if they are eligible for the health insurance exchanges. Families enrolling in exchanges will have to select among complex benefit levels and health plans. This complexity can be mitigated by designing accessible electronic enrollment systems and by offering families community-based enrollment assistance based on the CHOI model (2, 5). DPH and its network of community partners working on health insurance outreach, enrollment, utilization, and retention have laid the groundwork to implement new services and products under health reform.

CONCLUSIONS

- Significant improvement in children's health coverage requires informed access to medical insurance products and outreach, plus enrollment and retention help to ensure that families understand and use their benefits. The combination of the Healthy Kids insurance product, along with individual outreach and enrollment activities, increases success.
- Contractors provide the most value to families when they offer comprehensive enrollment and referral help, assessing all family members for all no- and low-cost programs for which they may qualify.
- Systems to simplify enrollment and renewal processes improve enrollment and retention rates.

- Ongoing training for CAAs is critical to ensure that they are current on eligibility rules and to enable them to assist families with lesser-known or under-utilized programs.
- Reevaluation of strategies for reaching and enrolling families can identify additional places to engage clients and more effective ways to support them.
- Systems approaches to outreach and enrollment can yield larger and faster results than one-on-one outreach. DPSS helped to enroll children with limited-scope (Emergency) Medi-Cal into Healthy Kids.
- Collaboration with other community partners can leverage outreach and enrollment and efficiently reach more families and children.
- Data collection, regular analysis, and reporting are crucial for program oversight, trending, and program evaluation.

REFERENCES

1. Hill I, Benatar S. What are the implications of losing healthy kids. Urban Institute. October 2009. Available from: http://www.urban.org/url.cfm?ID=412164 (accessed June 20, 2012).
2. A trusted voice: Leveraging the local experience of community-based organization in implementing the Affordable Care Act. California Children's Health Initiatives, April 2011. Available from: http://cchi4families.org/pdf/uploads/Executive%20Summary_new050411.pdf (accessed June 20, 2012).
3. Cousineau M, Wada E, Farias A, Raffi E, Carr C. State budget cuts threaten efforts in Los Angeles County to link uninsured children with health care. USC, Center for Community Health Studies, Policy Brief. August 2007. Available from: http://www.calendow.org/uploadedFiles/Policy_Brief_Governors_2007_Veto_re_OERU%20dollars.pdf (accessed June 20, 2012).
4. CHOI data system, Los Angeles County Department of Public Health, data from 2011.
5. Evaluation of the Los Angeles County outreach, enrollment, utilization and retention project. USC, Center for Community Health Studies, September 2007.

35 Partnering with Families

A New Service Delivery Model for Pediatric Physical and Occupational Therapy

WESLEY L. FORD, DEBRA RUGE, NANCY CAPPEL, TESS JENS O'HERN, AND SIDNEY ROTH

THE NATURE OF THE PROBLEM

The Los Angeles County (LAC) California Children's Services (CCS) Medical Therapy Program (MTP) is the largest physical and occupational therapy program for children in California. The program serves a medically and economically diverse population of more than 5,200 children up to age 21 who are diagnosed with lifelong disabilities.

An audit by California's Children's Medical Services Branch, found that the LAC MTP program was seriously understaffed, and had three major programmatic deficiencies: 1) major inequity in services provided to patients; 2) unacceptable delays in patient evaluations; and 3) a large and growing wait-list. In reviewing the findings, it also became clear that services were more therapist- than family-centered and the program's outcomes were not well-defined.

MTP staff found itself in a "Catch-22," needing to resolve program deficiencies linked to staff shortage when additional staff could not be afforded.

CONTEXT

The MTP program is run by the LAC Department of Public Health Children's Medical Services program and provides therapy to children who meet CCS eligibility criteria. There are no financial criteria for a child with a CCS-eligible condition for MTP services. Licensed physical therapists (PT) and occupational therapists (OT) evaluate, treat, consult and coordinate care for children enrolled in the program.

Overall management of MTP patients is complex. Therapists provide hands-on treatment, but also assess the need for, recommend, and order customized durable medical equipment (DME); assess home and classroom environments; and participate in medical therapy conferences (MTC) and individualized education planning (IEP) meetings. All services come under the prescription of a supervising physician coordinated by therapists at 23 therapy units, co-located in schools that comprise LAC's MTP program.

Two-thirds of children served by the program have cerebral palsy, a disorder of movement and posture, many of whom also have mental retardation, visual, hearing, speech, and swallowing issues. Others have congenital, genetic, or hereditary diseases of a neurological or musculoskeletal nature. They exhibit muscle wasting, limited sensation and/or movement, muscle contractures, respiratory difficulty, poor balance, frequent falls, and difficulty walking.

The children live at home and attend school, most in special education classes. Their abilities vary according to the severity of their condition. Many rely on a wheelchair or other equipment and need help to participate in everyday activities.

Physical and occupational therapists provide routine, multifaceted evaluations of patients when they first enter therapy and continue to do so until they turn 21 or are discharged from the program. Evaluations include review of the child's medical and therapy history, school placement, home environment and parental concerns, as well as a battery of objective assessments.

Evaluation goals are to identify physical functions that fall outside the range of normal parameters (see Table 35-1). This information is used by a therapist to determine whether the identified deficits are best addressed via therapeutic intervention, augmentative equipment, or referral to outside resources. A customized therapy plan is developed to include functional and measurable goals to address the identified deficits. The normal expectation is for prescribed functional goals to be met within one year.

After coaching by a therapist, many activities should be practiced at home by the patient with the help of a caregiver. As with a typical child, patients in the MTP program must constantly practice their developmental skills to perfect them. However, children with physical limitations usually need help practicing these skills. Caregivers provide the optimal opportunities for children to practice skills such as walking, eating, dressing, and grooming.

TABLE 35-1 *Objective Measures used in MTP Physical and Occupational Therapy Evaluations*

Objective Measure	Used to Address
Neurological Findings and Motor Control	Muscle tone, reflexes, movement disorders, sensation, proprioception, balance, equilibrium, coordination, motor planning, and voluntary motor control Oral control (swallow, cough, lip closure, tongue movement), speech, visual field, and auditory acuity
Respiratory Status and Endurance	Breathing pattern, vital capacity, and functional endurance
Musculo-skeletal	Range of motion, strength, structural and postural abnormalities
Developmental and Functional Skills	Developmental age and level of assistance needed in the areas of gross and fine motor skills, e.g., rolling, sitting, walking, transferring, and hand use for activities of daily living
Communication	Ability to interact with others verbally and non-verbally, and level of assistance or type of technology needed
Social Function	Social interaction and safety awareness in the context of daily routines, household chores, and interactions with family, peers, and others
Self-Care	Feeding, dressing, hygiene, grooming, bathing, and toileting

■ APPROACH TO THE PROBLEM

A Service Delivery Committee was established to evaluate how the program's three major deficiencies could be addressed without additional resources or negative outcomes. The Committee reviewed all program policies, evaluated the program's practice standards, analyzed program data, and reviewed the relevant literature.

After their assessment, the Committee found that the program's existing policies and practice standards encouraged outdated beliefs that children with lifelong disabilities should receive intensive long-term clinical interventions. However, ethical practice, as defined in the Physical and Occupational Therapy Practice Acts, urge services to be discontinued when they no longer maintain or enhance function (1, 2).

Data analysis demonstrated the degree to which this outdated belief was ingrained into the program. When the program's two distinct patient service groups—patients receiving intensive (i.e., one to five times per week) therapy versus those receiving less frequent, periodic therapy—were compared, the total prescribed hours for each group was the same. But therapists spent 80% of their time on the 20% of the patients (n = 1059) receiving intensive therapy, and only 20% of their time on the other 80% (n = 4235).

Families viewed therapists as experts who should address all of the patients' needs, enhanced by the perception that therapists were the "dream keepers" who gave parents hope that their child might someday be cured. Such convictions fostered many parents' feelings of dependence and helplessness, placing therapists in positions of power, and encouraging parents to passively rely on them to make appointments, request medical records, and navigate a complex medical system.

Most services were therapist-driven and planned around the school environment, with little expectation of family participation at home. Patients attending schools with co-located medical therapy units (MTUs) came to therapy directly from their classrooms; others were bused to the MTUs from nearby schools. Younger patients came to the MTUs with caregivers, who were not typically invited to participate in therapy. These practices minimized opportunity for family interaction and communication.

Most important, desired program outcomes were not well-defined or evidence-based. Review of the literature found that family-centered care and evidence-based practice were on the rise as gold standards of care for new service models across the country.

The LAC MTP program clearly needed a more family-centered model, with clearly defined evidence-based outcomes adherent to the newest PT and OT Standards of Practice. A new model had to be flexible to accommodate large numbers of stakeholders who need to be part of child-care delivery.

Four key principles formed the framework for a new "MTP Partnership Model" (1, 2, 3, 5, 6, 7, 8).

Family commitment and participation: Patients achieve more rapid progress when therapists and families partner through the therapy process. This requires therapist guidance and hands-on participation by parents in therapy sessions. Patient and family involvement in goal determination leads to the most effective and efficient attainment of the goals needed for patients to live as independently as possible.

The right level of therapy at the right time: A unique aspect of the MTP is its flexibility to provide episodic intensive therapy or less frequent periodic sessions tailored to each patient's progress. This is critical as patients grow through the many life transitions from infancy to adulthood. Intensive therapy can be scheduled all at once, weekly, or broken into separate bursts of therapy at varying times during the prescription period.

Skilled therapy when needed, discontinued when not needed: Therapy services that require the professional expertise and judgment of a licensed therapist are not needed for the *practice* of activities; the licensed therapist is responsible for determining the most appropriate service setting and provider, whether caregivers, therapy assistants, aides, or classroom personnel.

Patients and families empowered to practice in their natural environment: Empowering patients and families to reinforce skills in the natural environment yields more effective development of functional skills than does a clinical environment alone. Partnering with patients and families helps to communicate needs and identify activities that foster success.

■ IMPLEMENTATION

The new Partnership Model called for a number of changes to the existing program. Previously, length of prescriptive therapy for each patient was recommended by the patients' therapist. Now each patient is assigned to one of two patient service groups. Those determined to need services once per month or less were thought rarely to need more intensive therapy in later life stages. A new policy aligned available therapist hours with prescribed therapy hours. Therapists were now required to allocate time in proportion to the time prescribed to each of their patients, according to patients' current needs.

Documentation time lines were also tightened and strictly enforced. Previously, therapists had a month after evaluation of a child to complete written reports, which were now to be completed immediately after an evaluation. Paperwork thus was completed within 24 hours; therapy prescriptions were quickly approved and signed by the physician. This not only eliminated the long delays for children to receive care, but also improved the accuracy and thoroughness of reported documentation.

These two actions alone permitted therapists to better manage their caseloads, allowing the Committee to focus on issues of cancellation and no-show rates. Program staff were instructed to strictly enforce the patient and family attendance policy, not previously routinely enforced. Therapists thus could better manage their time and maximize therapy sessions.

The result of these system changes was a noticeable decrease in the number of children on the wait list, and a noticeable increase in the quality and frequency of services provided, more closely meeting the needs of the child. The next critical step was to redefine the roles of the therapist, patient, and family in goal setting and achieving desired outcomes. The literature strongly supported the notion that family participation was key to reaching patient goals and maintaining their functional skills (3, 4, 9, 10, 11, 12, 13). A family-centered approach creates strong partnerships with the therapist, and empowers patients and families to play important roles in their own health care.

The transformation from a therapist-driven culture to a partnership approach required a significant paradigm shift for both parties. Family participation was critical. Therapists alone no longer dictated the course of therapy. Instead. they were expected to collaborate. The therapist's role became more that of a coach than sole service provider, with the family having an active role in goal setting, planning, and parameters of treatment. Consequently, it also became necessary to implement accountability standards to consider family needs and goals.

At first, the Partnership Model met resistance all around. Ongoing training was provided to all internal stakeholders, such as supervisory and support staff, therapists, and all MTC physicians. Supervisors and senior therapists got leadership training on managing change, motivating staff, team building, effective communication, and conflict resolution. Therapists were trained on coaching and educating patients and families, effective communication, interviewing techniques, collaborative goal setting, providing effective home programs, and determining need for more skilled intervention. Support personnel were trained to use scheduling software to ensure family compliance with appointments through respectful but assertive communication. After receiving training, all employees were expected to apply what they learned.

The MTP Policy was updated to define clearly what families could expect and what the program expected from them: for example, attendance, participation, and responsibility for obtaining the medical records and prescriptions necessary for continued therapy services. Family schedules were taken into account when scheduling treatment sessions to improve compliance. Some cases were closed for non-compliance.

Many families were extremely motivated, but they too faced challenges. They needed training to perform therapeutic activities in their homes and communities. Therapists had to guide them through the process. Although it was stressful for some parents to learn these skills, both parents and patients benefited (3).

Materials were developed and distributed with uniform messaging. The *Family's Guide to Therapy* brochure, created with parental input, explains the Partnership Model and its therapy services, what to expect of an evaluation, and the roles and responsibilities of both therapist and family in a child's care. A *Personalized Therapy Worksheet* was developed as a tool for families to use in therapy evaluations to address the needs of their child and to aid family participation in goal setting. *Guidelines for Determining the Frequency of Therapy Services* explained when and why the different levels of services are recommended.

The model was introduced slowly, to new patients when they enrolled and to existing patients when reevaluated. The traditional way of providing services was very engrained, and the new system represented a significant paradigm shift, so we had to enforce compliance to the new system. Without enforced compliance there was too much risk of participants regressing to the familiar.

As staff implementation problems were resolved, the program moved toward full realization of the model. It then was necessary to educate the external stakeholders, for example, special education administrators, regional centers for developmental delays, medical facilities, and advocacy groups for children with special health care needs. All were educated about the major programmatic changes under way and how patients and families in their settings might be impacted. Their input was solicited.

Many were embarking on parallel changes in their own programs. A few misconceptions existed about the Partnership Model; by meeting with external stakeholders, we clarified them and alleviated concerns.

School personnel worried that the MTP Partnership Model would reduce needed services for which they would become responsible. School and regional center case workers were interested in the literature review and in improving parental involvement and accountability (see Table 35–2). Both agencies expressed concern over feasibility of parental involvement for all families and too rigid enforcement. The therapist's ethical and professional responsibility to provide therapy when needed (and to

TABLE 35-2 *Summary of Literature Review and Benefits of Including Families as Partners*

Professional paradigm shift from therapists as *experts* to parents as partners (9, 10).
Current practice focuses on motor learning in *functionally based* interventions (11).
Family participation and follow through is meaningful to the family and leads to better outcomes (4, 12).
If families don't perceive home programs as beneficial they will not follow through (3).
Mothers participated in *self-selected activities* if they were doable and could be integrated into daily routines and done in context of other home activities. Activities had to be enjoyable for the child and not stressful for mother or family (13).
Parent instruction is more stressful but is more beneficial to patients and parents in the long run (3).
Patients need less frequent visits to accomplish their goals with parent instruction and coaching by the therapist (3).
Being emotionally supportive, showing the parents that the therapist genuinely cares for the child and having an acceptable level of expertise fosters trust and partnership (9).

discontinue it when it was not needed) was discussed in detail. It was explained that family involvement could come from parents, adult siblings, or any other adult regularly present in the patient's life. The literature that showed outcomes improved with family participation, and as patients matured they were increasingly able to direct and practice their own therapy.

There was a misperception that the model was implemented to reduce the number of therapists to save money, which was not the case. A by-product of more frequent patient contact was the detection of equipment problems, allowing repairs rather than replacement. Patients with yearly therapy plans now were required to see their physician once a year as opposed to every six months, reducing clinic reimbursement costs. But financial benefits were secondary to the main goal of addressing the programmatic deficiencies identified in the audit without additional resources.

EVALUATION AND IMPACT

Many therapists were initially skeptical of the Partnership Model. They felt that the needs of patients on an intensive schedule were more important than those of the underserved, periodic patients who comprised the majority of their caseload. A key challenge was the need to change this mind-set.

As therapists began practicing the Partnership Model, they found they could provide required services and complete timely documentation for all patients. They discovered that underserved patients, many adolescents and young adults, had important needs not previously considered. Awareness grew that the needs of this group were significantly different from those of young children, especially when they transitioned into new life phases, such as going to high school, planning for college, and preparing to live independently.

Slowly, momentum began to shift toward total acceptance of the model. Supervisors reported more manageable caseloads. Families more actively participated in therapy sessions; adolescents and young adults began to receive the therapy they needed. Ongoing feedback revealed that the process was becoming mostly self-driven. Therapists realized that they had been clinging to an outdated pediatric rehabilitation culture. They found that patients and their families were fully capable of practicing therapy activities with ongoing coaching and therapist follow-up. When families were empowered and accountable, they had a better understanding of their child's diagnosis and equipment needs, expected developmental goals, and how to navigate the medical system. By redesigning the database as a scheduling tool, clerks could objectively prioritize scheduling needs. Patients with the most pressing needs were scheduled first. Starting each month, unit schedulers listed *all* patients due to be seen that month and fit them in according to their service codes. Patients who had received extensive weekly therapy were reassessed to see if less frequent skilled interventions were appropriate. This allowed therapists more time to see other children.

The outcomes from these changes were positive and encouraging; services were being more equitably distributed, evaluations were completed in a timely way, family participation increased, and the wait list decreased by 90% (see Figure 35–1).

Figure 35–2 shows that for many patients, traditional therapy sessions twice a year remained appropriate. Others needed more frequent traditional interventions, and after the new system was implemented, therapists could customize services to match a child's individual needs. For example, the adolescent and young adult population came to the therapy units more frequently than before to focus on the development of community skills and the ability to socialize.

Under the old system, only 22% of patients received therapy more than two times a year. Under the Partnership Model, 51% of patients are seen four times a year or more. The bars represent frequency of occupational and physical therapy prescriptions. Some called for therapeutic sessions only twice per year, while others required more frequent sessions. Almost all patients received more than one prescription per year, one each for physical and for occupational therapy.

To determine the Partnership Model's impact on patient's functional outcomes, the Functional Improvement Score (FISC) measured the amount of change a child achieved in a 6–12 month period. The FISC identified current functional ability using standardized measures. Items are scored on the level of independence demonstrated by the child, in three skill categories: general mobility, transfer, and activities of daily living. These represent most MTP therapy goals. The inventoried abilities were different for the physical and occupational therapy outcomes. Both versions are statistically reliable.

Preliminary results showed that the FISC average did not change when the program shifted to the Partnership Model (see Figure 35–3). Patient functions remained

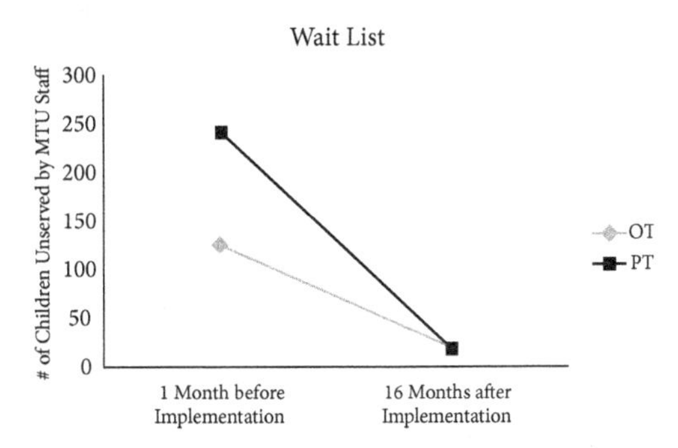

Figure 35–1 Wait List.

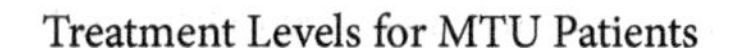

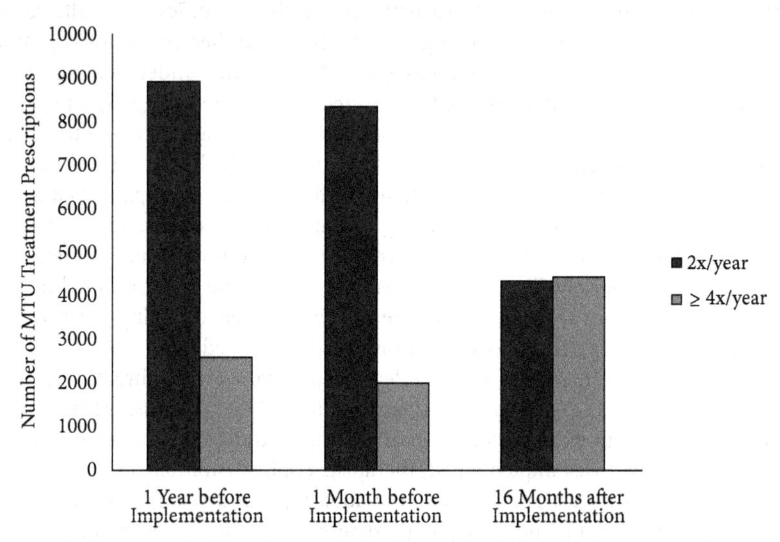

Figure 35–2 Frequency of Services.

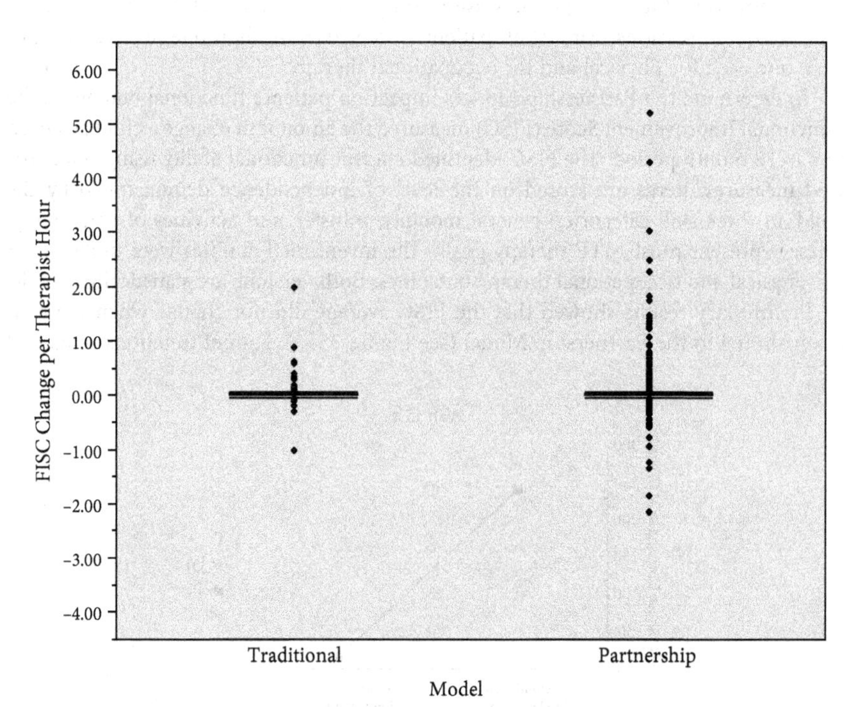

Figure 35–3 FISC Change for Individual Patients under the Traditional Therapy Model and the Partnership Model.

constant (p = .89), despite a decrease in direct therapy intervention. An increase in FISC variability (p<.001) was also observed. Many factors may have contributed to this, among them, the follow-through at home (or lack thereof), the ability of therapists to teach and coach families, and the ability of families to learn. Most patients receiving increased services were adolescents and young adults. The FISC could not adequately measure their change in function in the social and community domains.

To further evaluate the Partnership Model as it continues to evolve, the Canadian Occupational Performance Measure (COPM) and the Measure of Processes of Care (MPOC) are being used. These two tools were developed by the CanChild Centre for Childhood Disability Research, McMaster University, Canada (14, 15). The COPM is used to enhance collaboration between therapists and families via a semi-structured interview process designed to help patients and families identify and measure activities and goals that are important to them and their satisfaction with the performance of these activities. The MPOC is a two-part instrument—one for service providers and the other for families—used to measure provider and family perception of the Partnership Model's family centeredness. Results for these measures are pending.

■ CONCLUSION AND LESSONS LEARNED

By using the Partnership Model of service delivery developed for use in the MTP, we have:

- Provided equitable services to all patients based on individual needs;
- Incorporated family participation and values to optimize outcomes;
- Reframed our approach to pediatric rehabilitation in line with current literature;
- Found that with increased parent participation and more opportunities to practice in their natural environment, many patients can attain and maintain functional skills with less frequent formal therapy sessions;
- Discovered that many patients who previously received only semi-annual therapy later in life needed short-term intensive therapy as they transitioned through different life stages;
- Realized that empowered and accountable parents and caregivers are great partners with therapists and can do many things at home to augment therapy programs;
- Learned that this system must continue to be dynamic and evolve as new evidence arises.

■ REFERENCES

1. Bailes A, Reder R, Burch C. Development of guidelines for determining frequency of therapy services in a pediatric medical setting. *Pediatric Phys Ther.* 2008;20:194–198.
2. Guide to physical therapist practice. 2nd ed. *Phys Ther.* 2001;81:9–744.
3. Scales LH, McEwen IR, Murray C. Parents' perceived benefits of physical therapists' direct interventions compared with parental instruction in early intervention. *Pediatric Phys Ther.* 2007;19:196–202.
4. Novack I, Cusick A, Lannin N. Occupational therapy home programs for cerebral palsy: double-blind, randomized, controlled trial. *Pediatrics.* 2009;124:e606–14.

5. Campbell SK. Therapy programs for children that last a lifetime. *Phys Occup Ther Pediatrics.* 1997;17(1):1–15.
6. King S, Teplicky R, King G, Rosenbaum P. Family centered service for children with cerebral palsy and their families: A review of the literature. *Seminars in Ped Neurol.* 2004;11:78–86.
7. Palisano J, Murr S. Intensity of therapy services: what are the considerations? *Phys Occup Ther Pediatrics.* 2009;29(2):107–12.
8. Sumsion T. Pursuing the client's goals really paid off. *Brit J Occup Ther.* 2004;67(1):2–9.
9. Harrison C, Romer T, Simon MC, Schulze C. Factors influencing mothers' learning from paediatric therapists: a qualitative study. *Phys Occup Ther in Pediatrics.* 2007;27(2):77–95.
10. Piggot J, Paterson J, Hocking C. Participation in home therapy programs for children with cerebral palsy: A compelling challenge. *Qualit Health Res.* 2002;12(6):1112–29.
11. Levac D, Wishart L, Missiuna C, Wright V. The application of motor learning strategies within functionally based interventions for children with neuromotor conditions. *Pediatric Phys Ther.* 2009;21:345–55.
12. Valvano J, Rapport MJ. Activity-focused motor interventions for infants and young children with neurological conditions. *Infant Young Child.* 2006;19(4):292–307.
13. Hinojosa J, Anderson J. Mother's perceptions of home treatment programs for their preschool children with cerebral palsy. *Am J Occup Ther.* 1991;45(3):273–9.
14. Law M, Baptiste S, Carswell A, McColl MA, Polatajko H, Pollock N. Canadian Occupational Performance Measure©; Can Child Centre for Childhood Disability Research, McMaster University. Available from: http://www.canhild.ca/en/measures/copm.asp (accessed Aug. 9, 2011).
15. Woodside J, Rosenbaum P, King S, King G. Measure of Processes of Care©; Can Child Centre for Childhood Disability Research, McMaster University. Available from: http://www.canchild.ca/en/measures/mpoc20.asp (accessed Aug. 9, 2011).

36 Reducing Cases of HIV

Implementation of Post-Exposure Prophylaxis

JENNIFER N. SAYLES,
MARIO J. PÉREZ, GARY P. GARCÍA,
AND RAPHAEL J. LANDOVITZ

THE NATURE OF THE PROBLEM

A 26-year-old man presents to an outpatient clinic, reporting that 36 hours earlier he had receptive anal intercourse with no condom with a new male partner, who he just learned from a mutual acquaintance is infected with the human immunodeficiency virus (HIV). The patient has had several earlier negative HIV tests (the last, 6 months ago), and recently lost his job and health insurance. He asks if anything can be done to prevent HIV transmission from his recent exposure.

In 2010, an estimated 62,800 persons were living with HIV/AIDS in Los Angeles County (LAC). An estimated 2,000 new infections occur annually. Rates of new HIV infections nationally and locally show no decline since the early 1990s, despite intensive public health and community-based prevention efforts. Biomedical interventions to reduce HIV transmission are key to HIV prevention, particularly when combined with HIV and other sexually transmitted disease (STD) screening, risk-reduction efforts, and education for those at highest risk of infection. A 28-day course of antiretroviral therapy to prevent HIV infection, called HIV post-exposure prophylaxis (PEP), in observational studies reduces HIV transmission up to 81% when taken within 72 hours after exposure (1). While PEP for occupational HIV exposures is widely adopted in medical and occupational health settings, PEP to prevent HIV infection from sexual or injection drug exposure is difficult to access, and is underutilized by medical providers. Despite federal Centers for Disease Control and Prevention (CDC) and California Office of AIDS guidelines recommending the use of non-occupational post-exposure prophylaxis (nPEP) within 72 hours of a high-risk exposure to HIV, only a few U.S. jurisdictions receive public financing for identifiable coordinated programming to deliver nPEP services. When this patient presented in 2009 to an LAC clinic with no insurance, no programming existed to deliver a comprehensive nPEP HIV prevention intervention with risk screening and counseling, HIV and STD testing, clinical monitoring, and referral to related services.

CONTEXT

In 2006, recognition grew among LAC medical providers, public health officials, community advocates, and academics of the need for local comprehensive biomedical HIV prevention services. A gap existed for nPEP in many communities that had both high rates of HIV infection and under- and un-insurance. In several cases when nPEP was indicated and not available, public health leaders were sought out for assistance in addressing this need. The many challenges at the time to accessing nPEP in LAC are outlined below.

While state and national nPEP guidelines have been in place for many years, they are based on expert opinion but no rigorously conducted studies of efficacy. A 1997 case control study demonstrated that those who received the antiretroviral drug zidovudine after needlestick exposure were 81% less likely to have an HIV seroconversion. Despite the methodological limitations of this study (retrospective design, small sample, no uniform PEP protocol), these findings made a placebo-controlled study unethical, and a randomized comparative trial of various strategies (2 antiretrovirals vs. 3) economically infeasible to conduct, given low per-exposure seroconversion rates. Thus the evidence base for nPEP as a public health intervention with regard to efficacy remains modest. Additionally, observational data have been of limited use to bolster efficacy data (2).

To date, other than zidovudine to prevent perinatal HIV transmission, no antiretroviral agent has been approved by the Food and Drug Administration (FDA) to prevent HIV. This is likely due to the limited availability of PEP efficacy data and/or the low return on investment for pharmaceutical companies to seek this indication, given the limited additional market share that would be gained from nPEP use. The result is that use of antiretroviral therapy (ART) as PEP is considered an off-label use and subject to denied coverage by insurers, a potential barrier to access.

Both the literature and LAC Department of Public Health (DPH) experience suggest that the individuals at highest risk for HIV who would benefit from nPEP often are not aware of it or its benefits. A cross-sectional survey in California of gay and bisexual men found awareness and use of nPEP was modest (47%) (3). Similar findings from New York City report low knowledge of nPEP (36%) among men who have sex with men (MSM) (4).

In spite of widespread knowledge of PEP as an intervention after an occupational HIV exposure, many LAC providers are less familiar with nPEP as an HIV prevention intervention for patients with sexual or injection drug use exposure. A recent LAC survey found only 3% of primary care providers would provide nPEP (5). In the United States, HIV specialists almost always prescribe and manage ART, and occupational health professionals administer PEP in the setting of occupational HIV exposure, following established protocols. Thus many primary care providers may be unprepared to prescribe ART or to manage antiretroviral therapy–related complications that arise in the context of providing nPEP.

Finally, nPEP is time-sensitive. It is most effective when given as soon as possible after exposure, and always within 72 hours, creating additional access challenges. Both at-risk individuals and medical providers need to be aware of nPEP as an HIV prevention intervention, as well as the effective screening, triage, and provider flexibility needed to deliver it.

■ APPROACH TO THE PROBLEM

The LAC DPH's Office of AIDS Programs and Policy (OAPP), in collaboration with sister public health programs and key stakeholders, implemented an nPEP pilot program that serves the highest risk individuals and provides a comprehensive approach to HIV, STD, and viral hepatitis prevention. The conceptual framework guiding its development is "Highly Active HIV Prevention" (6), incorporating behavioral, biomedical, public health, and structural interventions for impact on the HIV epidemic

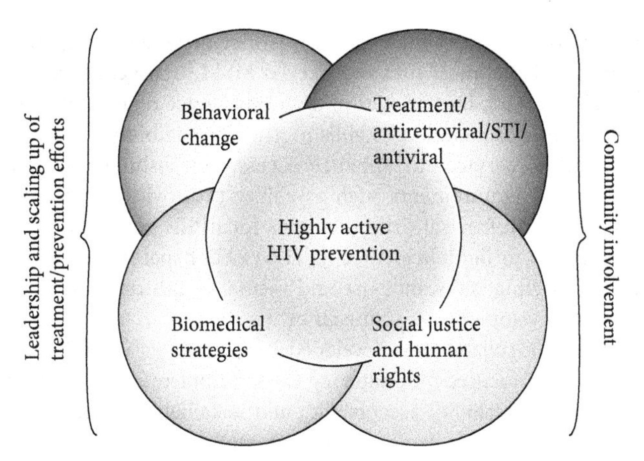

Figure 36-1 Highly Active HIV Prevention.
Adapted from Coates, Lancet 2008.

(see Figure 36-1). The longer term vision for a comprehensive nPEP program is to use it as an anchor for implementation of other emerging biomedical interventions. This would include delivering multifaceted combination HIV prevention approaches, such as integrated STD screening, behavioral, biomedical, mental health, and substance use interventions. Key components of the implementation plan were to engage key stakeholders in nPEP Workgroups, identify resources, define pilot program components and program evaluation, and build education/capacity as outlined below.

An nPEP Workgroup was formed to serve as an advisory committee to OAPP and to inform a countywide nPEP delivery model. The nPEP Workgroup drew a diverse set of stakeholders, including local HIV and primary care providers, academic HIV prevention experts, substance use and mental health providers, community members, and public health practitioners. They collaborated with OAPP to: 1) identify an overall model for nPEP in LAC; 2) outline pilot program components to be evaluated for feasibility, acceptability, and sustainability of nPEP services; and 3) select sites for the nPEP pilot program. This multidisciplinary workgroup proved critical to broad engagement and support for establishing an integrated biomedical and behavioral HIV prevention program.

Identifying resources to support a pilot program was particularly critical in planning. The goal was to develop a partnership financing model, whereby stakeholders and partners contributed direct funding, in kind services, medications, or testing. OAPP, with DPH endorsement, devoted resources for core delivery operations of the nPEP pilot and to evaluate its implementation. The OAPP investment was made from LAC general funds as contractual limitations prohibited use of existing federal funds. Medical providers at pilot sites provided in-kind staff time and resources to start the program, and community partners provided in-kind targeted outreach and education about nPEP. Academic partners provided technical expertise with protocol development, worked with DPH to train providers, and collaborated on program evaluation. Four pharmaceutical partners donated 300 courses of nPEP medications for the pilot, after which OAPP was responsible for establishing an ART procurement process.

A key step in planning for new evidence-based public health programming is defining and identifying the target populations for the intervention and experienced providers who know these populations. LAC's epidemic is concentrated in MSM and transgender communities, and several distinct geographic regions. Therefore, the nPEP pilot included clinical sites that served MSM, transgender individuals, and women at sexual risk, each located within high prevalence regions of LAC.

Program components included establishing nPEP eligibility criteria, identifying optimal placement of services to enhance access, establishing provider qualifications and operational requirements such as ability to provide services six days per week, determining antiretroviral drug regimens for nPEP, and defining the package of preventive services to be delivered (e.g., HIV/STD/hepatitis testing, vaccination, risk reduction counseling, substance use and mental health referral). An LAC nPEP protocol was then developed to describe all of the above.

OAPP and academic collaborators developed an evaluation plan, and vetted it with the nPEP Workgroup. This focused on evaluating the key implementation steps of an nPEP program, as well as the feasibility, acceptability, and sustainability of the intervention.

To support successful pilot program implementation, OAPP also developed education and capacity-building activities. This included orientation to the nPEP program protocol with providers at the selected nPEP sites, enabling them to deliver high-quality biomedical HIV prevention interventions. Outreach plans also were developed for medical and non-medical providers who serve high-risk individuals to increase awareness about nPEP as an intervention, and to assure that they could access the nPEP pilot program. A plan was synthesized to increase awareness of the nPEP pilot for individuals at risk, including a pamphlet about the service, a PEP "warmline" to provide non-urgent information and to direct patients to service sites through a phone tree, and targeted community presentations.

■ IMPLEMENTATION OF SOLUTIONS

The nPEP Workgroup proposed a "hub and spoke" model for implementing and delivering nPEP services (see Figure 36–2). Similar models have been implemented in Brazil and Amsterdam (7, 8). The model's core "hubs" would provide comprehensive biomedical prevention services. The "spokes" would be screening and referral sites, where individuals eligible for nPEP may be identified and evaluated, and given the first dose of nPEP on-site plus a three-day supply (enough to cover a weekend), and then referred back to the "hubs" for further evaluation to receive comprehensive HIV prevention programming and the remaining nPEP course. "Spoke" sites would include local community clinics, emergency departments, urgent care settings, substance use treatment sites with clinical care, and others. The workgroup's vision was that once "hubs" were implemented in the pilot project, attention would focus on establishing a larger network of "spokes." The goal was to increase access to sites capable of delivering nPEP in a time-sensitive way, relying on the "hubs" to deliver the integrated HIV prevention services.

The pilot program constructed two "hub" sites; "spoke" sites were not constructed as part of the initial pilot program. The "hubs" were outpatient clinics in LAC's highest HIV burden areas. One is a sexual health program serving a predominantly MSM and transgender populations; the second is an HIV clinic serving predominantly communities of color. Implementation of the sites was staggered to maximize attention to start up and technical assistance.

A program protocol helped to implement and assure fidelity to the agreed-upon program components. These included standardized eligibility criteria across sites consistent with CDC and California Office of AIDS guidelines (see Box 36–1). The

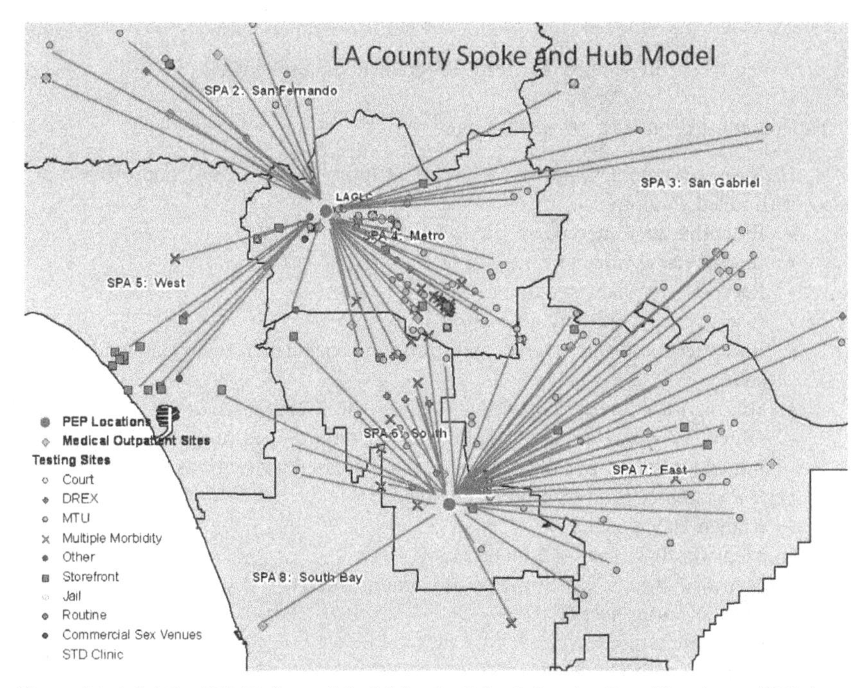

Figure 36–2 LAC nPEP Delivery Model for 7 of the 8 Service Provider Areas (SPAs) for LAC.
The "hubs" represent the two sites offering comprehensive nPEP services. The "spokes" leading toward the hubs represent pathways of referral for nPEP services from multiple entry points within the system of care, including publicly funded HIV prevention, testing, and medical care sites.

protocol standardized program components and assessments, such as intake procedures, ART regimens, laboratory monitoring, HIV, STD, and viral hepatitis screening, risk reduction counseling, follow-up visit procedures, and referral processes (see Box 36–2). Additional steps included intensive staff training for the pilot program, establishing a triage process and optimal clinical flow for nPEP patients needing a time-sensitive service, implementation of point-of-care rapid HIV testing as well as STD and hepatitis screening, coordination of stored samples for HIV nucleic acid amplification and resistance testing in case of seroconversion, and staff training to respond to PEP "warmline" calls.

Pamphlets for patients describing nPEP and the pilot program were disseminated to local providers, STD clinics, and at the PEP sites themselves. Community presentations by OAPP and academic project leaders reinforced these efforts.

Challenges to Implementation

Initially, 100 courses of antiretroviral agents were donated for nPEP and brisk enrollment and uptake of the intervention prompted donation of 200 more courses from pharmaceutical companies. All drugs were donated on condition that they be stored and dispensed under an FDA Investigational New Drug (IND) application (since

BOX 36–1 ■ nPEP Program Eligibility Criteria

Patients must be at least 18 years of age.

- *High-Risk Exposure Characteristic* (one or more of the below, unprotected or with failed condom use)
    - Receptive anal intercourse (RAI)
    - Insertive anal intercourse (IAI)
    - Receptive vaginal intercourse (RVI)
    - Insertive vaginal intercourse (IVA)
    - Receptive oral intercourse with intraoral ejaculation with known HIV+ source
    - Sharing injection drug works, which have been intravascular
    - Other exposures not listed above should be screened and eligibility determined by the on-site medical director on a case-by-case basis
- *High-Risk Source* (one or more of the below)
    - Known HIV positive
    - Men who have sex with men (MSM)
    - Men who have sex with men and women (MSMW)
    - Injection drug user (IDU)
    - Commercial sex worker
    - Sexual assault perpetrator
    - History of incarceration
    - From an endemic country (prevalence >1%)
    - Partner of one of the above
- *Exposure within 72 hours of presentation*
- *Not known to be HIV positive*
- *No countermanding concomitant medications or allergies*

nPEP is not an FDA-approved indication for antiretrovirals). Thus, additional regulatory and reporting procedures were required, including Institutional Review Board (IRB) approval, separate storage and dispensing of "research drug supply" from the pharmacy, and extensive reporting requirements for adverse events, among others. The subsequent additional workload on site staff was burdensome and substantially increased the time and resources needed to deliver nPEP services to patients.

OAPP reviewed program pilot data, determining that the program met implementation goals and addressed the need for a comprehensive biomedical HIV prevention intervention. When the supply of donated antiretrovirals was near depletion, OAPP began to finance the direct purchase of drugs used for the nPEP program, which decreased ART reporting and regulatory requirements. The drug purchase significantly increased the cost for the program: even when purchased at discounted safety net provider rates, a three-drug regimen costs twice that of a two-drug regimen. To date, no data show that a three-drug nPEP regimen is more effective than a two-drug regimen in preventing HIV transmission. Thus, OAPP, in consultation with the sites, offered a two-drug regimen once the donated supply of drugs had been exhausted. The unique circumstance of documented exposure to resistant virus allows the provision

BOX 36-2 ■ Schedule of Clinical and Lab Evaluations and Other Assessments

	Intake Visit	Week 2 Telephone Encounter	Week 4–6 Visit	Week 12 Visit	Week 24 Visit
Risk Assessment					
Sex, Drugs and Alcohol	X		X	X	X
HIV Diagnostic					
HIV ELISA[c]	X		X	X	X
HIV RNA to r/o AHI	X				
Stored HIV RNA and Genotype[d]			X	X	X
STD Diagnostic					
Urine/vaginal GC/CT	X				
Rectal GC/CT	X				
Pharynx GC	X				
Serum RPR	X			X	
Urine HCG[a]	X		X[b]	X[b]	
HBsAg	X				
HCV Antibody	X			X	
Safety Lab Diagnostic					
Cr, LFTs, CBC	X	X[b]	X[b]	X[b]	X[b]
Interventions					
Meds Dispensed	X				
Adherence Counseling	X	X			
Risk-Reduction Counseling (brief)	X	X	X	X	X
Referral to Services: (Intensive Risk-Reduction, Substance Abuse, Mental Health)—as needed	X[b]	X[b]	X[b]	X[b]	X[b]
HIV/STI Partner Services—as needed	X		X	X	X
Hepatitis A and B Vaccination (if indicated)	X		X	X	X

[a] Females of childbearing potential only
[b] If clinical and/or behavioral signs and symptoms direct, not routine
[c] Positive or indeterminate rapid HIV ELISA testing will be confirmed with a serum Western Blot
[d] Specimens will be drawn and stored at the indicated time points. If HIV seroconversion occurs, these samples will be run for HIV RNA (viral load) and genotyping.

of a third agent. It is notable that no instances of this type of exposure arose among the PEP participants treated in the pilot program. With the decision to use two-drug PEP, baseline HIV nucleic acid amplification testing was included in program baseline laboratory analyses, to identify patients seroconverting when starting PEP, who otherwise would be undetected by conventional HIV antibody testing. During the nPEP pilot, data emerged from a multinational randomized controlled trial of HIV pre-exposure prophylaxis (PrEP), demonstrating that exposure to a two-drug regimen in the case of acute seroconversion resulted in viral resistance within four weeks (9). A new CDC grant received by OAPP to enhance HIV prevention planning and programming became a resource for continuing nPEP locally, with PEP medications allowable expenses under this grant.

A consistent challenge throughout the program was developing a communication and outreach strategy for a pilot HIV prevention program that serves only those at highest risk of acquiring HIV *and* with an exposure in the past 72 hours. While it was imperative to make targeted individuals and providers aware of the service, it was also important not to overwhelm a new pilot program with a broad communication strategy that could result in a large number of low-risk individuals inquiring about services for which they were ineligible. Thus, a targeted communications and outreach approach was taken from the start. Despite a modest communication strategy, program enrollment was brisk (approximately 15 per month), and most referrals came through social networks and word of mouth. At the program's start, local providers were referring a number of patients who lacked high-risk exposures to the program, some of whom had been started on nPEP. After intensive community provider education about the program eligibility criteria, these referrals dramatically decreased.

Variations in demand and uptake for services between sites were another challenge. One site had much greater enrollment throughout the program, explained in part by more robust social networks and a densely concentrated urban community facilitating increased awareness of the program. The second site was located in a much larger and more demographically diverse catchment area. The limited enrollment may have been due to lower levels of awareness of the service, lower perceived need for the service, or the different social networks and community structures in the area. Additionally, the clinical site delivering nPEP services was a well-known HIV specialty clinic, and qualitative feedback from patients and providers suggested that the stigma of HIV may have deterred individuals from accessing services at this site.

■ EVALUATION STRATEGY

The evaluation strategy was to assess the implementation of a comprehensive nPEP program, not the efficacy of nPEP in reducing HIV transmission. Thus, the nPEP pilot had a structured pre-post quantitative evaluation of the implementation process and outcome measures. The measures included accrual of eligible participants and their completion of program visits, completion rates of the nPEP regimen for the first 100 patients, and the successful transition to a stable and sustainable intervention and drug supply for the program. Figure 36–3 describes the evaluation framework.

Evaluation data came from case reports completed at each visit and from laboratory results. Each patient was evaluated at visits at baseline intake, 2 weeks, 4 weeks, 12 weeks, and 24 weeks. The latter three visits followed completion of the 28-day

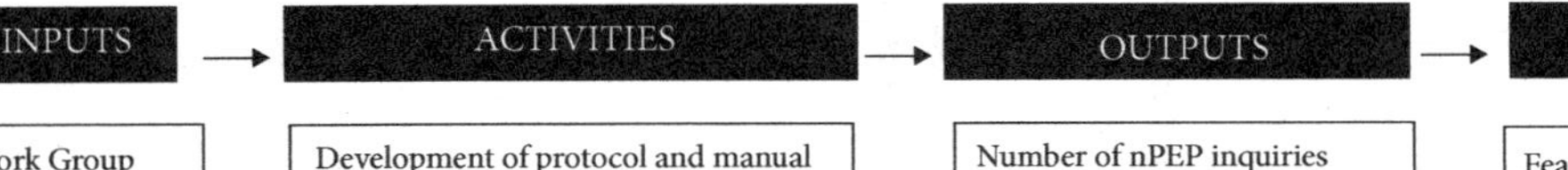

Figure 36–3 Logic Model for the nPEP Project Evaluation.

nPEP course with repeated HIV and STD screenings, risk assessment and counseling, and referral. Key process and outcome measures included program enrollment, time from exposure to receiving nPEP, adherence to nPEP medications, adverse events and toxicities experienced while on nPEP, program completion and retention rates, re-enrollments to nPEP after new exposure ("re-PEP"), HIV risk behavior, substance use, STI infections, and HIV seroconversions. While the pilot program did enroll patients already initiated on PEP from other resources, we were unable to assess how many individuals may have been given starter packs at other clinical sites and referred to the program, but failed to follow up at the nPEP clinical sites for the remainder of the nPEP course.

Two hundred and twenty-six participants met eligibility criteria and enrolled in the first 12 months (283 enrolled during the entire pilot program conduct period); program completion rates approximated 90%. The average time from exposure to receipt of nPEP services was 36.2 hours (range 2.0–71.7 hrs). Analysis of the first 100 patients revealed only two documented serious adverse events, both related to patients double dosing their medications, neither of whom discontinued the nPEP regimen. Mean self-reported adherence rates for nPEP was 98% at 2-week and 96% at 4- to 6-week follow-up. Though it has been well established that self-reported adherence often overestimates actual adherence, this was the best measure available at the time, and electronic drug monitoring (EDM) and/or drug levels were not economically or practically feasible for the pilot program. The mean number of participants' sexual partners in the 30 days before enrollment was 3.1. STD screening at baseline revealed that 12% of patients had *Neisseria gonorrhoeae* (5% pharyngeal, 5% rectal, 4% urethral), 7% had *Chlamydia trachomatis* (4% rectal, 3% urethral), and 3% had primary or secondary syphilis.

Two documented HIV seroconversions occurred among the first 100 patients enrolled, comparable to the 1–2% seroconversion rates reported in the few published nPEP studies in other jurisdictions. We do not know what the seroconversion rate would be in the absence of nPEP in this particular high-risk population. A local estimate of HIV incidence among MSM overall in LAC in 2007 has ranged from 0.7–1%. However, the MSM enrolled in the nPEP program report substantially more risk behavior than the general MSM population. The National HIV Behavioral Surveillance (NHBS) study conducted in LAC demonstrated that MSM sampled reported an average of 3.5 partners in 12 months, similar to the number reported in the past 30 days by nPEP patients. The available data suggests that MSM enrolled in nPEP are at higher risk for seroconversion compared to the general MSM population, and perhaps would have higher seroconversion rates in the absence of the nPEP intervention. However, conclusive evidence of this is not available, nor, as noted above, is proven efficacy of nPEP to reduce seroconversions in prospective trials.

In sum, the evaluation showed nPEP program implementation success, as measured by several process and outcome measures. While we lack a direct estimate of the number of individuals eligible at a given time for nPEP, data from the NHBS study sample from LAC can help to estimate those at risk in the MSM subpopulation who may need access to the service. NHBS data demonstrate that 1.3% of the MSM population reports being exposed to HIV in the past 12 months through unprotected sex with an HIV-positive individual. The MSM population in LAC is approximately 320,000. This suggests that some 4,000 MSM could need nPEP each year. However, it remains unclear what proportion of these at-risk individuals would be 1) aware of nPEP services, and 2) seeking nPEP services within 72 hours of an exposure in order to be eligible. Nonetheless, these estimates suggest that current nPEP services address only a fraction of the problem. A robust nPEP delivery model for LAC is needed to reach all the individuals eligible for nPEP.

IMPACT

The nPEP pilot program addresses a well-established need in HIV prevention services in LAC. It serves as a successful integrated, comprehensive platform for biomedical HIV prevention. It delivers nPEP packaged with screening and delivery of evidence-based interventions to address not only HIV, but also STDs, viral hepatitis, and substance use in a very high risk population. Critical factors for success of this program include continued engagement of key stakeholders in both development and implementation of the program, support from DPH leadership, increased awareness of the intervention and its goals among medical providers and communities at risk, and dedication of clinical site staff to a comprehensive biomedical HIV prevention program that includes risk reduction counseling and aligns with their mission and their patients' needs. The program continues, and is being scaled up to serve some 400 patients per year at the two sites. Patients entered the nPEP program with an average of 3.1 partners in the last month, and analysis revealed that at the 4- to 6-week visit, patient reports averaged 0.7 partners. This suggests that during the time that patients received the comprehensive nPEP intervention, risky behavior declined. However, a rigorous risk analysis across the longitudinal time points assessed in the program is in progress, and will help to clarify short- to medium-term changes in risk behavior among those receiving the intervention.

The pilot program provided several lessons:

- Community, provider, public health department, and academic partnerships are critical to successful development and implementation of innovative public health programming;
- Models of "highly active HIV prevention" that integrate biomedical, behavioral, public health, and structural interventions are an important approach to the HIV epidemic and move prevention programming forward;
- Starting a comprehensive biomedical HIV prevention intervention such as nPEP for individuals at highest risk is acceptable and feasible. Sustainability of nPEP services is being evaluated for cost at full implementation;
- The development of detailed protocols that include eligibility, treatment, and monitoring standards, additional STD and viral hepatitis screening and prevention, risk reduction counseling, and follow-up activities are critical to successfully implementing this comprehensive and high-quality HIV prevention intervention;
- The process, key components, and structure of the nPEP program can inform other jurisdictions aiming to implement nPEP or other biomedical HIV prevention programs.

REFERENCES

1. Cardo DM, Culver DH, Ciesielski CA, Srivastava PU, Marcus R, Abiteboul D, Heptonstall J, Ippolito G, Lot F, McKibben PS, Bell DM. A case-control study of HIV seroconversion in health care workers after percutaneous exposure. Centers for

Disease Control and Prevention Needlestick Surveillance Group. *N Engl J Med.* 1997 Nov 20;337(21):1485–90.

2. Roland ME, Neilands TB, Krone MR, Katz MH, Franses K, Grant RM, Busch MP, Hecht FM, Shacklett BL, Kahn JO, Bamberger JD, Coates TJ, Chesney MA, Martin JN. Seroconversion following nonoccupational post-exposure prophylaxis against HIV. *Clin Infect Dis.* 2005 Nov 15;41(10):1507–13.
3. Lui AY, Kittredge PV, Vittinghoff E, Raymond HF, Ahrens K, Matheson T, Hecht J, Klausner JD, Buchbinder SP. Limited knowledge and use of HIV post- and pre-exposure prophylaxis among gay and bisexual men. *J Acquir Immune Defic Syndr.* 2008 Feb 1:47(2):241–47.
4. Mehta SA, Silvera R, Bernstein K, Holzman RS, Aberg JA, Daskalakis DC. Awareness of post-exposure HIV prophylaxis in high-risk men who have sex with men in New York City. *Sex Transm Infect.* 2011, Jun;87(4):344–8.
5. Landovitz RJ, Combs KB, Currier JS. Availability of HIV postexposure prophylaxis services in Los Angeles County. *Clin Infect Dis.* 2009 Jun 1;48(11):1624–7.
6. Coates TJ, Ritcher L, Caceres C. Behavioural strategies to reduce HIV transmission: how to make them work better. *Lancet.* 2008 Aug 23;372(9639):669–84.
7. Schechter M, do Lago RF, Mendelsohn AB, Moreira RI, Moulton LH, Harrison LH, Praca Onze Study Team. Behavioral impact, acceptability, and HIV incidence among homosexual men with access to postexposure chemoprophylaxis for HIV. *JAIDS.* 2004. Apr 15;35(5):519–25.
8. Sonder GJ, Regez Rm, Brinkman K, Prins JM, Mulder JW, Spaargaren J, Coutinho RA, van den Hoek A. Prophylaxis and follow-up after possible exposure to HIV, hepatitis B virus, and hepatitis C virus outside hospital: Evaluation of policy 2000–2003. *BMJ.* 2005 Apr 9; 330(7495):825–29.
9. Grant RM, Lama JR, Anderson PL, McMahan V, Liu AY, Vargas L, et al. Preexposure chemoprophylaxis for HIV prevention in men who have sex with men. *N Engl J Med.* 2010 Dec 30;363(27):2587.

37 STDs/HIV in the Adult Film Industry

Public Health, Workplace Hazards, and the Need for Worker Protection

JANE STEINBERG, REBECCA BUTLER, MARK ROY MCGRATH, AND PETER R. KERNDT

NATURE OF THE PROBLEM AND CONTEXT

While sexually transmitted diseases (STDs) are a major public health problem in California and nationwide, especially among youth, occupations with potential exposure to STDs in legally sanctioned business establishments are limited to Nevada brothels and the adult film industry (AFI). The legality of California's AFI was established in 1988 after the California Supreme Court ruled in the case of *People v. Freeman* that the production of non-obscene pornography did not meet the criminal definitions of pandering or prostitution, and is protected by the guarantee of free expression under the First Amendment (1). With this decision and the subsequent development of media technology, adult film production in California rapidly grew to a multibillion-dollar industry. However, despite legalization, government regulation of the adult film industry with regard to worker safety has proved to be elusive. Unlike legal commercial sex work in Nevada, the adult film industry was legalized in California through case law, not by statute, and has, for the most part, not had strict governmental oversight (2). Regulation of the industry has been largely limited to prevention of child pornography. Title 18, Section 2257 of the U.S. Code of Regulations explicitly prohibits performers under the age of 18 and provides for civil and criminal prosecutions for any violation (3). As such, under federal law, adult film production companies and distributors are required to have a Custodian of Records to document and retain records of the age of all performers in order to enforce the age restriction.

The U.S. adult film industry produces 4,000 to 11,000 films and earns an estimated \$9 to \$13 billion in gross revenues annually (4). California is the largest center for adult film production worldwide, although adult film production occurs throughout the United States. An estimated 200 production companies in Los Angeles employ up to 1,500 workers (5). Approximately 75% of all workers in the industry are female. By contrast, the number of mainstream Hollywood motion pictures released per year is estimated at 500 to 550, and mainstream performers are protected by stringent union-enforced regulation (6).

According to the California Occupational Safety and Health Administration (Cal/OSHA), some workers in the adult film industry are paid as employees, where they receive a paycheck and receive an IRS W-2 form, with taxes and other deductions withheld by the employer. Other workers are paid as independent contractors and receive an IRS 1099 form at the end of the year (7). Even workers who are paid as independent contractors under one law may be considered employees under another law. In California, the Division of Labor Standards Enforcement provides guidance for determining whether someone is an independent contractor. Although determinations about whether a person is an employee or an independent contractor are made based on the circumstances of each case, an employer-employee relationship has been found in similar circumstances, including in the mainstream film industry and exotic dance establishments (8).

■ WORKPLACE HAZARDS IN THE ADULT FILM INDUSTRY IN CALIFORNIA

Throughout the course of their employment, adult film performers are routinely exposed to extreme and unhealthy working conditions, such as 1) multiple and concurrent sex partners over short time periods, which increases the risk of transmission and acquisition of sexually transmitted diseases (STDs) and HIV; 2) an industry trend toward riskier types of sexual contact, such as anal or double anal and penile penetration and internal ejaculation, which increases the potential for rapid spread of STDs (9); 3) prolonged intercourse that may result in inadequate lubrication and anogenital trauma or bleeding, resulting in exposure to semen, seminal and vaginal/cervical fluids, and blood; and 4) lack of condoms or other barrier methods for reducing exposure to infectious bodily fluids or fecal pathogens (10). STDs are often asymptomatic or "silent" and hence undiagnosed, but can result in significant morbidity if treatment is delayed or does not occur. Additionally, the presence of STDs increases the likelihood of HIV transmission during sexual contact (11).

While condoms are an effective means to prevent the transmission of STDs, use in the heterosexual segment of the adult film industry is infrequent. An analysis of condom use found that condoms are used only 3% of the time for penile-vaginal intercourse in the heterosexual industry (12). As of 2010, only one of the estimated 200 adult production companies in Los Angeles County required their performers to use condoms (13). In February 2006, one of the last two remaining adult production companies to require performers to wear condoms during their sex scenes changed their policy, allowing performers to choose whether they wanted to wear condoms (14). According to many workers, if they insist on using a condom in an adult film, they will not be employed (15). Lack of barrier protection significantly increases the risks to workers for acquiring and transmitting HIV and other STDs, which have serious health consequences for workers and the community.

Founding of Adult Industry Medical Clinic

The adult film industry had tried to address performer workplace safety issues through self-regulation. In response to a 1998 outbreak of HIV that resulted in the infection of five female performers (16), the industry assisted in the creation of the Adult Industry Medical (AIM) Health Care Foundation. The purpose of AIM was to provide STD/HIV testing and information to performers. AIM also kept a database of these test results of performers in order for adult film production companies to determine whether the performer had recently tested positive for an STD. In 1998, the industry's protocol was to ask performers to show up on set with a copy of a negative HIV test within the past 30 days.

AIM created a new industry "standard," which required adult performers to have a verified negative HIV PCR test performed at AIM within the 30 days prior to a shoot. Later urine-based testing for chlamydia, gonorrhea, and, less frequently, for other STDs, was added to the screening panel of tests prior to adult film production. Positive test results for reportable infections of performers tested at the program began as an effort to reduce transmission of infections through early diagnosis, treatment, and to "quarantine" any performer who tested positive for HIV (17).

In 2011, AIM filed for bankruptcy and closed. It is believed that the closure was due, in part, to a privacy lawsuit challenging AIM's handling of patient records after the clinic was converted from a non-profit to a private clinic and reopened two months after its shutdown by state and county health officials (18). This shutdown was due to AIM's business practices, such as operating without the correct licensure and the clinic's lack of a required agreement with a hospital where patients could be transferred as needed (19). Following AIM's closure, it was replaced by Adult Production Health and Safety Services (APHSS), an industry-sponsored testing program (20). It appears that, similar to the AIM model, most performers are required to pay for their own screening tests per the APHSS website.

HIV/STD Morbidity in the Adult Film Industry

In April 2004, four outbreak-related cases (one male, three females) of HIV were identified among performers in Los Angeles County's (LAC) AFI. The LAC Department of Public Health (DPH), in conjunction with Cal/OSHA, the Centers for Disease Control and Prevention's (CDC) Division of HIV/AIDS, and the National Institute for Occupational Safety and Health (NIOSH), launched an investigation. The male performer had tested negative for HIV in February and March 2004, then tested positive for HIV in April 2004. During the time interval between the negative test results, he experienced a flu-like illness after performing unprotected vaginal and anal intercourse for an adult film produced in Brazil.

After returning to California, he performed unprotected sex acts for adult films with 13 female partners who had all tested negative for HIV in the preceding 30 days; three subsequently tested positive for HIV, yielding a 23% attack rate (see Figure 37–1). Sexual contact histories were obtained and subsequent gene sequencing strongly supported workplace transmission of HIV (21–23). All three HIV-positive females had unprotected double-anal intercourse with the index case. The outbreak demonstrated that screening for HIV alone, without requiring the use of condoms, is insufficient to prevent disease transmission. A performer could be exposed to an STD infection immediately after testing, have no symptoms, be highly infectious, and unknowingly transmit the infection to others.

In 2009, a female performer tested positive for HIV (24) and in October 2010, another performer was acutely infected with HIV (25). A CDC Epidemic Intelligence Service Officer assisted the DPH with the 2010 investigation. The performer identified 14 occupational and one non-occupational sexual contacts, including 5 men and 10 women, during the eight-week period preceding the October diagnosis (26). Occupational exposures involved 12 filming locations and 10 production companies. The actor reported having used condoms in productions involving anal exposure, but not during vaginal or oral exposures. Contact investigation was completed among 5 of 14 occupational sexual contacts. One non-occupational contact had

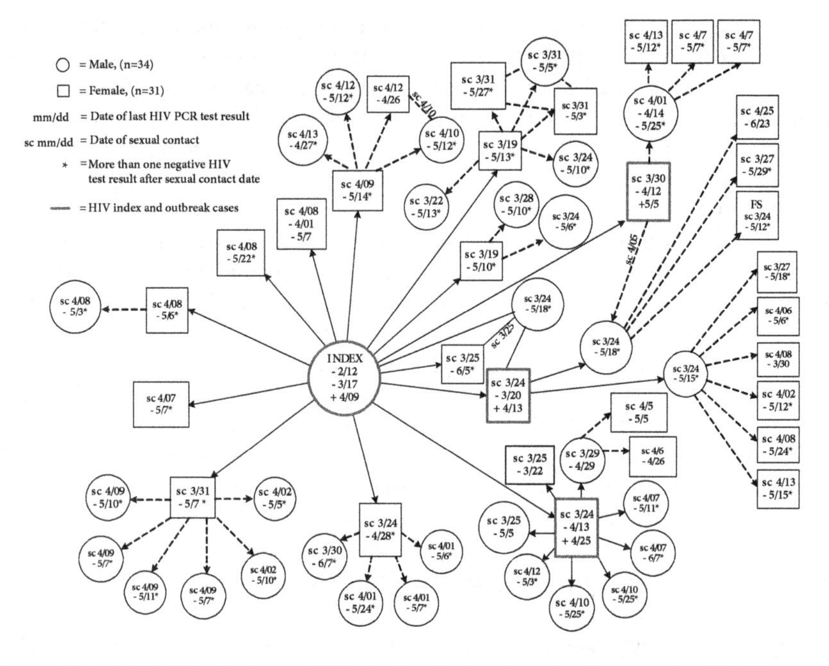

Figure 37–1 Adult Film Industry HIV Outbreak, Los Angeles County, April 2004.

pharyngeal gonorrhea; two occupational contacts were HIV-infected; three contacts were HIV-uninfected; and 9 had unknown status.

Outbreaks of other STDs have been well documented among persons involved with the AFI. A recent study by the DPH's STD Program found that between 2004 and 2007, 2633 chlamydia and/or gonorrhea cases were reported among 1849 performers. Seventy-two percent of cases (n = 1903) were reported among females. Chlamydia was the most frequent diagnosis (57%), followed by gonorrhea (35%) and co-infection with both STDs (8%) (27). The annual cumulative incidences of chlamydia and gonorrhea were estimated to be 14.3% and 5.1%, respectively. The reinfection rate within one year was 26.1%; female performers were 27% more likely to be reinfected than males.

Figure 37–2 shows the annual number of chlamydia and gonorrhea cases among AFI performers reported between 2004 and 2008. The number of chlamydia cases generally increased, with a drop in 2006 and 2008, whereas the number of gonorrhea cases increased between 2004 and 2005 and steadily declined thereafter, decreasing nearly 60% between 2005 and 2008. This decrease is likely due to one or a combination of multiple possible factors: 1) a reduction in STD testing among performers due to lower demand in the AFI or decreased compliance with the "voluntary" testing standard; 2) increased use of self-medication or empirical treatment by providers; 3) a true decrease in STD reports, likely due to expanded efforts of case investigations, interviews, and partner referrals for treatment; and 4) less frequent reporting from laboratories of performer testing facilities.

The ranges for annual cumulative incidences of chlamydia and gonorrhea among AFI performers (based on a performer population range of 2,000–3,000 performers

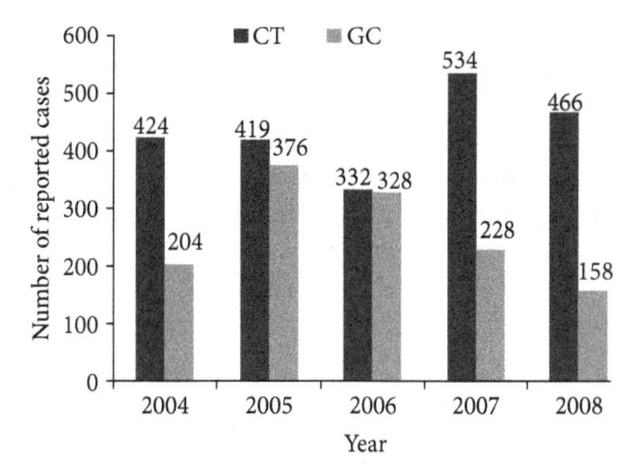

Figure 37–2 The Annual Number of Chlamydia (CT) and Gonorrhea (GC) Cases among AFI Performers Reported Between 2004 and 2008.

using 2008 data) are shown in Figure 37–3. Between 14% and 21% of performers had one or more chlamydial infections reported, and 5% to 8% had at least one gonorrhea infection reported in 2008. While these data suggest higher rates than among the general population, the rates cannot be directly compared since rates among performers are based on more frequent testing.

■ INDUSTRY PRACTICES REGARDING WORKER SAFETY AND PUBLIC HEALTH

Testing Not a Substitute for Prevention

The industry's response to outbreaks of STDs and HIV among performers in the heterosexual segment of the AFI continues to be voluntary STD/HIV testing and quarantine of performers with retesting. Although testing can reduce the spread of disease, it does not stop it. The 2004 HIV outbreak occurred when three

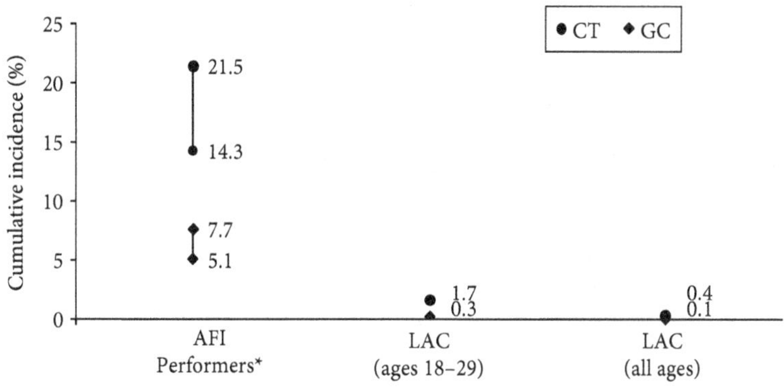

Figure 37–3 Estimated Range of Chlamydia (CT) and Gonorrhea (GC) Annual Cumulative Incidences among Adult Film Performers Compared to the Los Angeles County (LAC) General Population (2008).

performers who had been compliant with monthly screening contracted HIV (28). At that time, a male performer who had tested HIV negative only three days earlier infected three of 14 female performers.

Another limitation of the testing policy is the time period of STD/HIV testing (29). As noted previously, the current industry testing standard is to conduct urine-based tests for chlamydia and gonorrhea, but performers are not routinely screened for oral and rectal infections. Since oral and anal sex are common practices in the AFI, many cases of orally and rectally acquired chlamydia and gonorrhea are likely missed, with potential continual exposure and transmission of infections to others.

Further, current screening among performers is not comprehensive. Performers are not routinely tested for fecal-oral pathogens, or other viral pathogens such as Hepatitis A, B, and C. Although HIV and syphilis are typically included in the screening panel, many other reportable and non-reportable STDs, such as herpes, human papillomavirus (HPV), *Trichomonas*, and bacterial vaginosis, are not, thus underestimating the true prevalence and health impact of the full range of sexual transmitted infections. Infections among performers may also be underreported due to either prophylactic self-medication or presumptive empirical treatment without testing. Due to these limitations, the reported rates of STDs and reinfections likely underestimate the true rates of disease in this population.

■ INDUSTRY VIOLATION OF WORKER HEALTH AND SAFETY PRACTICES

Since 2004, throughout the course of disease investigations of AIM by the DPH, a number of worker health and safety violations have occurred. Most performers are required to pay for their own screening tests and to sign a consent form that permits disclosure of their test results to other performers and producers before filming. Both of these practices are explicitly prohibited under Cal/OSHA regulations that require employers to pay the costs of their health and safety program (30) and to maintain a confidential medical record for all employees. Performers are also required to sign a waiver releasing the employer from liability if the performer contracts HIV or an STD in the workplace while not providing adequate protection through the use of administrative, personal, or engineering controls, as is required by Cal/OSHA.

■ APPROACH TO THE PROBLEM

Public Officials' Recommendations, Worker Health, and Safety in the Adult Film Industry

In 2003, the *Los Angeles Times* published a detailed report on the incidence of HIV and other STDs among AFI workers and the lack of condom use in the AFI (31). In response, an LAC Board of Supervisors member made the following Board Motion:

> Last weekend the *Los Angeles Times* reported on the increasing incidence of HIV/AIDS and other sexually transmitted diseases among workers in the adult film industry. The lack of education and oversight of this industry is troubling. These actors and actresses engage in unsafe behavior with infected individuals and then often

unknowingly go on to spread these diseases to their partners. Improved education is one step toward reducing the incidence of infection.

I therefore move that the Board of Supervisors instruct the Director of Health Services (DHS) to consult with County Counsel to determine the appropriate regulatory entity at either the State or County level to oversee this industry to ensure the protection of its workers and limit the spread of communicable diseases, such as HIV, hepatitis, and other sexually transmitted diseases, and to work with the Chief Administrative Office and the County's legislative advocates to advocate for any State legislation needed to implement regulation. (32)

On March 25, 2003, the supervisors passed a follow-up motion instructing the Board to send letters to the governor and the director of Cal/OSHA, requesting Cal/OSHA to: 1) review the applicability of designated sections of the California Labor Code (Title 8) that may be applicable to the adult film industry and to worker health and safety issues, specifically §5193, Bloodborne Pathogens, and §3203, Injury and Illness Prevention Program; 2) review the need for a new standard to protect sex industry workers from occupational exposure to sexually transmitted diseases and other health risks; and 3) require a written industry plan for worker health and safety either under applicable authority of Title 8 or under new regulations. Also included in the motion was that the Board instruct the county's legislative advocates to consult with Cal/OSHA and, if necessary, to pursue a legislative remedy. Cal/OSHA determined that the sections of Title 8 did apply to the AFI and that a new standard was needed to protect AFI workers from occupational exposure to STDs and other health risks (33).

Legislative Hearing

In June 2004, the California Assembly Committee on Labor and Employment convened a legislative hearing in the San Fernando Valley to consider the feasibility and potential impact of mandating HIV/STD screening and condom use in the AFI (34). Participants included officials from Cal/OSHA, the LAC DPH, the California Department of Health Services, the American Civil Liberties Union, and the industry trade organization, the Free Speech Coalition. The Director of Public Health testified in support of legislation to regulate and require the industry to: 1) require condom use for all high-risk sexual encounters; 2) have screening requirements for STDs set by the state with screening costs paid by the industry, and offer vaccinations for appropriate preventable conditions; 3) mandate education and training of all AFI performers; and 4) ensure AFI compliance with reporting and regulations by state and local health departments. Following the hearing, an assemblyman sent a letter to 185 adult film production companies, urging them to adopt condoms or face legislative action (35). Additionally, the Los Angeles County Health Officer sent letters to 760 adult film corporate entities statewide that held a Custodian of Record in California, reiterating these recommendations.

■ CAL/OSHA RESPONSE

The California Occupational Safety and Health Act, enacted in 1973, requires employers to: provide a safe and healthful workplace for employees, pay the costs of their health and safety program, and not discriminate against employees who complain about safety and health conditions. This same act gives Cal/OSHA jurisdiction over most private employers in California, including employers in the AFI. Employers must comply with all relevant regulations, which are contained in Title 8 of the California Code of Regulations. Two key provisions that apply to the AFI are the Injury and Illness Prevention Program (IIPP) (36) and the blood-borne pathogens standard (37). For the IIPP, each employer must establish, implement, and maintain a written safety and health program. An IIPP identifies potential hazards specific to the workplace and ways to protect workers from those hazards.

The Cal/OSHA blood-borne pathogens standard requires employers to protect workers from exposure to serious diseases, including HIV, hepatitis B, and hepatitis C, which can be transmitted through exposure to blood and other potentially infectious materials (OPIM).The employer must also develop a written exposure control plan that describes the types of engineering and work practice controls that will be used to protect employees from contact with blood or OPIM. This would include simulation of sex scenes or ejaculation outside the partner's body. Performers must also be made aware of the risks associated with participation in various sexual acts and how to fully benefit from preventive practices. Also included in the exposure control plan is a procedure for exposure incidents when an employee has contact with potentially infectious material. Employers are also required to provide post-exposure prophylaxis. Universal precautions, which assume that all material is potentially infectious, are part of the blood-borne pathogens standard.

Additional requirements of the Standard that apply to employers include: 1) employees' use of personal protective equipment and other barrier methods in the production of all films (e.g., condoms, dental dams, eye protection); 2) medical evaluation (e.g., HIV/STD testing, follow-up, and providing hepatitis B vaccinations and follow-up) at no cost to the employee if an exposure to pathogens occurs; 3) employer-sponsored training on blood-borne pathogens, including how employees can protect themselves against infection, and what to do if they are exposed; and 4) maintenance of confidential employee medical records.

Cal/OSHA Involvement in Worker Health and Safety, Adult Film Industry

Cal/OSHA has jurisdiction over "places of employment" (38). It has no jurisdiction unless an employer-employee relationship exists. Once this relationship exists, Cal/OSHA has jurisdiction over every employment and place of employment in California. The California Labor Code and Title 8 of the California Code of Regulations (CCR) set forth the means by which Cal/OSHA exercises its authority to ensure employee safety. This is generally done through issuing citations that include administrative penalties for violating one or more of the Title's workplace safety standards (39). These penalties can be appealed to the California Occupational Safety and Health Appeals Board (40).

Following the 2004 outbreak, Cal/OSHA developed a web page for adult film employees and employers to inform them of the requirements of the blood-borne pathogens standard and IIPP regulations and key elements of a model exposure control plan (41). A dedicated phone line was also established to receive complaints and inquiries from people involved in this industry. In response to the HIV outbreak, Cal/

OSHA issued citations against two companies for failure to comply with the blood-borne pathogens standard, failure to report a serious work-related illness, failure to record injuries and illnesses, and failure to prepare and follow a written injury and illness prevention plan. As of January 2010, Cal/OSHA has conducted 44 investigations of workplace violations since the HIV outbreak (42). Although some of these cases are still under investigation, citations have been issued for violations of the blood-borne pathogens and Injury and Illness Prevention Standards in eight of these investigations. All citations were initially appealed, most citations have been settled, and no appeal has yet been heard by the OSHA Appeals Board.

■ INDUSTRY RESPONSE

Following the 2004 HIV outbreak, the industry temporarily suspended filming while AIM notified and tested all known partners of the infected individual. After the latest HIV outbreak in October 2010, several production companies temporarily suspended filming, while the AIM clinic said it would notify and test all partners of the infected individual, as it had done in the prior outbreak. AIM's investigation, however, could not be verified because of the refusal by AIM to cooperate with the DPH by providing any information on the source individual, other performers exposed, test results, or the production companies involved. The refusal to cooperate compromised public health efforts to deliver partner services and contain disease transmission in the AFI and obstructed the investigation of Cal/OSHA by shielding the identity of the involved production companies. Notification with the immediate offer of postexposure prophylaxis, which has been shown to prevent HIV in people with known exposures, needs to be provided with 72 hours of an exposure (see Chapter 36) (43).

One of the largest producers of adult film in the United States temporarily implemented a condom-only policy after the initial outbreak, only to reverse itself in 2006. Industry members have maintained their position that self-regulation still works and that testing is sufficient for reducing the transmission of STDs/HIV (44). Spokespersons for the adult film industry have consistently opposed greater regulation of health and safety standards for performers (45). The CEO of one of the companies has stated that: 1) audiences do not want to watch condoms and therefore companies will lose business if they have to use condoms; 2) as a result of the potential loss in revenue, the industry will go "underground" or leave California entirely; and 3) the industry's voluntary testing program works well, given that so few people have tested positive for HIV (46, 47, 48).

Regarding this last point, the fact that there is such high STD morbidity within the AFI underscores the limitations of a testing program. Although there may be far fewer cases of HIV infection in the AFI, this is likely due to other factors (e.g., persons with HIV are excluded from performing and thus may not be counted; AFI performers in the heterosexual AFI may not be at highest risk for HIV).

While there are no large studies that assess whether audiences would reject adult films if condoms were used, one of the longest running and largest production companies became a condom-only company after the HIV outbreak. In addition, Brazil boasts a high condom usage rate in its adult films while still maintaining a large share of the international market as the world's second largest adult film industry, suggesting that condom use in adult films does not have to erode profitability. Filming techniques can also be used to reduce the visual effect of condoms by using flesh tone–colored condoms or by digitally removing them after production. Facial ejaculations could be simulated through the use of inert materials such as liquid antacids combined with filming techniques, which would eliminate any health risk to the performer. Likewise, "ass-to-mouth," a common genre in adult films, could be produced using simulated methods and eliminate any exposure to fecal pathogens.

■ CURRENT WORK PRACTICES: "BUSINESS AS USUAL?"

Despite multiple outbreaks of HIV and STDs in the AFI and repeated recommendations from public officials on how to make the adult film industry safer, it is believed that industry practices continue to be out of compliance with Cal/OSHA worker protections (49). Performers are still required to pay for STD screening tests—a violation of Cal/OSHA standards, which requires the employer to pay for needed medical monitoring. Since the closure of the AIM clinic, it is currently unknown to what extent the industry has improved its worker health and safety standards, although information posted on the web site for the new industry testing program, APHSS, provides some insights. Their website states that there is a "secure database that ensures performer privacy" yet it also states that "[p]erformers can complete a release waiver at the time of testing; to specify any parties they wish to have access to their medical records. Performers that choose to, should list producers, agents and APHSS.org on the waiver, to give permission for access." This violates a worker's right to medical confidentiality per the blood-borne pathogens standard.

■ NEVADA AS A MODEL OF SUCCESSFUL REGULATION

The state of Nevada has demonstrated the feasibility of lowering STD rates among sex workers through strict regulations for its legal brothel industry. The mandatory use of condoms in brothels was instituted in 1988. The sex workers in brothels are tested for chlamydia and gonorrhea on a weekly basis and syphilis and HIV on at least a monthly basis. Since the implementation of these regulations, not a single individual has tested positive for HIV while working in the brothel (50). Of more than 7,000 STD tests conducted between 1982 and 1989 among brothel workers, only 20 positive STD cases were diagnosed, all of which occurred before implementation of the mandatory condom law (51). Because of the Nevada regulations, sex workers have become virtually free of STDs, and the few who do contract them do so primarily before entering the industry or from sexual partners when on leave from the brothel (52). Regulation of the Nevada brothel system is a feasible model for the adult film industry. Sex workers in both industries typically stay in the business for only a brief time, and they do similar types of work.

■ ENFORCEMENT CHALLENGES: CAL/OSHA

Although Cal/OSHA has jurisdiction over places of employment in California, monitoring and enforcement capability is limited because of the small number of enforcement officials who must serve all the employers and employees in the state. Workers may also not be aware of their rights, or may be reluctant to file a complaint for fear of loss of employment or employer retaliation. In addition, Cal/OSHA can only regulate events that occur in the context of an employer-employee relationship, and thus it cannot regulate treatment of independent contractors. As noted previously, some performers in the AFI are treated as employees, and others are treated as independent contractors; this creates challenges to the universal enforcement of health and safety standards in the adult film workplace.

In 2008 the Workers' Compensation Appeals Board, in response to a claim, found that an adult film performer who had contracted HIV during the production of a film was an employee of the film production company, rather than an independent contractor. The Board relied on facts that the production company controlled all meaningful aspects of the business relationship and had the primary power over work safety, including the types of HIV tests for performers, the collection of test results, the use of condoms, and directing the production of the film (53). Thus, the adult film performer's contraction of HIV, as an employee, was deemed to be a compensable workplace injury. This type of ruling may assist Cal/OSHA in the workplace regulation of the adult film industry.

Cal/OSHA's ability to investigate workplace transmission of disease may be impeded by California's HIV confidentiality laws. In 2009, Cal/OSHA investigated a potential workplace blood-borne pathogens violation after the news media reported that a female performer had tested positive for HIV. When AIM, which was the testing agency, learned of the positive HIV result, it notified the industry in order to enact a quarantine of the performers. In response to this information, Cal/OSHA conducted an unannounced inspection of AIM facilities, and requested to review medical records of the female performer and other AIM patients. AIM refused to produce the patients' medical records. In response, Cal/OSHA served a subpoena on AIM seeking information regarding patients who have tested positive for HIV and other STDs from 2004–2009, as well as the test dates, names, and contact information for each production company for which the patient worked and the dates of work. AIM objected (54).

The female performer, anonymously called Patient Zero, sued Cal/OSHA. The trial court ruled that Cal/OSHA's actions of seeking to compel the disclosure of Patient Zero's medical information violated her rights to privacy under the United States and California Constitutions. Specifically, the Court ruled that Cal/OSHA's subpoena illegally sought HIV test information in violation of Health and Safety Code § 120975. Cal/OSHA further could not state a compelling governmental reason to override Patient Zero's privacy interest in her own medical records. As a result, the Court issued a permanent injunction against Cal/OSHA prohibiting it from seeking to compel the disclosure of personally identifying HIV test information or other information that would identify Patient Zero or other patients of AIM as HIV positive without the specific authorization of such patients.

■ ENFORCEMENT CHALLENGES: LOCAL HEALTH DEPARTMENTS

Local health departments monitor STD/HIV treatment and follow-up of exposed and infected persons for disease investigation and control purposes. Local enforcement of the AFI, however, has been met with significant barriers in LAC, where the industry in the United States is primarily based. Disease investigators have routinely been unable to establish contact with exposed and infectious performers to initiate timely treatment and partner services and to contain the spread of infectious diseases to performers and their partners. After the 2010 HIV outbreak, when the AIM clinic refused to provide performer contact information to the local health department for disease investigation, the DPH could not identify the source of the disease outbreak and mount a rapid public health response. Public health departments need to be able to quickly identify people known to have been occupationally exposed to STDs/HIV for treatment, follow-up, and partner management to control further spread of disease to others in the community.

Another challenge in local enforcement of the adult film industry is that local health departments are bound by state laws that require communicable diseases to be reported to the health jurisdiction in which care is provided (55); optimally, that information would be provided to the jurisdiction where transmission is suspected to have occurred. The transient nature of adult film work often results in performers being diagnosed with a communicable disease in one health jurisdiction and then relocating to another jurisdiction before the local health department is made aware of the incident. As a result, disease investigation and follow-up often does not occur in these circumstances. Partner management in the AFI is particularly important because workers are considered "core transmitters" due to extensive sexual networks with multiple and concurrent sexual partners. There are many barriers to AFI disease investigations, including the transient nature of the workforce, a lack of cooperation with investigations by STD testing sites, talent placement agencies and production companies, and a reluctance of performers to cooperate with public health investigations for fear of future hiring difficulties. It is often difficult to identify the source of potential disease outbreaks and mount a rapid public health response when an outbreak occurs in the AFI. In addition, local public health officials have also expressed concerns about the staffing resources needed to effectively monitor and enforce regulation of the approximate 200 adult film production companies and have called for statewide legislation to increase staffing (56, 57).

■ IMPLEMENTATION OF SOLUTIONS

Legislation and Regulation of the Adult Film Industry

Lacking the will or ability to regulate itself beyond a regular HIV/STD testing protocol, the adult film industry must be compelled through state legislation to enforce health and safety standards for adult film performers. Despite repeated recommendations from local public health officials, Cal/OSHA, and a legislative hearing on how to make the adult film industry safer, it appears that industry practices remain unchanged. At the same time, no California legislator has authored a bill to protect AFI performers. Legislation should clarify that all workers in the adult film industry should be considered employees for purposes of protecting the public's health.

Public health agencies and organizations including the American Public Health Association (58), the American Medical Association (59), the California Medical Association, the Los Angeles County Medical Association, the California Conference of Local Health Officers (60), the California Conference of Local AIDS Directors (61), the California STD Controllers Association, the County of Los Angeles (62),

Planned Parenthood Affiliates of California, Beyond AIDS, and the American Sexual Health Association, support improved workplace protections for adult film performers and mandatory and enforced condom use (63).

Another way to improve worker health is through regulatory changes. In December 2009, a community-based HIV medical provider, AIDS Healthcare Foundation, submitted a petition to the California Occupational Safety and Health Standards Board (OSHSB) to amend California's Blood-borne Pathogens Standard to clarify required protections for workers in the adult film industry and include a section that would specifically address health hazards in the adult film industry (64). An excerpt from their petition follows:

> Although workers in adult films should enjoy protections under the current phrasing of the regulation, as well as the Board's determination that adult film workers are employees, the adult film industry has steadfastly refused to take any steps to protect its workers from diseases spread by blood borne pathogens, resulting in thousands of employees becoming infected with sexually transmitted diseases. Clarification and enhanced enforcement of the rules are called for.

In response to the petition and after a hearing of the OSHSB in March 2010, Cal/OSHA initiated seven public statewide meetings to discuss whether the regulations should be amended to specifically address the adult film industry (65). The LAC DPH agreed with the proposed change to the regulations and developed a set of recommendations for consideration by the OSHSB (see Table 37.1). Two subcommittees were formed by Cal/OSHA on disease control measures and on medical issues; these consisted of health experts, industry personnel and talent, and other

TABLE 37–1 *Los Angeles County Department of Public Health Recommendations to Protect Workers in the Adult Film Industry**

1. Mandatory condom use for all penetrative sex acts, including oral sex.
2. Routine screening of performers for HIV infection and other STDs.
3. Universal vaccination of non-immune performers against hepatitis A and B, and HPV vaccination.
4. Mandatory education and training for all AFI performers on work-related health and safety hazards in this industry.
5. Medical monitoring by periodic screening at all appropriate anatomic sites for HIV infection and other STDs.
6. Requirement that production companies that make or buy adult films maintain and produce upon demand the information necessary to enable local health departments to investigate and control occupational exposures to infectious pathogens.
7. Requirement that any person, clinic, or other organization that provides testing services or refers performers to employment in the adult film industry (i.e., talent agents/agencies) maintain and produce upon demand information necessary to enable local health departments to investigate and control occupational exposures to infectious pathogens.

*Adapted from Los Angeles County Department of Public Health Recommendations to the Cal/OSHA Advisory Committee on Blood borne Pathogens, June 29, 2010

http://www.dir.ca.gov/dosh/doshreg/comments/Statement%20from%20the%20Los%20Angeles%20County%20Department%20of%20Public%20Health%206-29-10.pdf

interested parties. Topics of discussion in these meetings included health hazards in the adult film industry and workable methods for addressing prevention and control strategies. Topics covered included the use of condoms and other barrier protection and simulation, risks associated with different routes of exposure to blood-borne pathogens and other STDs, how to identify these risks and implement controls for different sexual acts, issues related to the intermittent workforce, the provision of hepatitis B vaccine, training issues, post-exposure prophylaxis, confidentiality issues, periodic testing, primary and secondary producers, and record-keeping issues.

Based on the outcomes of these meetings, Cal/OSHA held a pre-rulemaking public meeting in Los Angeles. Draft language was provided that included a proposed new section in the CCR that would specifically address STDs in the adult film industry. Also provided was a draft that contained modifications that could be made to the proposed language if a proposal were to permit the use of alternative control measures for oral sex (neither of these documents represents a rulemaking proposal from Cal/OSHA).

■ LITIGATION TO SPUR REGULATORY ACTION

Litigation is sometimes used to spur regulatory action by a governmental entity. In 2009, the AIDS Healthcare Foundation (AHF), dissatisfied with the public health response, sued the LAC DPH and alleged that county public health officials had a mandatory legal duty to require adult film producers and performers to ensure that condoms be used during the filming and production of adult films in LAC. AHF's petition requested the Superior Court to order the county's health officer to require condom use in adult-film production, and that the failure of the county's health officer to unilaterally impose such an industry-wide regulation would be an abuse of his discretion (66). The Superior Court dismissed the case, ruling that the county health officer had broad discretion over how he managed public health matters (67). AHF appealed. In 2011, the Court of Appeal upheld the dismissal (68), ruling that California communicable disease control laws gave local health officers discretion to act in a particular manner depending on the circumstances presented. Accordingly, the county's health officer could not be required to issue a regulatory order mandating condom use for performers in the adult film industry. The court specifically commented that it could not compel the county to implement AHF's policy agenda, and that AHF's public policy advocacy was better directed at lawmakers to change the workplace regulations. Ultimately, AHF's request for review by the California Supreme Court was denied (69).

■ LOCAL EFFORTS

Los Angeles City Council Motion

In an effort to address the high incidence of STDs within the AFI, in March 2011 the Los Angeles City Council unanimously passed a motion requesting that the City Attorney's Office report on the mechanisms necessary to implement improved health and safety measures for permitted adult productions within the city's jurisdiction (70). The city attorney rendered an opinion that the city does not have the power to adopt such conditions because they are preempted by state occupational safety and health standards. Cal/OSHA issued a follow-up opinion that state law does not preempt such action by the city because the city was not seeking to enact an occupational health and safety standard, but rather a public health standard applicable to any film activity, where the purpose of the city's permit process is to protect public health and safety regardless of employment relationship, within the city boundaries (71). The city attorney's office issued a response letter in December 2011 to Cal/OSHA refuting the Cal/OSHA opinion.

At a subsequent meeting, the Los Angeles City Council passed a resolution to include in its 2011–2012 State Legislative Program two key provisions that apply to the AFI: 1) support for legislation or administrative action requiring Cal/OSHA and the LAC DPH to enter into an agreement to create a mechanism of local enforcement in the administration/enforcement of any occupational safety and workplace standards for the AFI, as covered in the California Labor Code; and 2) support for legislation to amend Section 5193, Title 8 of the CCR to specifically include the word "condoms" as a form of barrier protection, which would be required by adult film performers in situations covered by this code section.

Local Ballot Initiative

In the summer of 2011, AHF developed a City of Los Angeles ballot initiative that would allow Los Angeles City voters to vote on a proposed ordinance that would formally condition the issuance of adult film permits by the City of Los Angeles to companies that maintain engineering and work practice controls, including the provision of and required use of condoms, sufficient to protect employees from exposure to blood or other potentially infectious materials consistent with state law within the Los Angeles City limits. The proposed ordinance also would require that any film permit issued under the authority of the City of Los Angeles for commercial filming of an adult film be conditioned on the compliance with this requirement and include language regarding the obligation to comply with applicable workplace health and safety regulations. The proposed ordinance also would require the city to charge applicants seeking permits for production of adult films a fee sufficient to pay for periodic inspections. The proposed ordinance would amend the Los Angeles City Municipal Code (72). In response, the Los Angeles City Attorney's office filed a lawsuit seeking judicial review of the merits of the proposed ballot measure. According to the lawsuit, the initiative is preempted by existing state laws mandating workplace safety, which address the need for protective barriers to be used when workers are exposed to blood-borne pathogens, such as HIV and other sexually transmitted diseases (73).

On January 10, 2012, the Los Angeles City Council voted to approve the initiative petition to require condom usage in the adult film industry and related permitting requirements, subject to the approval of the mayor. On January 23, 2012, the mayor of Los Angeles signed the measure. Following this action, officials in Simi Valley, a nearby community, were considering a similar rule out of a concern that adult film producers could move location to their more suburban community, fleeing the condom requirement in Los Angeles City. The city's condom requirement only applies to adult film productions that apply for a permit, but officials said a permit was not required when filming in a soundstage. AHF is gathering signatures for a ballot measure that would go before Los Angeles County voters and, if approved, would force adult film companies to obtain health permits. If that happens, it would increase the burden on adult film companies, wherever they shoot in Los Angeles County, to comply with existing California workplace laws.

LA Film Board

Within Los Angeles, all film production companies are required to obtain a permit for insurance underwriting and to satisfy local and state health and safety standards. The City of Los Angeles contracts out the permitting process to Film LA, Inc., a private nonprofit organization that coordinates and processes permits for on-location motion pictures. When production companies apply for a film permit, they sign an explicit statement agreeing to follow local and state occupational and health and safety laws. Furthermore, film permits have conditional language prohibiting a variety of activities. For producers of adult content, permits are issued on the condition that all "interior and exterior nudity or sexual activity must not be visible or audible by the public," though city officials believe many adult films do not obtain the required permits (74).

As noted earlier, Cal/OSHA has determined that producers of adult content must comply with all relevant regulations contained in Title 8 of the CCR. These require barrier protection to limit exposure to infectious materials, health and safety training, vaccinations for employees, and an injury prevention plan to be followed in the event of unforeseen exposure. Nonetheless, these requirements have not been very effectual. First, only a limited number of adult film production companies purchase permits. Second, while production companies agree to follow applicable laws, the contractual language is vague and there is no specific language referencing the blood-borne pathogens standards or Title 8 of the California Labor Code. Finally, adult content is primarily produced in obscure localities where inspections and proper enforcement do not occur.

■ EVALUATION AND IMPACT

Methods for evaluating the success of improved health and safety in the AFI have focused on three key process measures: 1) enhanced surveillance; 2) multi-sector collaboration; and, 3) legislative/regulatory advocacy. Through case reports, the DPH has been able to establish high rates of STDs within this industry to make the strong case for the need to take action to address the occupational risks and prevent the spread of disease. These surveillance data have been utilized by Cal/OSHA to justify the need for proposed changes to the blood-borne pathogens standard as described previously. Cross-sector collaboration is ongoing and has consisted of meetings within and between health department staff, women's health organizations, performer groups, AIDS service organizations, other community-based organizations, and Cal/OSHA. Meetings have focused on educating and informing these groups about occupational health issues within the industry.

These collaborations have extended to state and national organizations through policy development related to the industry, educational sessions, fact sheets, and disease updates. These have led to policy recommendations by local, state, and national organizations for improvements in worker health in this industry, as discussed previously. In the area of regulatory and legislative advocacy, the health department has played an active role in the Cal/OSHA hearings in addressing proposed changes to the blood-borne pathogens standard. The DPH has, along with other health advocates, sought to sponsor legislation in California to directly address the health risks to workers in this industry.

CONCLUSIONS

While there have been a number of attempts to reduce the workplace health hazards associated with communicable diseases in the adult film industry, significant challenges remain. As noted previously, the public health strategy to improve worker health and safety in the adult film industry has centered on three key strategies: 1) using surveillance data to document the high disease burden; 2) working at local, state and national levels for regulatory and legislative change; and 3) strengthening collaborations with internal and external stakeholders. These strategies can serve as a model for addressing related occupational health and public health issues of our time.

REFERENCES

1. *People v. Freeman* (1988) 46 Cal.3d 419, 425–27.
2. Grudzen CR, Kerndt PR. The adult film industry: Time to regulate? *PLoS Med.* 2007 Jun;4(6):e126.
3. Title 18, 2257. Record keeping requirements. Legal Information Institute, Cornell University Law School. Available from: http://www.law.cornell.edu/uscode/18/usc_sec_18_00002257----000-.html (accessed Jan. 28, 2012).
4. Schlosser E. *Reefer Madness: Sex, Drugs, and Cheap Labor in the American Black Market.* New York: Houghton Mifflin; 2003.
5. Kaiser Family Foundation. Group says HIV "outbreak" contained among adult film actors; L.A. health officials obtain workers' medical records. *Kaiser Daily HIV/AIDS Report.* 2004 (April 23). Available from: www.kaisernetwork.org/daily_reports/rep_hiv_recent_rep.cfm?dr_cat=1&show=yes&dr_DateTime=23-apr-04#23346 (accessed July 5, 2011).
6. De Cesare MR. Note. Rxxx resolving the problem of performer health and safety in the adult film industry. *South Calif Law Rev.* 2006;79:667–710.
7. Division of Industrial Relations, California Occupational Health and Safety Administration. Available from: http://www.dir.ca.gov/dlse/faq_independentcontractor.htm (accessed Dec. 12, 2011).
8. Division of Occupational Safety and Health.Vital information for workers and employers in the adult film industry. Available from: www.dir.ca.gov/DOSH/AdultFilmIndustry.html#PPE (accessed Aug. 8, 2011).
9. Grudzen 2007 (see number 2 above).
10. Grudzen CR, Ryan G, Margold W, Torres J, Gelberg L. Pathways to health risk exposure in adult film performers. *J Urban Health.* 2009;86(1):67–78.
11. Fleming DT, Wasserheit JN. From epidemiological synergy to public health policy and practice: The contribution of other sexually transmitted diseases to sexual transmission of HIV infection. *Sex Transm Infect.* 1999;75(1):3–17.
12. Grudzen CR, Elliott MN, Kerndt PR, Schuster MA, Brook RH, Gelberg L. Condom use and high-risk sexual acts in adult films: A comparison of heterosexual and homosexual films. *Am J Public Health.* 2009; 99(suppl 1):S152–6.
13. Barrett B. Porn industry dropped condom policy. *The Boston Globe.* 2007. Available from: www.natap.org/2007/newsUpdates (accessed Dec. 15, 2011).

14. Fishbein P. Vivid entertainment quietly goes condom-optional. *Adult Video News.* Available from: http://business.avn.com/articles/video/Vivid-Quietly-Goes-Condom-Optional-47646 (accessed Nov. 15, 2011).
15. De Cesare 2006 (see number 6 above).
16. Mark Wallice. Available at: http://en.wikipedia.org/wiki/Mark_Wallice (accessed July 5, 2011).
17. Grudzen 2007 (see number 2 above).
18. Romero D. Porn clinic aim closes for good: Valley-based industry scrambles to find new STD testing system. May 3, 2011. Available from: http://blogs.laweekly.com/informer/2011/05/porn_clinic_closed_aim_testing.php (accessed Dec. 15, 2011).
19. Hennessey-Fiske M. Porn industry clinic in Sherman Oaks is closed by L.A. County. December 10, 2010. Available from: http://articles.latimes.com/2010/dec/10/local/la-me-porn-hiv-20101210 (accessed Dec. 1, 2011).
20. Adult Protection Health and Safety Services. Available from: https://aphss.org. (accessed Dec. 1, 2011).
21. Brooks JT et al. Molecular analysis of HIV strains from a cluster of worker infections in the adult film industry, Los Angeles 2004. *AIDS.* 2006;20:923–8.
22. Centers for Disease Control and Prevention. HIV transmission in the adult film industry—Los Angeles, California, 2004. *Morb Mortal Wkly Rep.* 2005;54(37):923–6. Available from: www.cdc.gov/mmwr/preview/mmwrhtml/mm5437a3.htm (accessed June 29, 2011).
23. Taylor MM, Rotblatt H, Brooks JT, et al. Epidemiologic investigation of a cluster of workplace HIV infections in the adult film industry: Los Angeles, California, 2004. *Clin Infect Dis.* 2007;44(2):301–5.
24. Lin II, RG, Yoshino K. Porn actress tests positive for HIV. *Los Angeles Times.* Available from: http://articles.latimes.com/2009/jun/11/local/me-porn-hiv11 (accessed July 27, 2011).
25. Hennessy-Fiske M, Rong-Gong L II. Porn film performer tests positive for HIV. *Los Angeles Times.* 2010. Available from: http://articles.latimes.com/2010/oct/13/local/la-me-porn-hiv-20101013 (accessed June 29, 2011).
26. Meza F. Investigation of HIV and gonorrhea transmission in the adult film industry, Los Angeles, California, 2010. Paper presented at the American Public Health Association Annual Meeting, 10/30/11. Available from: http://apha.confex.com/apha/139am/webprogram/Paper250239.html (accessed Jan. 27, 2012).
27. Goldstein BY, Steinberg JK, Aynalem G, Kerndt PR. High chlamydia and gonorrhea incidence and reinfection among performers in the adult film industry. *Sex Transm Dis.* 2011Jul;38(7):644–648. Available from: http://journals.lww.com/stdjournal/Abstract/2011/07000/High_Chlamydia_and_Gonorrhea_Incidence_and.12.aspx (accessed June 29, 2011).
28. Grudzen 2007 (see number 2 above).
29. Testimony by Robert Kim Farley, MD, MPH, to the Cal/OSHA Standards Board. STD and HIV and health risks among workers in the adult film industry. June 29, 2011. Available from: http://www.dir.ca.gov/dosh/doshreg/comments/STD%20and%20HIV%20Disease%20and%20Health%20Risks%20Los%20Angeles%20County%20DPH.pdf (accessed Aug. 5, 2011).
30. Division of Occupational Safety and Health.Vital information (see number 8 above).
31. Huffstutter PJ. See no evil. *Los Angeles Times Magazine.* 2003;Sect 12. Available from: www.aegis.com/news/Lt/2003/LT030110.html (accessed June 27, 2011).
32. Transcript, meeting of the Los Angeles County Board of Supervisors, January 14, 2003. Available from: http://file.lacounty.gov/bos/transcripts/01-14-03%20Board%20Meeting%20Transcript.pdf (accessed June 28, 2011).

33. Division of Occupational Safety and Health.Vital information (see number 8 above).
34. Committee on Labor and Employment. Worker health and safety in the adult film industry. 2004. Available from: http://www.lapublichealth.org/std/docs/afi/koretz_posthearingreport.pdf.
35. Madigan N. Sex-film industrythreatened with condom requirement. *New York Times.* August 24, 2004. Available from: http://query.nytimes.com/gst/fullpage.html?sec=health&res=9803E2DF153EF937A1575BC0A9629C8B63 (accessed June 29, 2011).
36. Calif. Code of Regulations, Title 8. 2007. §3203. Injury and Illness Prevention Program. Available from: www.dir.ca.gov/title8/3203.html (accessed June 29, 2011).
37. Calif. Code of Regulations, Title 8. 2007. §5193. Bloodborne Pathogens. Available from: www.dir.ca.gov/title8/5193.html (accessed July 5, 2011).
38. California Labor Code §6307.
39. California Labor Code §6317.
40. California Labor Code §6319.
41. Division of Occupational Safety and Health.Vital information (see number 8 above).
42. Personal communication, Cal/OSHA staff, January 27, 2011.
43. Centers for Disease Control and Prevention. Updated US Public Health Service guidelines for the management of occupational exposures to HBV, HCV, AND HIV and recommendations for postexposure prophylaxis. *Morb Mortal Wkly Rep.* [online] Recomm Rep. 2001; 50(RR-11):1–52. Available from: www.cdc.gov/mmwr/preview/mmwrhtml/rr5011a1.htm (accessed June 29, 2011).
44. Memo from Len Welsh to the California Occupational Safety and Health Standards Board. February 16, 2010. Available from: www.dir.ca.gov/oshsb/petition513_DOSH_eval.pdf (accessed June 15, 2011).
45. Romero D. Porn industry argues that regular STD tests are as good as condoms. November 10, 2011. Available from: http://blogs.laweekly.com/informer/2010/11/porn_industry_tests_condoms.php (accessed Nov. 10, 2011).
46. City of Los Angeles Files Complaint Against AHF on Validity of Condom Ballot Measure. December 10, 2011. Available from: http://www.freespeechcoalition.com/pressreleasesmedia/185-city-of-los-angeles-files-complaint-against-ahf-on-validity-of-condom-ballot-measure.html (accessed Dec. 11, 2011).
47. Cohen A. In porn industry, many balk at condom proposal. National Public Radio. 2010. Available from: www.npr.org/templates/story/story.php?storyId=126289177 (accessed June 29, 2011).
48. Yoshino K, Rong-Gong Lin II. Porn stars at L.A. convention defend HIV tests. *Los Angeles Times.* June 13, 2010. Available from: http://articles.latimes.com/2009/jun/13/local/me-porn-hiv13 (accessed June 29, 2011).
49. Policy Statement, American Public Health Association: Prevention and control of sexually transmitted infections and HIV among performers in the adult film industry. Policy number 20102; November 9, 2010. Available from: http://www.apha.org/advocacy/policy/policysearch/default.htm?id=1396 (accessed Jan. 5, 2011).
50. Reade R, Richwald G, Williams N. The Nevada legal brothel system as a model for AIDS prevention among female sex industry workers [abstract]. IntConf AIDS. 1990;6:267 (abstract no. S.C.715) Available from: http://gateway.nlm.nih.gov/MeetingAbstracts/ma?f=102196554.html (accessed July 5, 2011).
51 Unpublished surveillance data, Nevada State Health Division, Office of Health Statistics and Surveillance. Overview of STD/HIV Prevention in the Brothels, 2010.
52. Huffstutter PJ. See no evil (see number 31 above).
53. 2 Cal.WCC 1025, 2008 WL 4191236 (Cal.App.2 Dist.)
54. *Patient Zero vs. California Division of Occupational Safety and Health, et al.*; County of Alameda Superior Court Case No.: RG09463124; Final Judgment; September 22, 2011.

55. California Health and Safety Code (17 CCR 2643.5(c).)
56. Memo from Jonathan Fielding to Los Angeles County Board of Supervisors, October 17, 2009. Available from: http://file.lacounty.gov/bc/q3_2009/cms1_137588.pdf (accessed June 16, 2011).
57. Lin II RG. LA County can't require condoms for porn actors, officials say. *Los Angeles Times*. February 10, 2010. Available from: http://latimesblogs.latimes.com/lanow/2010/02/la-county-cant-require-condoms-for-porn-actors-officials-said.html (accessed June 29, 2011).
58. APHA 2010 (see number 49 above).
59. American Medical Association House of Delegates, 2010. Available from: http://www.msmaonline.com/Docs/Annotated%20Report%20of%20Reference%20Committee%20D.pdf (accessed July 6, 2011).
60. Communicable Disease Control and Prevention Committee, California Conference of Local Officers. February 19, 2009, agenda. Available from: http://www.cdph.ca.gov/programs/cclho/Documents/CDCPAgendaFebruary192009.pdf (accessed Mar. 5, 2009).
61. California Conference of Local AIDS Directors, Position Statement. Worker health and safety in the adult film industry. Available from: http://publichealth.lacounty.gov/std/docs/afi/CCLADAFI.pdf (accessed July 6, 2011).
62. Los Angeles County Chief Executive Office, Update to the county's state legislative agenda for the second year of the 2009–2010 session. Available from: http://ceo.lacounty.gov/igr/PDF/Adopted%20State%20Legislative%20Agenda%20for%20the%20Second%20Year%20of%20the%202009–10%20Session.pdf (accessed July 6, 2011).
63. Klausner JD and Katz KA. Editorial: Occupational health and the adult film industry: Time for a happy ending. *Sex Transm Dis*. 2011 Jul;38(7):648–9.
64. Occupational Safety and Health Standards Board Petition File No. 513: Bloodborne Pathogens. Available from: www.dir.ca.gov/oshsb/petition513.html (accessed July 5, 2011).
65. Division of Occupational Safety and Health. Bloodborne pathogens in the adult film industry—advisory meetings. Available from: http://www.dir.ca.gov/dosh/doshreg/5193Meetings.htm (accessed July 6, 2011).
66. Yoshino K. Lawsuit lays burden on county to curb AIDS in porn industry. *Los Angeles Times*. July 17, 2009. Available from: http://articles.latimes.com/2009/jul/17/local/me-porn-hiv17 (accessed July 27, 2011).
67. Yoshino K. Judge dismisses petition requiring the use of condoms in porn films. Los Angeles Times. December 23, 2009. Available from: http://articles.latimes.com/2009/dec/23/local/la-me-porn23-2009dec23 (accessed July 27, 2011).
68. Weiss KR. L.A. County does not have to require condoms for porn actors, court rules. *Los Angeles Times*. July 15, 2011. Available from: http://latimesblogs.latimes.com/lanow/2011/07/condoms-porn-industry-aids.html (accessed July 27, 2011).
69. Hennessy-Fiske, M. Porn trade group to revive performer STD database. *Los Angeles Times*. July 27, 2011. Available from: http://www.latimes.com/health/la-me-porn-0110727,0,6343044,print.story (accessed July 27, 2011).
70. City of Los Angeles. Available from: http://clkrep.lacity.org/onlinedocs/2011/11-0002-S75_ca_05-25-11.pdf (accessed June 15, 2011).
71. Romero D. Porn industry (see number 45 above).
72. AIDS Healthcare Organization. Sixty-four thousand signatures send porn initiative to a vote in Los Angeles. November 30, 2011. Available from: http://www.aidshealth.org/archives/2961/ (accessed Dec. 10, 2011).
73. Pardon R. L.A. files suit to block porn-condom referendum. *XBiz*. December 9, 2011. Available from: http://newswire.xbiz.com/view.php?id=141944. (accessed Dec. 13, 2011).
74. Hoffman C. Porn shoots get under their skin. *Los Angeles Times*. April 30, 2006. Available from: http://articles.latimes.com/2006/apr/30/local/me-nimby30 (accessed July 27, 2011).